gii Medicorum Philadelphiensis

ÆC PERVENERINT

em

ood Gerhard Virum doctum et

secundo septemb 1834 adscriptum fuisse, om-

consecutum esse. In cujus Rei Fidem

stra subjecimus.

Aprilis Anno Domini 1835

Tho. C. James Praeses

Thomas T Hewson V. Praes.

A BICENTENNIAL HISTORY

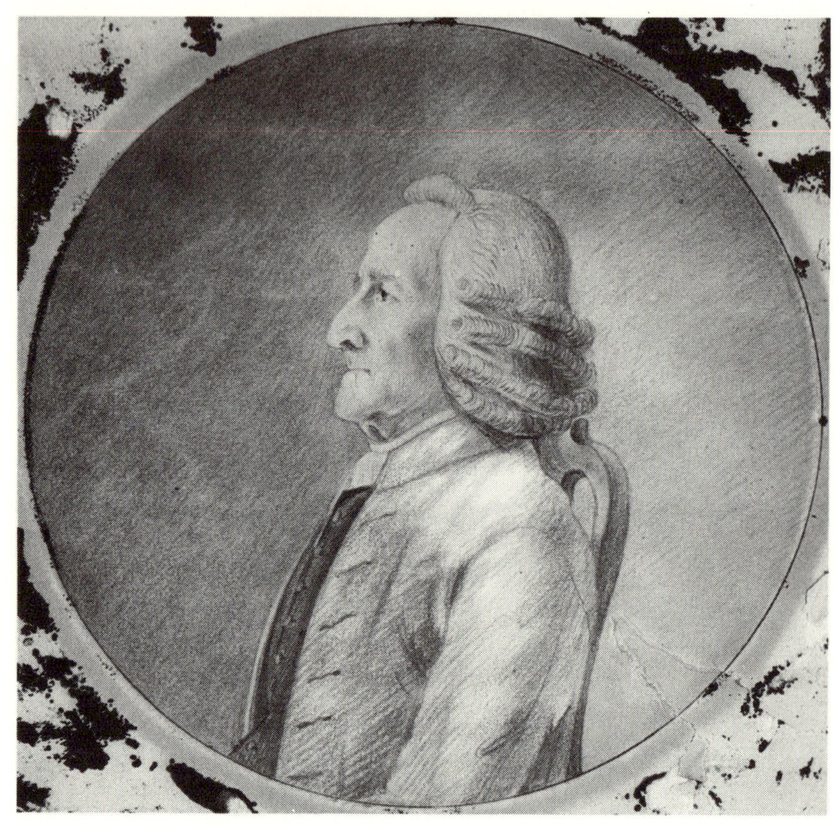

John Redman, (1722–1805). President of the College, 1787–1805. Crayon; miniature by an unknown artist, c. 1790.

# The College of Physicians of Philadelphia

## A BICENTENNIAL HISTORY

*Whitfield J. Bell, Jr.*

SCIENCE HISTORY PUBLICATIONS, U.S.A.

1987

First published in the United States by
Science History Publications, U.S.A.
a division of
Watson Publishing International
Post Office Box 493, Canton, MA 02021


Library of Congress Cataloging-in-Publication Data
Bell, Whitfield J. (Whitfield Jenks)
The College of Physicians of Philadelphia.

Includes index.
1. College of Physicians of Philadelphia—History.
2. Mitchell, S. Weir (Silas Weir), 1829-1914. I. Title.
[DNLM: 1. Mitchell, S. Weir (Silas Weir), 1829-1914.
2. College of Physicians of Philadelphia. 3. Physicians—biography. 4. Societies, Medical—history—United States.
WB 1 AA1 B43c]
R15.C6373B44 1987 610'.60748'11 87-20570
ISBN 0-88135-003-6

# *Contents*

# *Preface*

THE HISTORY of the College of Physicians of Philadelphia is an integral part of the history of medicine in that city, and it has sometimes been a vital part of the national story as well. Its history is not, of course, the whole of either the national or local history. The College never sought a national role, and in its early years it shared authority and prestige with the University of Pennsylvania Medical School and the Pennsylvania Hospital. After the middle of the nineteenth century it was one of several institutions—medical schools, hospitals, the County Medical Society, for examples—that made Philadelphia a great medical center. Throughout the years, however, the College Fellows in general have been the best educated doctors, the most successful practitioners, and the most influential teachers, and many had national influence and reputation. One Fellow was called to attend President Garfield, another operated on President Cleveland, a third on President Eisenhower. Although Weir Mitchell, himself a scientific investigator, urged his fellow physicians to join research and practice, and at the end of his life was hoping that a research institute, like the Rockefeller Institute in New York, might be established in Philadelphia, the lasting contribution of the Fellows was to their patients as clinicians. It was such as they whom John Redman, first president of the College, had in mind when he offered a toast

> To the individual practitioner, who makes the health, comfort & happiness of his fellow mortall one of the chief ends & delights of his life; and acts therein from motives that render him superior to all difficulties he may have to encounter in the pursuit thereof.

This history rests principally on the minutes, reports, publications and other records of the College. Biographical information on many Fellows is to be found in obituary memoirs printed in the *Transactions,* a source too seldom used. There are, I suspect, many references to, and even reflections on, the College in the pages of Philadelphia's medical journals, especially in the nineteenth century, when editors were less inhibited and more unmannerly than in our own day. I have been able to examine only a few of these publications, and then only on specific points. Of personal correspondence regrettably little seems to have survived—but, then, as the College was a local institution and the Fellows regularly saw one another on Spruce and Pine Streets, it is unlikely that they would have discussed College business in private letters. Weir Mitchell's diaries and correspondence, in possession of descendants as recently as 1950, I have not located.

*Acknowledgments.* Thomas A. Horrocks made bibliographical and biographical searches for this book when it was begun; after becoming Curator of Historical Collections of the Library, he continued to be helpful in other and broader ways. I am grateful also to his assistants Jean P. Carr and Brenda L. Galloway for their detailed knowledge of the collections, both catalogued and "unaccessioned." The staff of the Reading Room were also always prompt and cheerful when fetching books from the general collection.

I owe a particular word of thanks to Annette Miller, who took my manuscript, done in the old-fashioned way, put it on her word-processor, then corrected the tape repeatedly as I revised, expanded, and rewrote.

Diana E. Long, director of the Francis C. Wood Institute for the History of Medicine, and William F. Chaveas, formerly executive director of the College, provided a room to work in. John M. O'Donnell, now executive director, has always been interested and helpful. He read the entire manuscript; Samuel X Radbill read most of it before his recent death. Both made useful comments and corrections, but neither responded to my pleas for rigorous criticism as fully as I—and my readers—might wish. Gerald Lombardi edited the manuscript for the press; and I appreciate, as doubtless the College does, the zeal and forebearance of the publisher.

*Publisher's Note.* Except as noted, illustrations are from the College Collections and the Mütter Museum of the College of Physicians of Philadelphia, by courtesy of Gretchen Worden, curator; and from the Library's Historical Collections, by courtesy of Thomas A. Horrocks, curator. The end papers are a Certificate of Fellowship in the College, issued in 1835 to William Wood Gerhard, elected in 1834. Blind embossed on the front cover is Dr. John Redman, after a picture in the former Ridgway Branch of the Library Company of Philadelphia, reproduced in J. Thomas Scharf and Thompson Westcott, *History of Philadelphia 1609–1884* (Philadelphia, 1884), II, 1592.

CHAPTER I

# *The Founding and Founders*

THE American Revolution, Dr. Benjamin Rush of Philadelphia was fond of saying, gave a "spring" to men's minds in scientific and moral enterprise, creating a national determination to complete the act of independence.[1] Men believed the "revolution" would be fully achieved only when all American institutions were separated from their British foundations and American culture and customs were planted in native soil. So the Anglican Church, for example, separating itself from the Church of England by changes in organization and liturgy and by the ordination of bishops in America, became the Protestant Episcopal Church in the United States in 1787. Similarly the General Assembly of the Presbyterian Church, the first ever held, created the Presbyterian Church in the United States of America in 1786. In the same year the Grand Lodge of Masons in Pennsylvania, originally chartered by the Grand Lodge of England, declared itself independent. On another level, histories of the new states and of the war by David Ramsay and others helped to establish the sense of national independence and identity. Jedediah Morse's *American Geography* (1789) and Humphry Marshall's *American Grove* (1785), a catalogue of native trees and shrubs, had the same effect. Noah Webster undertook to fashion an American language and speech; while earnest reformers and light-hearted satirists, decrying foreign manners, called on Americans to adopt customs and a national costume suitable to republican simplicity. "Let us not weakly, and meanly, and treacherously, and impiously, neglect the opportunity, given to us, by

God," one such patriot implored his fellow-citizens, "of showing, by our example, to our fellow-citizens of the world, how FREEMEN ought to live."[2]

The new "spring" that Rush described manifested itself in a score of institutions, some new, others reorganized, designed to complete "the American revolution."[3] The American Philosophical Society, which had achieved international reputation by its observations of the Transit of Venus in 1769, erected a meeting hall in 1785, resumed in 1786 publication of its *Transactions* (interrupted by the war), and was urged by some members to become the center of a national association of state and local scientific societies. The abolition of slavery and the education of free blacks, as logical consequences of the "revolution," were promoted by voluntary associations in the larger cities and in a few small towns. The Philadelphia Society for Alleviating the Miseries of Public Prisons (1787) pioneered in obtaining humane treatment for prisoners; its work soon became and long remained an object of interest, study, and imitation by European reformers.

Nothing was more important for securing the blessings of liberty won by the revolution than education. Rush played a decisive role in founding Dickinson and Franklin Colleges in Pennsylvania (1783 and 1787 respectively), championed the education of women, and sketched a system of higher education for the new nation—colleges, state universities, and professional schools, and at its peak a national university where citizens would be trained for public office. In politics the "spring" produced two incomparable lasting achievements in the summer of 1787—the Federal Constitution and the Northwest Ordinance—which were to be the twin pillars of the American democratic empire.

Medicine too was caught up in the intellectual and institutional ferment of the first decade of peace. It was not surprising, Rush wrote, that "before the human faculties had contracted to their former dimensions, a college of physicians, formed upon principles accommodated to the present state of society and government in America," should be established "in the capital of the United States."[4]

## *Predecessors*

The College of Physicians of Philadelphia was not the first medical society in the city—or in the nation for that matter. For some years societies of physicians in several towns had met more or less regularly. In Boston before mid-century there was a "Physicall Club," to which the autocratic but able William Douglass, a Scotsman with a medical degree from Utrecht, read a paper on scarlet fever in 1736 and with which Alexander Hamilton of Annapolis spent an evening in 1744.[5] "A Weekly Society of [Medical] Gentlemen" met in New York in 1749; it may have been the same group which twenty years later proposed that a medical school be established in connection with King's College.[6] In Philadelphia in 1749 the doctors joined in warning that the copper machinery used in distilling spirits created a danger to health.[7] Before the war, in 1767, thirty-one physicians of Litchfield County, Connecticut, formed a medical society, and in 1779 some of them organized another, under the grandiose title of "The First Medical Society in the thirteen United States of America since their Independence." This society proposed to examine "every Candidate for Practice, either Apprentice or any Physician, or Surgeon within this County, or Foreigner, coming into the County." It solicited the help of Benjamin Franklin in Paris to open a correspondence with the French Royal Society of Medicine.[8]

In Philadelphia, the largest city in the colonies after mid-century and for twenty-five years until 1800 the seat of government of the new nation, physicians and medical students established several professional societies in the two decades before the founding of the College of Physicians. One of these, significant but short-lived, usually called the Philadelphia Medical Society, was founded by John Morgan in 1766. A Fellow of the Royal College of Physicians of Edinburgh and a licentiate of the Royal College of Physicians of London, Morgan cherished high aspirations for his profession, hoping that the Philadelphia society might become a college on the model of the Royal Colleges, with power to examine and license physicians throughout the colonies. Others, however, feared that Morgan's society would devalue the degrees of the new medical school of the College of Philadelphia. John Fothergill, the London Quaker physician who was a friend of Franklin and of Pennsylvania, strongly advised Thomas Penn not to grant it a charter on the ground that such a society with such powers would lead to monopoly of the kind he had fought in the Royal College in London. Fothergill's opposition was decisive, and the society was absorbed soon afterwards into the American Society for Promoting Useful Knowledge, its members becoming the standing committee on medicine and anatomy.[9]

The medical students also had a society. It held its meetings in the Pennsylvania Hospital, most likely under the patronage of Thomas Bond, a physician to the Hospital, whose clinical lectures were required of candidates for the medical degree of the College of Philadelphia.[10] This hospital medical society seems to have merged with the American Medical Society, which was founded in Philadelphia in 1770. With its mixed membership of students and physicians the American Society was patterned on the medical societies clustering about Edinburgh University, especially the Medical (after 1778 the Royal Medical) Society. Although its work was suspended during the war, the American Medical Society was again active in the 1780s, when papers read at its meetings were published in Philadelphia magazines.[11]

Most of these societies and clubs depended on the ideas and enthusiasm of individuals, and withered away with hardly a trace. A few that were more broadly based, however, survived and were flourishing in the 1780s. The medical societies of New Jersey (1766), Massachusetts (1781) and New Haven County, Connecticut (1784), drew members from a wider area than a single town; the New Jersey doctors, for example, held their annual meetings alternately in New Brunswick and Burlington. These state and county societies received and published observations and reports from their members' practices and, addressing professional concerns, tried to do something about the "illiterate, vain pretenders to physic," as Litchfield's "First Medical Society" called them, who abounded throughout the country and brought medicine into disrepute and contempt.[12]

These words were hardly too strong to describe the medical profession at the time. Outside the larger towns only a handful of practitioners had received any formal training. In the country a few clergymen cared for the bodies as well as the souls of their parishioners. Pastor Heinrich Melchior Muhlenberg, for example, attended courses in medicine at Halle before going out to Pennsylvania to serve the Lutheran churches there; and the Reverend Mr. Robert McKean, a missionary of the Society for the Propagation of the Gospel, was sufficiently respected as a physician to be elected the first president of the New Jersey Medical Society.[13] But they were exceptions. Most physicians, whether in town or country, had learned their medicine as apprentices for a season or two to an older physician; others were wholly self-taught. Most sick and injured persons had to depend on family and folk traditions, prescriptions in almanacs, the advice and concoctions of local goodwives, and the healing power of nature. "Few Physicians amongst us are eminent for their Skill," wrote William Smith in his history of New York in 1757:

> Quacks abound like Locusts in Egypt, and too many have recommended themselves to a full Practice and profitable Subsistence. This is the less to be wondered at, as the Profession is under no Kind of Regulation. Loud as the Call is, to our Shame be it remembered, we have no Law to protect the Lives of the King's Subjects, from the Malpractice of Pretenders. Any Man at his Pleasure sets up for Physician, Apothecary, and Chirurgeon. No Candidates are either examined or licensed, or even sworn to fair Practice.[14]

Nevertheless, under such conditions several medical societies in the United States before 1787 were actively promoting medical science and the interests of the profession. They, as well as those which had languished and died, afforded encouragement and a pattern, were any needed, to prospective founders of yet another society.

### *Rush and the College*

One physician with hopes and plans for another such society was Benjamin Rush, a graduate of Edinburgh University, professor of chemistry in the first faculty of the medical school of the College of Philadelphia, for a short time a member of the Continental Congress, physician-general of the Middle Department of the Continental Army, and a tireless and imaginative advocate of a score of movements to improve men and society. That he now contemplated a college of physicians with licensing powers may be inferred from the letter a young American medical student, Samuel Powel Griffitts, wrote him from London in the summer of 1783:

> Your idea of an American College of Physicians is what has several times occurred to me. I have often been asked, what it is that gives a Licence to practice Physic with us;

> I have answered by saying what ought to, but to say what really does, would make Physic appear rather in a low State in America. Your Plan would effectually remedy this Evil.[16]

At the same time Francis Rigby Brodbelt of Jamaica, Rush's fellow-student at Edinburgh fifteen years before, was under the impression there was already a college of physicians in Philadelphia:

> When you have time let me know how the College goes on in Physic & every other kind of Study. I wish much to belong to your Philosophical Society at Philadelphia, and to be an honorary or ordinary fellow of your College of Physicians. . . . I will thank you to get me chose[n] a member of your Society as well as of your College, & let me know the expence & will immediately send you the money.[17]

Both Griffitts and Brodbelt may have learned about Rush's aspirations for the American profession from John Coakley Lettsom. This benevolent London Quaker doctor, who considered himself an American because he was born in the West Indies, was a warm friend of Rush and of America and American institutions. "I want to see America great in every thing," he exclaimed.[18] Like Rush, he was full of ideas for the promotion of science and learning in the New World.

> I hope now Peace is yours, that you will cultivate the Arts of peace. . . . I think were I in Philadelphia, I should not only have a philosophical Society like our Royal Society or the French Acad. des Sciences; but likewise a medical college taking in likewise Foreign Members . . . . Your Medical College might include Natural history, which you have so many opportunities of improving by forming a public Cabinet. I do not know that any of the performances I have sent you would assist in the Institution of such societies, but I thought the perusal might afford an hour's employment. Should not you likewise establish a Society for the recovery of the drowned, the frozen & of sudden deaths?[19]

Although he appreciated Lettsom's interest and encouragement, Rush judged the time not ripe:

> The state of our country for some years past has been unfavorable to improvements of every kind in science. I approve of your plan for instituting a medical society in Philadelphia, and am not without hopes of seeing it carried into execution as soon as the minds of our literati are more perfectly detached from the political subjects that have swallowed up all the ingenuity and industry of our country.[20]

But Lettsom did not stop pressing his American correspondent. Applauding Rush's "desire to improve the healing art," he pointed once more to the unique opportunities of American philosophers. "You have such an extent of novelty in your Soil, produce, improvement &c, as must stimulate genius, and gratify invention and study."[21] A few months later he gave Rush another nudge by having him elected a member of the Medical Society of London; Rush responded with a paper on the cause and cure of tetanus. In 1789 the Society voted Rush a silver medal.[22] Two other Philadelphians, Adam Kuhn and Benjamin Say, were also in correspondence with Lettsom at this time; both became founding members of the College of Physicians.

Lettsom continued to shower ideas upon his American friend: "Set your Men of Science upon studying your own Country—its native improveable productions. Your resources would influence Europe—Your reflections would instruct her."[23] In some irritation Rush replied on October 26, 1786:

> You have suggested a number of excellent hints for the improvement and extension of knowledge in America. But, my friend, who shall undertake to carry such hints into execution? Philosophy does not here, as in England, walk abroad in silver slippers; the physicians (who are the most general repositories of science) are chained down by the drudgery of their professions; so as to be precluded from exploring our woods and mountains. Besides, there are not men of learning enough in America as yet, to furnish the stimulus of literary fame to difficult and laborious literary pursuits. I have felt the force of this passion;

> Alas! my friend, I have found it in our country to be nothing but 'avarice of air.'[24]

The tone of this letter is puzzling. Although Rush was a man of rapidly changing moods, it is strange that he should have seemed so discouraged, so subdued, at the very moment when the first firm steps had been taken to establish the College of Physicians of Philadelphia.

### *Founding the College*

The earliest recorded meeting of the College is that of January 2, 1787.[25] At least three meetings were held before that date, however; and, if they were held a month apart, as the first by-laws prescribed, the College could not have been organized or the first officers elected later than October 1786. The evidence is in the inaugural address of John Redman as president. Redman spoke of his election as having taken place "at our first meeting to form a Society," and he expressed regret that he had been prevented from attending "your next meeting." Thus, there were two meetings before that at which Redman spoke; and as he did not address the College in January—at least the minutes of that date record neither an election nor Redman's address—he probably spoke to the College in December; the meeting he had been unable to attend was November's, and the meeting at which he was elected, October's. As there must have been one or more preliminary meetings to agree on College purposes and an agenda and to select the founding members, the earliest meetings were probably held during the late summer of 1786. No matter whether or when such earlier meetings occurred, there can be no doubt about January 2, 1787; and that is the date the College has accepted and celebrated in its centennial, sesquicentennial, and bicentennial years.

The objects of the College were set forth in its constitution:

> to advance the science of medicine, and thereby to lessen human misery, by investigating the diseases and remedies which are peculiar to our country; by observing the effects of different seasons, climates and situations upon the human body; by recording the changes that are produced

> in diseases, by the progress of agriculture, arts, population, and manners; by searching for medicines in our woods, waters and the bowels of the earth; by enlarging our avenues to knowledge, from the discoveries and publications of foreign countries; by appointing stated times for literary intercourse and communications; and by cultivating order and uniformity in the practice of physic.[26]

The original membership of the College, agreed upon in the fall of 1786, was composed of twelve senior and eleven junior Fellows. The seniors were in fact just that—the youngest was thirty-five, and none of the juniors had yet attained that age. Moreover, all but one of the senior Fellows had studied in Edinburgh, London, or some European university, and most had the degree of doctor of medicine. The rest were bachelors of medicine from the College of Philadelphia, and one had been admitted into the Company of Barber-Surgeons of London. The senior and junior Fellows, although they comprised less than half the practicing physicians of Philadelphia, were the best educated, the most experienced, and most favorably known.

Both senior and junior Fellows were required to be residents of the city of Philadelphia, the borough of Southwark, or the Northern Liberties. Juniors, of whom there might be any number, were expected to be "of good capacity, of good Moral Character, and decent deportment," and must be at least twenty-four years old. "Persons of Merit in the profession" who lived beyond these geographical limits might be elected Associate Fellows. Only the seniors could hold office. When a vacancy occurred in their ranks, they might elect one of the juniors to fill it, a vote of three-quarters of the whole number of seniors being required. Stated meetings were to be held on the first Tuesday of every month, but special meetings might be called by the president or on petition of any six Fellows. The admission fee was $8 and the annual subscription was $2.[27]

Its constitution gave the College a much less expansive role than Rush once had in mind for it. The number of senior Fellows was limited to twelve, and all Fellows had to come from the narrow limits of the old city and its two neighboring sections. After some years the number of Fellows was increased and the area from which they might come was extended to seven miles (but not including the east side of the Delaware River). Attitudes and habits of exclusion, persisting for many years, severely limited the usefulness and influence of the College. Nothing in the constitution hinted at a representative *American* college of physicians or even a *Pennsylvania* medical society like those of New Jersey and Massachusetts; and the College never asserted a claim to enforce professional standards by examination and license. The institution taking form in the fall of 1786 fell far short of Rush's original aspirations; perhaps that is why in his letters to Lettsom he sounded frustrated and discouraged.

Because of the similarity of names, it has often been assumed and sometimes stated that the College was consciously patterned on the Royal College of Physicians of London. That seems unlikely. None of the founders made that claim. It is true that John Morgan was a licentiate of the London College, and that both he and William Shippen, Jr., were Fellows of the Royal College of Edinburgh; but neither knew much about the work of either institution: licentiates did not attend meetings, and neither Morgan nor Shippen was elected a Fellow of the Scottish institution until after he had left Edinburgh. In any event, it was the power to examine and license physicians that distinguished the Royal Colleges from all other British medical societies, and that power was not given to, or ever sought by, the Philadelphia college. Nor did the American college resemble other possible British prototypes in any essential respect. It was unlike the Royal Medical Society of Edinburgh (of which Rush, Morgan, and Kuhn were members, and Caspar Wistar was student president in 1785) because it did not include students in its membership; and it differed from Lettsom's Medical Society of London because it did not include apothecaries.[28] There were sufficient precedents for Rush and his fellow-founders, had they needed any; but they knew what they wanted and what was feasible, and did not copy any foreign model.

### *The Officers*

As their president the Fellows elected John Redman, at sixty-five one of the oldest physicians in the city.[29] Some of his colleagues, such as Morgan and Rush, had been his apprentices, and he could address most of them as "my professional Children." He had studied medicine at Edinburgh and taken his degree at Ley-

# Form of the Constitution of the College of Physicians of Philadelphia.

The Physicians of Philadelphia influenced by a conviction of the many Advantages that have arisen in every Country from Literary institutions, have associated themselves under the Name and Title of the College of Physicians of Philadelphia.

The Objects of this College are, to advance the Science of Medicine, and thereby to lessen Human Misery, by investigating the diseases and Remedies which are peculiar to our Country, by observing the effects of different seasons Climates and situations upon the Human Body, by recording the changes that are produced in diseases by the progress of Agriculture, Arts, Population and Manners, by searching for Medicines in our Woods, Waters, and the bowels of the Earth, by enlarging our Avenues to knowledge from the discoveries and publications of foreign Countries, by appointing stated times for Literary intercourse and communications, and by cultivating Order and uniformity in the practice of Physick.

For the purpose of obtaining these Objects the

Constitution of the College of Physicians. Preamble, 1787.

5

Two fifths of the Fellows shall be a quorum for all Business except the Election of Members, the expenditure of Money, the Making of Laws, or the altering of the Constitution, in the three last cases, a Majority of the Fellows shall be a Quorum.

15 Every Fellow upon his Admission, shall subscribe to the above Rules, as a Testimony of his consenting to be bound by them. He shall at the same time, pay into the Hands of the Treasurer, the Sum of eight Dollars towards establishing a fund for the use of the College; he shall likewise pay two Dollars annually for the same purpose. —

John Morgan
John Redman
John Jones
William Shippen jr
Adam Kuhn
Benjn Rush
Gerardo Clarkson
Samuel Duffield
Thomas Parke
James Hutchinson
George Glentworth
Abra: Chovet

Constitution of the College of Physicians. Subscribers, 1787.

den in 1748. In Philadelphia he soon acquired a large practice and was elected a member of the first medical staff of the new Pennsylvania Hospital. During a long professional life, however, he published almost nothing. For many years Redman was a trustee of the College of Philadelphia and of the College of New Jersey at Princeton, and throughout his life was a devout and active member of the Second Presbyterian Church. He resigned his Hospital appointment after twenty-nine years' service in 1780 and retired from practice a few years afterwards to devote himself to religious reading and contemplation. He had taken no part, and apparently expressed no judgment, in the bitter quarrels among Morgan, Shippen, and Rush over the Medical School and the administration of the Medical Department of the Continental Army. Trusted and respected by all in the disputatious and divided profession, Redman was someone on whom all could unite. He was chosen president "at our first meeting to form a Society" and acknowledged his election presumably in the meeting of December 1786.

The statement was highly personal.[30] Except for tributes to his friends Thomas Cadwalader, who had died in 1779, and Thomas Bond, who died in 1784, whom he wished might have lived to be presidents of the College, Redman's address was entirely an apology for "growing infirmities of body and mind" and a confession of general incapacity to discharge the duties of the office. He regretted "the loss of that Spirit of Business, and that activity & Vigour of Body & mind, with their several faculties (such as they were) which I was once possest off [sic];" he assured his colleagues that his ambition was merely to behave "rather with integrity & usefullness than Eclat," appealed for their understanding and support, and promised to resign if unable to continue. In a postscript he called on the Fellows "to Acknowledge the Supreme Being to be our Sovereign, Lord & Ruler" in this enterprise, with all that that implied. There was not a word about medicine, the medical profession, or the duties and opportunities of the College.

John Jones was elected vice-president. The son and grandson of Philadelphia Quaker physicians, apprenticed as a youth to his cousin Thomas Cadwalader, he studied medicine in London, Edinburgh, and Paris, and received his medical degree from the University of Rheims in 1751. Settling in practice in New York, he acquired the reputation of a skillful lithotomist and was elected a member of the faculty of the medical school of King's College. At the outset of war in 1775, he wrote a useful manual entitled *Plain*

*Concise Practical Remarks on the Treatment of Wounds and Fractures,* which was reprinted twice in Philadelphia the next year. Although he served as a surgeon in the Continental Army, Jones was not involved in the controversies that swirled around its Medical Department. After New York came under British Army control in 1776, Jones moved to Philadelphia, where he was promptly elected one of the physicians to the Pennsylvania Hospital, and soon numbered both Franklin and Washington among his patients.[31]

James Hutchinson, at thirty-five the youngest of the senior Fellows, was elected secretary of the College. A birthright Friend who was disowned for unacceptable military and political activity during the war and for marrying out of meeting, he had received the degree of bachelor of medicine from the College of Philadelphia, where he was also awarded a gold medal for distinction in chemistry. In London Dr. Fothergill strongly advised him to make surgery his specialty; accordingly, he took a ticket for Percival Pott's lectures at St. Bartholomew's Hospital and attended the lectures of William Hunter and the anatomical class of Hunter's brother John. Hutchinson returned home somewhat dramatically in the winter of 1777, carrying dispatches from Dr. Franklin to the Congress. He was elected a physician to the Pennsylvania Hospital, was appointed a surgeon in the Flying Camp, served at Valley Forge, and held a variety of military medical posts. A radical in politics, he was a supporter of the Pennsylvania Constitution of 1776 and served in the State Assembly.[32]

Like Jones, the treasurer Gerardus Clarkson was a native of New York. After his father's death and his mother's remarriage, he was brought to Philadelphia, where he studied medicine with Thomas Bond. He then went abroad for further study. Clarkson was a member of John Morgan's proposed college of physicians in 1766. He was appointed physician to the Almshouse in 1772 and to the Society for Inoculating the Poor in 1774, but he declined an invitation to become a physician to the Pennsylvania Hospital. He was one of the original trustees of the University of the State of Pennsylvania in 1779.[33]

Four censors were charged with wide and varied oversight of College business, including responsibility for publications and library. They were John Morgan, William Shippen, Jr., Adam Kuhn, and Benjamin Rush. All were graduates of Edinburgh University, were or had been physicians to the Pennsylvania Hospital, and had some acquaintance with the social and learned world of Europe. Morgan's tour, for example, was famous: he visited Holland with James Boswell, travelled in Italy in the party of the Duke of York, had a private audience with Pope Clement, and spent an afternoon with Voltaire at Ferney. Both Shippen and Kuhn became presidents of the College, Shippen succeeding Redman in 1805, and Kuhn Shippen three years later.[34]

The four remaining senior Fellows were Abraham Chovet, Samuel Duffield, George Glentworth, and Thomas Parke. Chovet, a man of eighty-three, had been a demonstrator in anatomy in the Company of Barber-Surgeons of London. He had made a famous collection of "Anatomical Preparations," which he exhibited throughout England before moving to Jamaica, where the *Gentleman's Magazine* in 1759 identified him as "surgeon of Kingston . . . a Dr. of physick." He finally settled in Philadelphia, where for several years after 1774 he offered private lectures in anatomy. His "Skelletons" and wax models were judged "most admirable" by John Adams, being "exquisite Representations of the whole Animal Æconomy."[35] A Tory during the war, despite his age and good humor he narrowly escaped a suit of tar and feathers at the hands of the rebel mob. He died in 1790.

Glentworth and Parke had studied in Edinburgh, although neither took a degree there. Glentworth on his return home became a member of Morgan's Philadelphia medical society. Both Glentworth and Duffield were physicians to the Almshouse, and both took active parts in the smallpox epidemic of 1773-74, Duffield as a physician to the Society for Inoculating the Poor, and Glentworth as conductor of an inoculation hospital. Parke succeeded Morgan as a physician in the Pennsylvania Hospital in 1777. Glentworth was interested in botany and horticulture and imported bulbs each year from Holland. Duffield was active for many years in the American Philosophical Society, where he was curator from 1773 to 1792. None of these three taught in the Medical School or offered private lectures, but probably all had apprentices from time to time.

The College completed its organization during the first months of 1787. Fourteen Fellows—nine seniors and five juniors—signed the constitution at the January meeting; and the secretary was directed to publish the document in the newspapers, "together with a Note inviting communications from such friends of Medical science throughout the United States who may be disposed to promote the important designs of this institution." Drs. Shippen, Kuhn, and William W. Smith were named to draft by-laws; they reported them on April 1, 1788. Another committee, composed of Rush, Griffitts, and Benjamin Duffield, was named to design a seal and form of diploma. They reported promptly at the February meeting, when the College amended the motto they proposed—*Non Sibi Sed Aliis*—to *Non Sibi Sed Toti,* which were the words the famous Dr. Richard Mead of London had chosen for his own motto—an improved sentiment, but not better Latin.[36] Both seal and certificate were engraved by Robert Scott, who a few years later was to engrave plates for Dobson's *American Encyclopedia.* At the same February meeting five new junior Fellows were proposed; one of them was Caspar Wistar, Jr.

### *On the Objects of the Institution*

The principal business of the meeting of February 6, however, was Benjamin Rush's address on the aims of the College.[37] Although he repeated and expanded on the purposes set forth in the constitution, Rush nonetheless revealed uncertainty about the character of the institution. Perhaps this confusion reflected his and other members' unresolved views about its proper role. Assuring his colleagues that the new institution would benefit both the profession and the public, Rush tried to distinguish between a *college* of physicians and a medical *society* and claimed that the new organization would embody functions of both.

As a *college,* he said, the institution would address principally matters of public concern. Thus, it might undertake a national dispensatory and offer advice to legislative bodies on matters affecting the health and happiness of the citizens, as the Royal College of Physicians of London had formerly borne "testimony against the pernicious effects of distilled spirituous liquors." As a *college* it would create and maintain order and uniformity in the profession, not through examinations and licenses, but "by establishing incentives and rewards for character." Although professional rivalries in Philadelphia were so acute as to be the butt of satirists,[38] Rush counted heavily on the sense of collegiality:

> The reception we shall meet with from each other in our meetings will serve to correct or to improve our conduct.

> If we are as chaste as we should be in the admission of members, a fellowship in our college will become in time, not only the sign of ability, but an introduction to business and reputation in physic.

As a *society,* Rush went on, a wide field lay open to the members to collect and publish medical observations and inquiries. He offered a long list of specific topics, many in his view of a peculiarly American nature: the influence of climate, diet, occupation, dress, and manners on health and disease; the effects of agriculture, horticulture, manufactures, commerce, and civilization upon human life and health; the effects of clearing forests; the influence of American laws and government. "Are madness, melancholy, the hysteria and hypochondriasis more frequent in republics than in monarchies?" he asked. The causes of tooth decay, "so frequent in the middle and eastern states of America," the consequences of drinking cold water, and the effects of coal fires should each be investigated. Meteorological records and improved mortality statistics should be kept so that the society could correlate climate and disease. "The reason why the suburbs and south end of our city are more subject to autumnal fevers than its centre and north end, and why those fevers are less frequent within these three years than formerly, deserve our attention," Rush told his colleagues. To further these goals and inquiries the College as a *society* should hold meetings, cultivate a botanic garden, and collect a library. "It is a general opinion that the condition of man in our world is mending," Rush concluded in the tone appropriate to his soaring vision of the expanding future:

> The conveniences and pleasures of life, are daily multiplying by the inventions of philosophy. Many disorders, once deemed incurable, now yield to medicine. No wonder then that a general expectation prevails—that a revolution is soon to take place in favour of human happiness. Natural means appear to be the instruments designed by heaven to fulfil its purpose of mercy and benevolence to mankind. I am fully persuaded that there does not exist a disease in nature, that has not an antidote to it. And when I consider the influence of liberty and republican forms of government upon science, and the vigour which the American mind has acquired by the events of the late revolution, I

am led to hope that a great portion of the honor and happiness of discovering and applying these antidotes may be reserved for the physicians of America.

With such thoughts and hopes proudly borne in mind, the Fellows of the College, led by President Redman and followed by the students of medicine, marched in the Grand Federal Procession in Philadelphia on July 4, 1788, celebrating the ratification of the Federal Constitution, the completion of independence, and the establishment of the American federal republic.[39] On April 21, 1790, twenty Fellows in a body, representing the College, attended the great public funeral of Benjamin Franklin. A few months later, in yet another corporate appearance that brought it to public attention, the College held a memorial service for Dr. William Cullen of Edinburgh, teacher of some of the older Fellows. All the physicians and medical students in the city were invited, and Rush delivered the eulogy.

### *College Business*

Within a short time of the inauguration of the College, several changes in the nature of its membership were made. The distinction between senior and junior Fellows was eliminated by amendment on November 6, 1787. The 1788 by-laws provided that seven members should be a quorum for transacting ordinary business, and eleven for making or amending the by-laws and for electing members, "provided always that in the election of Members three fourths of the Members present must Concur."

In another change the rank of Associate was clarified. The College voted on May 4, 1790, that Associates should be persons "of well known & established character in medicine," at least thirty years of age, and that their numbers should not exceed forty, of whom ten might be residents of foreign countries. This amendment opened the way to creating a national constituency, but the opportunity was not taken. James Tilton, president of the Medical Society of Delaware, Nicholas Way, also of that state, and Isaac Senter of Newport, Rhode Island, were elected Associates. In the remaining years of the century, only five others were proposed, and two of these were rejected. Associates had to be nominated by three Fellows; aspirants to resident Fellowship had to apply individually in writing; and all were chosen "by ballotting into a covered box"—which cost the College £1 4s. 6d. (about $4).

On May 1, 1787, John Morgan suggested that the College should petition the Pennsylvania Assembly for a charter of incorporation. While the appeal was being prepared, Morgan made another suggestion. The geographical limitation on membership was, he thought, too restrictive; the area of eligibility should be extended to seven miles, as was the case with the Royal Colleges of London and Edinburgh. This, Morgan argued, would "add to the respectability, nay to the dignity & usefulness of the College in a future day. I foresee *even* a Necessity for it," he continued. "That distance is not too far for such fellows to attend who are zealous for its Welfare . . . ."[40] But the College disagreed. A simple charter of incorporation was voted by the Assembly on March 26, 1789. The College printed the charter, constitution, and by-laws in 1790.

Thus encouraged, the College on April 7, 1789, sent an address to "the most respectable Medical Characters in the United States" requesting communications on "Medical Subjects" and, more particularly, cooperation in preparing a national pharmacopoeia "adapted to the present State of Medicine in America." The appeal continued:

> When we consider the great Number of Publications of this kind, which Europe has been, and is annually producing, we think no doubt can arise, of the absolute Necessity of some Standard amongst ourselves, to prevent that Uncertainty and Irregularity, which, in our present Situation, must infallibly attend on the Compositions of the Apothecary, and the Prescriptions of the Physician.[41]

Congratulating the College on its initiative, Isaac Senter expressed confidence that the proposed pharmacopoeia would "undoubtedly be highly beneficial to the practice of physick in this *New Empire* & will be further beneficial in lessening our dependance [sic] on foreign Countries for the advancement of Medical Science." Other responses came from the New Haven County and Delaware medical societies.[42] Several physicians sent papers for presentation to the College; but on the whole the response was disappointing. Nonetheless, the committee appointed in 1788 to prepare a pharmacopoeia "for the use of the College," continued its work, at least in a desultory way; and in 1797 it voted "that an enumeration be made of all such medicinal substances & pharmaceutical processes as shall appear useful and proper to compose the intended Pharmacopoeia—that all the chemical processes be made in a laboratory at the expence of the College . . . ."

### *Public Health*

In his address on the objects of the College, Rush had promised that as a *college* the institution could address legislative bodies on matters of public health. Its first act of the kind was a memorial to the State Assembly in November 1787 on behalf of temperance, a favorite reform of Quakers, Methodists, and Benjamin Rush. The draft is in Rush's hand. Saying nothing about "the baneful effects" of excessive consumption of spirituous liquors on private economy and morals, but citing principally its effects on health (it was pronounced a cause of dropsy, epilepsy, palsy, apoplexy, melancholy, and madness), the physicians called for laws "for the checking the improper use of distilled Spirituous liquors." Nothing came of this petition, but the reform continued to gain support, and in 1790 the College appealed to the national Congress with stronger arguments, asking specifically for heavy duties to discourage consumption. Distilled spirits, the memorial claimed, produce "a great proportion of the most obstinate, painful and mortal Disorders which affect the human body" and are "not only destructive to Health and Life, but . . . impair the Faculties of the Mind, and thereby tend equally to dishonor our character as a Nation, and to degrade our species as intelligent Beings." This memorial, like that to the Pennsylvania Assembly, was tabled, with no other comment than that of Mr. Jackson of Georgia, who, disapproving what he considered interference in congressional business, expressed the opinion that the doctors might "with equal propriety interpose their offices to prevent the use of other articles which are deemed pernicious or of a poisonous quality," such as mushrooms.[43]

On other occasions as well, the College expressed its view on matters of public health. It called the attention of the Supreme Executive Council of Pennsylvania, as the City Councils did that of the mayor, to "the disagreeable Consequences to health" from the "general Illumination" planned to greet Washington on the way to his inauguration as president in April 1789. "A handsome display of fireworks" took place, nonetheless; whether this was what had alarmed the College is not clear.[44] A committee was appointed to consider establishing hot and cold baths in the city, an innovation Rush had recommended in his discourse and one that was to engage the attention of the College off and on for at least a century. In 1789 the Pennsylvania Assembly asked the College to recommend measures to prevent contagious diseases from being brought into Philadelphia. The College advised that a certificate of health be required of every vessel coming from a Mediterranean port, but reckoned that no other addition to the laws was required. On the other hand, the College made no comment on the city streets, where "dead dogs, cats, fowls, and the offals of the Market, are among the cleanest articles that are to be found"—conditions so offensive that a grand jury in 1786 charged the Street Commissioners with neglect.[45]

### *Unethical Conduct*

At least twice in its first five years the College was disturbed and tested by issues of ethics. Of the charges brought against a Fellow, John Linn, it is known only that he described them as "ill founded, groundless, & malicious" and denounced the College's action in striking his name from the roll, apparently without a hearing, as "unconstitutional, cruel, and unprecedented."[46] More details appear in the case of John Foulke, whom William Currie charged with unprofessional conduct in violation of Article 6 of the 1788 by-laws, which read as follows:

> To promote Order and Uniformity in the practice of Medicine, it is agreed by the fellows of this College, that they will not attend or prescribe for any patient who hath previously employed another fellow of the College in the same illness, unless it be in Consultation with the first Physician or in case of Sudden emergency, where the said Physician cannot be found.
>
> In all such cases of Emergency, when any fellow of this College is called to a Family, because the Family Physician is not at hand—the Fellow thus called in shall resign the patient to the Family Physician . . . .

The facts are these: Jacob Meyer fractured a leg.[47] He was treated by Drs. Currie and Jones. On an occasion when Currie was out of town, Jones was attending another patient, and the dressing needed to be changed, Meyer sent for Foulke. The latter hesitated to act in the absence of one of the principal physicians. "My God," cried the patient, "must i fall a sacrafice [sic] to the disease because those two gentleman cannot be Present. No," he told Foulke, "i insist uppon [sic] your attendance." Foulke proved eminently acceptable to Meyer, who informed Currie that he wanted Foulke to remain on the case. Understandably, Currie believed Foulke had acted improperly, charged him with using "some rash & ungenerous exclamations," and laid the matter before the College at its next meeting. Foulke responded with a number of witnesses who testified that his conduct had been "gentlemanly and delicate." After hearing the evidence, the College concluded that Currie had been misinformed and that there was no ground for action. In consequence of the Linn and Foulke cases, the College amended its by-laws to provide that thereafter charges against Fellows should be heard by the Censors, with the right of appeal to the College at large. Subsequently, most cases of unprofessional conduct were heard and decided in private.

### *Garden and Library*

Rush had proposed that the College create a botanic garden "to furnish us with an opportunity of cultivating that part of the Materia Medica which is derived from the vegetable kingdom." To this end the College asked the General Assembly for a piece of land in the city. Not only was the study of botany essential to the progress of medicine, the petitioners asserted, but

> a Botanical Garden in this new country is rendered more necessary, in order to preserve and transmit to posterity many plants, which, in the progress of improvements and cultivation of the earth, cannot fail of being lost, or of existing under circumstances less profitable, than may be expected from being cultivated in a spot appropriated to that purpose.

This petition was signed by Redman on March 3, 1788, presented and read to the Assembly on March 14, and ordered to lie on the table, where it remained.[48]

The College was more successful with another of Rush's desiderata. A library, he told his colleagues, would "help diffuse knowledge among us upon easy terms." As the history of other societies showed, such tangible property held in common might also help keep the College together. In the spring of 1788, Drs. Jones, Griffitts, and Wistar were named a committee to draft a plan. After some delay the College simply recommended that Fellows present volumes from their own libraries for the purpose. None did so until December, when Morgan, possibly partly to move his colleagues to action, donated sixteen volumes, including the works of Aristotle and manuscript notes of anatomical lectures of Professor Monro of Edinburgh. A few months later Shippen gave half a dozen volumes. The committee on a library plan then came forward with several recommendations: that the censors should collect books, provide a suitable place to keep them, and enact borrowing regulations, and that a part of any annual surplus should be spent "for the Service of the Library" in the ensuing year. Accordingly, on July 7, 1789, with £64 3s. 4 1/2d. in hand, the College authorized that £50 be spent for the library. A list was drawn up and the order sent to Amsterdam. The books arrived in sheets, were directed to be "bound in plain Calf, and lettered," and placed in cases "in the Room we meet in." Counting it an honor to serve a learned institution such as the College, the purchasing agent refused his usual commission. Meanwhile, a dozen more volumes came to the College as a bequest from Morgan, among them an edition of the works of William Harvey and a handsome copy of Morgagni's *De Sedibus et Causis Morborum,* which the great pathologist had given him personally.

Even this small collection began to crowd the Fellows in the room they occupied in the old College building at Fourth and Arch Streets. Furthermore, the University of Pennsylvania, formed by the union of the University of the State of Pennsylvania and the restored College of Philadelphia, needed the space. In the spring of 1791 the College began to look for "a proper room for their meetings and for the reception of the books," and accordingly approached the American Philosophical Society about renting a room in the Society's new hall on South Fifth Street. The Society, whose resources were limited, wanted its tenants to complete the rooms they rented with whatever carpentry, plastering, and painting were necessary. The College, however, preferred a fixed annual rental, and agreement was reached for the use of the southeast room on the second floor for £12 a year. To furnish this the College spent £27 6s. 8d., which included the cost of "1 large Rittenhouse fire place" with andirons, tongs, and shovel, eighteen chairs and two arm chairs, a table, bench, and, at a cost of £6, a book case.[49] To meet the increased expenses, the admission fee was raised to £10 (about $25) and the annual dues to $4.

Now in possession of the nucleus of a library, the College on May 1, 1792, appointed its first librarian, Nicholas B. Waters, who had volunteered for the post. He was a recent graduate of the University of the State of Pennsylvania and had edited a volume of extracts from the writings of the British surgeon Benjamin Bell. After eight months Waters resigned and was succeeded by Michael Leib, who was an attending physician at the Philadelphia Dispensary. Neither Waters nor Leib was kept very busy. The borrowing record, begun in 1792, shows that in the ensuing three years twenty-five books were taken out. Only two Fellows borrowed more than two volumes—Benjamin Smith Barton borrowed nine, and Adam Kuhn six.[50]

### *Transactions*

The presentation and exchange of scientific information was, of course, a principal object of every medical society. As a *college,* Rush told his colleagues, their stated meetings could promote inquiries and observations on the prevailing diseases of the city; as a *society,* they could collect and publish such observations and inquiries. Whatever this apparent distinction meant, Rush clearly regarded the publication of scientific papers as a major activity of the College.

The New Haven County Medical Society published a volume of *Cases and Observations* in 1788, and the Massachusetts Medical Society issued the first of its *Medical Communications* in 1790. In Philadelphia at this time medical papers were printed, if they appeared at all, in newspapers, magazines, and the *Transactions* of the American Philosophical Society. The *Columbian Magazine* published papers read to the American Medical Society, "inaugural dissertations" written as a requirement for the degree of doctor of medicine, and letters on medical subjects by local doctors or their correspondents. In a letter to Rush printed in the *American Museum,* for example, Jacob Hall, principal of Cokesbury College in Maryland, recounted a hard and painful ride to his institution to be treated with its electrostatic machine for an obstruction in the biliary tract.

The first paper read to the College was a communication on September 4, 1787, from Thomas Dolbeare of London to Rush describing "a Singular Case of the Curvature of the Spine." In the ensuing five years, several score papers were presented. Fellows read their own papers; others were sent from distant places; and many were letters or extracts from letters addressed to Fellows, principally to Rush, who had the widest professional correspondence of all. At least four were on tetanus, one by Thomas Noble Stockett of South River, Maryland, who also sent along "An Account of an Headache cured by the discharge of a worm from the nose." The influenza epidemic of 1789–90 elicited observations from Chester County, Pennsylvania, and Georgetown, Maryland. Rush wrote on measles, Isaac Cathrall on aneurism, John Jones on anthrax, and James Durham of New Orleans on "putrid sore throat"—diphtheria. Isaac Senter of Newport and Benjamin Duffield reported on cases of inverted uterus. Hydrocephalus drew a good deal of attention in the eighteenth century: Rush, Currie, and Leib reported cases under their observation. A special meeting was called so that Dr. Foulke might exhibit a young man, aged twenty-five, with a hole in his trachea "thro' which he appeared to respire." Of special interest is the report by Joseph Capelle on a parasite he found in the livers of nineteen rats. Capelle had come to America with the French forces during the American Revolution, married an American, and settled in Wilmington, Delaware. On April 9, 1790, John Mitchell's account of his experiences with yellow fever in Virginia in 1737–41 was presented;[51] it was to play a significant role in the treatment of that disease in Philadelphia three years later.

Out of forty-eight papers, twenty-five were selected to be printed. There were delays. The Committee on Publication, for example, was uncertain of its authority. (The College resolved the question by ruling that the censors and the president and vice-president should make the selection; the committee was merely to see the papers through the press.) Currie's strictures on Cullen's theory of fevers was judged "inadmissible," and there was hesitation about including Rush's "Discourse" in a volume of scientific papers. (It appeared as the introduction.) There were also money problems. Not until the late summer of 1793 were the *Transactions* printed. It was numbered, hopefully, Volume I, Part I—'a *pledge* to our medical brethren" that the College would issue more volumes as often as material offered. The pledge was not redeemed for nearly half a century.

Copies were sent to the medical societies of the United States and to the Medical Society of London and the Royal Colleges of London and Edinburgh. In Germany the volume was translated by Christian Friedrich Michaelis of Leipzig—he had been a surgeon with German troops in America during the Revolutionary war—and published in 1795 as *Medizinische Verhandlungen des Kollegiums der Aerzte zu Philadelphia.*

The printer delivered the first printed copies of the *Transactions* on September 3, 1793. The event was hardly noticed. Ten days before, on August 25, a special meeting of the College had been called—the first of many that summer—'in consequence of the prevalence of a fever of a very alarming nature in some parts of this city." It was the yellow fever.

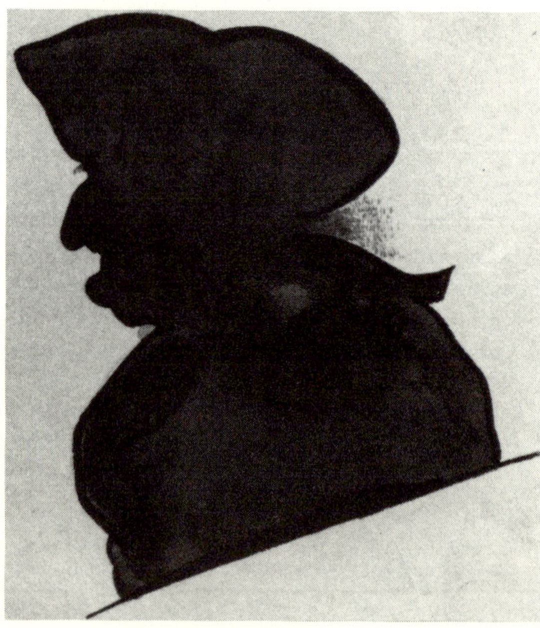

Abraham Chovet, (1704–1790). Silhouette by Joseph Sansom, 1790?

CHAPTER II

# *Yellow Fever*

ONLY six Fellows attended the regularly scheduled meeting of the College on August 6, 1793. As that was not a quorum and there was no business to consider, the Fellows only exchanged professional and social chat.[1] Perhaps Rush, who was present, told them that the day before he had visited young Dr. Hugh Hodge's daughter, "ill with a fever of the bilious kind." Two days later she died. In the ensuing week or ten days Rush treated other patients similarly ill. One displayed "all the symptoms of a bilious fever," some died within a few hours or a day or two, others recovered. To Rush these cases appeared no different from those he saw every summer in Philadelphia, and they excited no unusual interest. But on August 19, in a consultation with Hodge and John Foulke on a woman "in the last stage of a highly bilious fever," Rush reviewed the cases he had seen, and suddenly realized there was an epidemic in the city.[2] He pronounced it yellow fever and located its source as Water Street.

Not everyone agreed. In the first place, the appearances were equivocal; in the second, there were strong reasons for not wanting to admit that it was the same fever that had swept through the city with alarming consequences thirty years before, or that it was of local origin. Most preferred to believe that the fever had been imported in the privateer *Sans Culottes,* which had arrived in Philadelphia on July 22 "in a foul, dirty condition." If yellow fever was imported, then quarantine was the indicated means of confining it; but if it was of local origin, then sanitary measures needed to be adopted. There were profound constitutional and philosophical implications here: quarantine would require only customary minimal intervention by government—the local authorities were already reasonably familiar with such measures; but the adoption of sanitary measures would require those powers to be expanded in unacceptable ways.[3]

In this climate of uncertainty Governor Thomas Mifflin asked James Hutchinson, the port physician, to tell him whether the disease was in fact contagious and what its source might be. Hutchinson inquired of his medical brethren, interviewed some citizens and a number of fever victims, and reported that "a malignant fever" was indeed about and that it was of domestic origin. Pointing to the filthy streets and gutters, he suggested that decaying coffee on the docks might be the probable cause. Mayor Matthew Clarkson accordingly ordered the streets cleaned at once. But the disease intensified and spread. "The fever has assumed a most alarming appearance," Rush wrote his wife on August 25. "It not only mocks in most instances the power of medicine, but it has spread through several parts of the city remote from the spot where it originated."[4]

On that same day, a Sunday, the Fellows of the College of Physicians at the request of the mayor met in special session "to consider what steps should be taken by them on the occasion consistent with their duty to their fellow citizens." Sixteen Fellows were present. After "a free communication of sentiment," a committee of Rush, Hutchinson, Benjamin Say, and Caspar Wistar was appointed to report on the best means to prevent the spread of the disease. Rush drafted the recommendations that night. They were submitted to the College, revised, and adopted at another special meeting next afternoon; and a copy was sent to Mayor Clarkson.[5] The recommendation read as follows:

> The College of Physicians having taken into consideration the malignant and contagious fever which now prevails in this city, have agreed to recommend to their fellow citizens the following means of preventing its progress:
>
> First. That all unnecessary intercourse should be avoided with such persons as are infected by it.
>
> Second. To place a mark upon the door or windows of such houses as have any infected persons in them.
>
> Third. To place the persons infected in the center of large and airy rooms, in beds without curtains, and to pay the strictest regard to cleanliness, by frequently changing

their body and bed linen; also by removing, as speedily as possible, all offensive matters from their rooms.

Fourth. To provide a large and airy Hospital in the neighbourhood of the City, for the reception of such poor persons as cannot be accommodated with the above advantages in private houses.

Fifth. To put a stop to the Tolling of the Bells.

Sixth. To bury such persons as die of this Fever in carriages, and in as private a manner as possible.

Seventh. To keep the Streets and Wharves of the City as clean as possible. As the contagion of the disease may be taken into the body, and pass out of it without producing the Fever, unless it be rendered active by some occasional cause, the following means should be attended to, to prevent the contagion being excited into action in the body.

Eighth. To avoid all fatigue of body and mind.

Ninth. To avoid standing or sitting in the Sun, also in a current of air, or in the evening air.

Tenth. To accommodate the dress to the weather, and to exceed rather in warm than in cold cloathing.

Eleventh. To avoid intemperance, but to use fermented liquors, such as wine, beer and cyder, with moderation.

The College conceive Fires to be [a] very ineffectual if not dangerous means of checking the progress of the Fever. They have reason to place more dependance [sic] upon the burning of Gunpowder. The benefits of Vinegar & Camphor are confined chiefly to infected rooms, and they cannot be used too frequently upon handkerchiefs, or in smelling bottles, by persons whose duty calls them to visit or attend the sick.

The advices were sound as far as they went, but even the committee had no confidence the measures were anything but palliative. "I fear no efforts will totally subdue the fever," Rush confided to his wife that evening, "before the heavy rains or frosts of October."[6] His fears were well founded. The mortality steadily increased. By the end of August 325 were dead; in Water Street alone thirty-nine persons in eleven families had succumbed in nine days.

On August 26 the College resolved to meet weekly thereafter "to confer upon the treatment of the existing malignant fever" as long as the fever prevailed. At the next weekly meeting, September 3, Redman read a paper on the epidemic of 1762, which he remembered.[7] Other Fellows discussed their cases and, as the disease was worsening, voted to meet twice a week.

In their treatments the physicians tried everything, but with little success, and concluded there was no remedy. On August 29 Rush wrote his wife:

> The common remedies for malignant fevers have all failed. Bark, wine, and blisters make no impression upon it. Baths of hot vinegar applied by means of blankets, and the cold bath have relieved and saved some. . . . This day I have given mercury, and I think with some advantage. . . . I have advised all the families that I attend that can move to quit the city. There is but one preventative that is certain, and that is 'to fly from it.'[8]

A week later, however, Rush thought he had an answer—mercury administered liberally, especially in the first stage of the fever, to which should be added bleeding. Adam Kuhn took a contrary view, relating successful treatments with camomile tea, bark or laudanum, wine, lemonade, fresh fruits, and baths of cold water. Replying to Kuhn in a letter to the College on September 12, Rush stoutly defended mercury purging and copious bleeding: "I have bled twice in many, and in one acute case, four times, with the happiest effects. I consider intrepidity in the use of the lancet at present to be as necessary, as it is in the use of mercury and jalap, in this insidious and ferocious disease."[9]

Certain that bleeding and purging were the only sound treatment—ten ounces of blood and ten grains of calomel (mercury)—Rush claimed that four-fifths of his patients treated in this way from the first day recovered. There was, he assured the public, "no more danger to be apprehended from it [this treatment], when those remedies are used in its early stage, than there is from the measles or influenza."[10] He regretted the "contrariety of opinion" among the Fellows—differences which arose, he conceded, from the yellow fever's being confused with jail or hospital fever.

The "contrariety of opinion" persisted, and the College found itself involved in the dispute, as many of the arguments in support of one treatment or another were addressed to it. Alexander Hamilton, Secretary of the Treasury, publicly recommended his physician Edward Stevens, a practitioner from the West Indies, whom he credited with bringing both him and Mrs. Hamilton through the fever; and Stevens, on the eve of his departure for New York, described his treatment—like Kuhn's, opposed to evacuation and bleeding—in a letter to the College. Rush responded promptly, again defending his own vigorous therapeutics which, if followed, he said, would reduce the danger and mortality of the fever "to a level with a common cold." To add to the uncertainty, William Currie, a Fellow of the College, asserted in a public letter that the disease had "greatly abated" and would "most certaintly be entirely eradicated in a few days." He endorsed Kuhn and Stevens, rejected bleeding and all but the mildest purges, and even questioned whether the disease was yellow fever at all.[11]

Meanwhile inquiries and advice began to reach the College from other cities—from the president of the Medical Society of New York, from John Warren and the Massachusetts Medical Society, from George Buchanan in Baltimore, from their Associate Fellow James Tilton of Delaware, and from others. The Fellows were now too busy with patients, sick themselves, or even out of the city, to attend meetings, much less reply to even well-meaning letters. Only two members appeared on September 17, and Redman decided to call no more meetings. Ten days later he too was down with the fever.

September had 1,442 deaths, and as summer passed into early fall, the disease increased in virulence. In the second week of October 720 died. Hutchinson, Linn, Pennington—all Fellows—and John Morris, a former Fellow, were dead. Kuhn, Griffitts, Gibbon, Leib, and Wistar were felled. Rush was stricken twice, once for nearly three weeks in October. Three of his pupils died, and two others became ill. "Hardly one of the practicing doctors that remained in the city, escaped sickness," wrote Mathew Carey, "—some were three, four, and five times confined."

As the epidemic progressed, Rush grew increasingly confident of his treatment and increasingly intolerant of anyone who questioned it. He charged Wistar with betrayal because, taken sick in October when Rush himself was seriously ill, Wistar had called in Kuhn, under whose mild regimen—Rush would have said, *despite* whose mild regimen—he recovered. Attacking the "Kuhnians" as "enemies," Rush compared himself with David standing against the armory of Saul. Physically and emotionally exhausted, he replied angrily to every expression of difference or doubt, taking each as a personal affront and insult. Redman did not put him on the committee to prepare a reply to the questions Governor Mifflin put to the College on October 30:

> Was the disorder imported or not? If imported, when, by what means, and from what place? If not imported, what were the probable causes that produced it? What measures ought to be pursued to purify the city from any latent infection; and what precautions are best calculated to guard against the future occurrence of a similar calamity?

"I am persuaded, "the Governor concluded,

> that the public spirit and benevolence of the College of Physicians will induce them chearfully [sic] to excuse and to comply with this request, which is intended to establish a foundation for regulations, that may co-operate with their professional labours, in preserving to their fellow citizens the invaluable blessing of health.[13]

Apparently the members of the committee could not agree, and three more Fellows were added to their number. The enlarged committee was also unable to reach a conclusion and was discharged. A third committee, composed of Parke, John Carson, and Samuel Powel Griffitts, none yet a leader of the profession, was chosen. After "several readings & alterations," the College on November 26 approved the following text:

> No instance has ever occurred, of the disease called the Yellow Fever, being generated in this city, or in any other part of this state, as far as we know; but there have been frequent instances of its having been imported, not only into this, but into other parts of North-America. . . . We are of opinion, that this disease was imported into Philadelphia by some of the vessels which arrived in the port after the middle of July. This opinion we are further confirmed in by the various accounts we have received from the best authorities we could procure on the subject.

To destroy the contagion the College recommended that every house, particularly those in which there had been sickness, should be "thoroughly cleansed and kept open, so as to admit fresh air through every aperture," the walls whitewashed, and gunpowder burned in every room. The beds and woollen apparel of the sick should be destroyed, or smoked with gunpowder in a closed room, and then hung out in air and rain. Unslaked lime should be thrown into privies and the streets should be kept clean. The College concluded with the hope that the legislature would enact laws to protect the port from future importations of disease and with the assurance that "on such an occasion the College will ever cheerfully co-operate with them in their endeavours to prevent, avert, or, remove those dangerous calamities."[14]

Mifflin cited the opinion of the College in his address to the General Assembly on December 5:

> That the disorder was not immediately engendered by any noxious quality of our soil, or climate, but was brought hither from a foreign port, is a circumstance, which, being supported by the opinion of the College, affords a very serious consolation to the mind of every lover of his country.

He then called for a stricter examination of the health of foreign vessels:

> every vessel from beyond [the] sea should be liable to examination before she shall anchor near the city, whatever may be the number, or condition, in point of health, of the persons on board: that a competent allowance should be made, for fixing the residence of a Health-officer, and a Physician, contiguous to the place appointed for such examination; and that a Pest-house should be constantly supplied with a Steward, a Matron, and proper Houses. If, in addition to an institution, thus regulated, an Hospital, easily accessible by land or water, and situated in the neighbourhood of the city, were established, for the accommodation of those, who may, at any future period, be attacked by a contagious disease, the danger . . . would, in a great measure, be removed.[15]

Meanwhile Rush found himself increasingly alone in his views on the domestic origin and heroic treatment of the disease. Excluded from the committee that drafted the College's reply to the Governor, disregarded and repudiated by many of his fellow physicians, supported only by a handful of the younger doctors, Rush submitted his resignation as a Fellow on November 5, the first meeting of the College after the fever disappeared. He accompanied the letter of resignation with a copy of Wallis' edition of the works of Thomas Sydenham, a final testimony, he wrote afterwards,

> to convey to the College a defense of the principles which had regulated my practice in the yellow fever, and a rebuke of the ignorance of many of the members of the College, of the most common laws of Epidemicks which are recorded in almost every page of that author.[16]

Opening his lectures at the Medical School that fall, Rush deliverd a moving account of the epidemic and of the behavior of the College and individual physicians towards him. He carried on an unremitting correspondence with friendly colleagues and admiring students like John Redman Coxe,[17] and in the summer of 1794 published a full *Account of the Bilious Remitting Yellow Fever, as it appeared in the City of Philadelphia, in the Year 1793.*

The "contrariety of opinion" between Rush and the other physicians created confusion and uncertainty among public officials and other laymen no less concerned than he for the health of the citizens. It also created a division in the profession, so long vexed by the rivalries and antagonisms of Shippen and Morgan and their partisans, which the existence of the College had largely healed. Rush's resignation was a sharp blow to the College's reputation in the medical world, for, as the Fellow best known to medical men throughout the United States and abroad, he had attracted correspondence and learned papers to its *Transactions* and had given it a kind of recommendation to the profession.

## *Yellow Fever, 1794–1802*

The yellow fever reappeared in 1794. Calling it by its right name, bleeding and purging his patients, Rush again summoned the authorities to clean up the city. For this he was strongly attacked—by physicians, who denied it was yellow fever, and by editors, merchants, and public officials because the charge was bad for business, public morale, and the city's reputation. A correspondent in the *Gazette of the United States* confidently asserted that "the yellow fever is not in our city, nor is it possible for it to be generated in it, in its present situation." The people and some of the doctors knew differently.

The Board of Health asked the College whether a hospital for contagious diseases should be erected. The College, warmly approving, offered its opinion "that the building ought to consist of one continued range, fronting the south, and should be so constructed as to admit of a free passage for the air through every room."[18] Shortly afterwards, on January 26, 1795, the College called on the General Assembly to reform and strengthen the Board, in particular by the addition of two consulting physicians—the port physician's associates did not have to be physicians—who, with the Board's own appointee, should be consulted on all matters respecting quarantine, fumigation of vessels, and the construction and operation of a city hospital. Furthermore, the College advised, the Board should be empowered to remove from their houses both the sick and those exposed to the contagion. The bill, which the legislature passed, authorized the governor to appoint four physicians, Fellows of the College. Instead of selecting the four as the governor asked, the president of the College submitted the entire membership roll.[19] The governor named the physicians, but the law was repealed after the new Board had held only one meeting, thus excluding the Fellows from any further authority or responsibility.[20]

The summers of 1795 and 1796 saw only a handful of yellow fever cases; but in 1797 the fever returned in strength. It began in the usual way: one of the physicians saw one case at the end of July, then two more; and on August 15 he reported on them to the College.[21] By then the fever had taken at least ten lives. As he had done in 1793, Governor Mifflin on August 14 turned to the College for facts and "an opinion upon the best mode of averting the calamity threatened." The College replied with its familiar recommendations. In particular the sick and their families should be isolated, and all contact between them and the city suspended. "For this purpose," the College warned, "Mercantile business must, of course, be suspended there, and the vessels removed from the adjoining wharves." The citizens were also advised to be temperate, take exercise, avoid fatigue and exposure to sun and night air, and to keep their clothing clean. To prevent the introduction of contagious diseases in the future, the College recommended that quarantine requirements be strengthened and that the Board of Health be reformed with "full power to do everything necessary respecting the quarantine to be performed by vessels arriving in this port, as well as to direct the removal of any vessels, after their arrival at the city, which may be found or suspected to be unhealthy." A physician should be in constant attendance at State Island from June through September.[22]

The governor forwarded the College's recommendation to the Board of Health, which published it. But the Board, which lacked the powers to cope with an epidemic in the way that the College suggested, could only assure the public that the fever was limited and unlikely to prove dangerous and ask the College to meet daily to prepare and publish "such information and advice to the citizens of Philadelphia, as they may judge will tend to check the progress of contagion."[23] The College accordingly on August 25 offered its customary advice about fumigation, removal of the sick, and burial of the dead.

> It cannot be repeated too often, that the sick should be placed in large airy apartments, which should be constantly ventilated: Their cloathing and bed linen changed daily and washed in cold water. Half an ounce of strong oil of vitriol poured upon an equal quantity of powdered saltpetre, in China or glass vessels, produces a vapour that has been found very beneficial in destroying contagion in sick rooms.[24]

Although the epidemic subsided with the coming of cool weather, nearly 1,100 persons had died.

As the fever abated, Governor Mifflin from his refuge in Germantown once more appealed to the College, asking the same questions he had put before and receiving much the same answers. "What measures ought to be pursued to purify the City from any latent infection?" he asked. "And what precautions are best calculated to guard against the future occurrence of a similar calamity?"[25] The College recommended sanitation and fumigation, as formerly. "These, with the frost, we believe, will be found

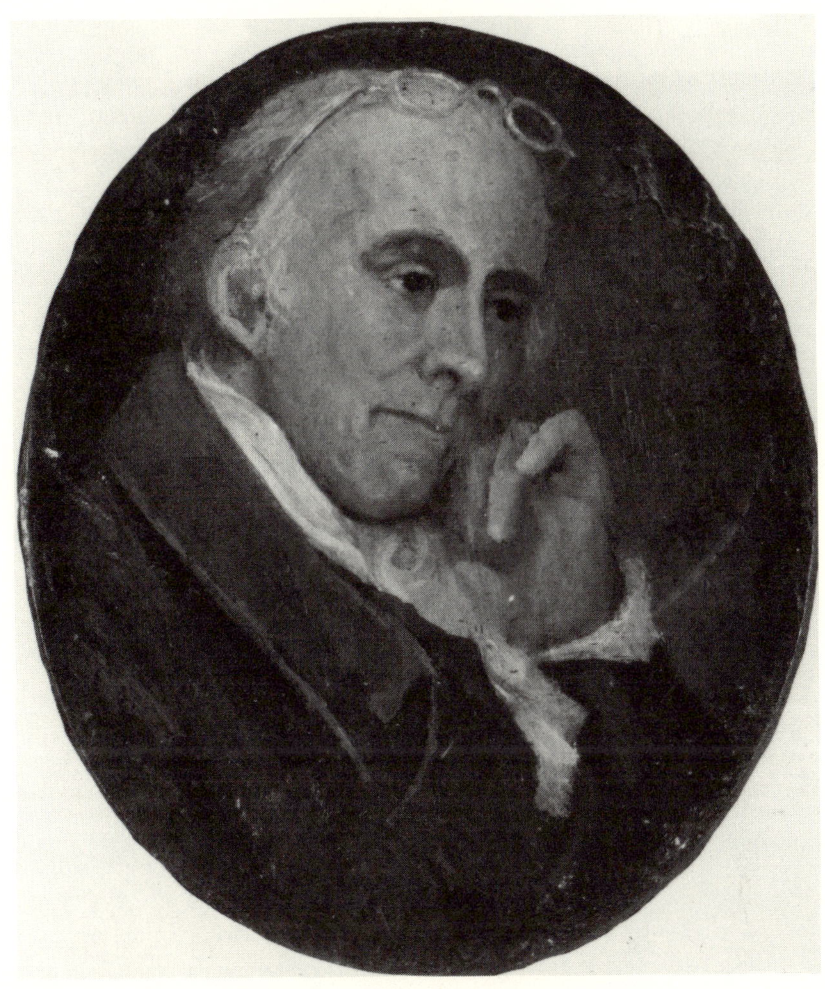

Benjamin Rush, (1746–1813). Miniature; copy by an unknown artist after Thomas Sully.

sufficient entirely to destroy any latent contagion."[26] As for preventing a recurrence, the College enlarged upon the advice it had given two months before.

> Let an entire new health-law, be made, constituting a Board of Health, to consist of five persons, two of whom to be practitioners of physic. The smallness of the number will ensure responsibility, and a constant residence in the city, and the professional knowledge of the medical characters will be necessary to assist in directing the measures of the Board. Let no person whose private interest may be affected by quarantine laws, be a member of this Board.

Penalties for violating the quarantine law should be severe. "Let the punishment of a master of a vessel, who evades the law, by landing cargo, crew or passengers, contrary to the intent and meaning of it, be the same as for murder of the second degree." The College recognized that the cooperation of neighboring states or of Congress must be procured if Pennsylvania's quarantine laws were to be effective. "Let the Board of Health have power, with the concurrence of the Governor, to cut off intercourse with infected persons and places. Let the long projected Hospital be erected."[27]

The College reinforced its recommendations to the Governor by a strong appeal to the General Assembly. Its memorial of December 5, 1797, presented reasons for believing that the yellow fever was of foreign origin, imported principally from the West Indies; it repeated its conviction that the existing health laws were deficient and urged their amendment. Having thus tendered their views, the physicians held themselves "discharged from all responsibility, on account of the evils which may arise from the present imperfect state of the legislative arrangements respecting this important subject."[28]

In January 1798 the College published a summary of its *Proceedings . . . relative to the Prevention of the Introduction and Spreading of Contagious Diseases* since 1793. Five hundred copies were printed, and copies were sent to President John Adams, Governor Mifflin, and members of the Pennsylvania and federal legislatures.

Governor Mifflin had also asked Rush for his opinion, understanding, as he put it diplomatically, "that you and many other learned members of the Faculty do not attend the deliberations of that institution."[29] The "others" included John Redman Coxe, the grandson of the president of the College of Physicians, Philip Syng Physick, William Potts Dewees, Felix Pascalis, and Francis B. Sayre. They were at this time engaged with Rush in organizing a medical society whose principal purpose was to demonstrate the falsity of the College's views and the correctness of their own. Of the thirteen members of the Academy of Medicine only Charles Caldwell was a Fellow of the College, and he held that institution in no high regard. Of the remaining twelve, only John C. Otto ever became a Fellow—and that was more than twenty years later, when time and his unassailable achievements had effaced the memory of his challenge to the physicians' majority view. The Academy was similar to the College in general organization and in the residence requirements of members, but it also required each member in turn to write and deliver a medical or scientific paper.[30] The Academy's *Proofs of the Origin of the Yellow Fever . . . in the year 1797, from Domestic Exhalation* refuted the College's *Facts and Observations* on the question of origin and urged such measures as removal, sanitation, and temperance. As the 1798 epidemic gained strength, the Board of Health authorized publication of a communication from the Academy strongly rejecting the contagion theory.[31] As for the Academy itself, despite Rush's confident prediction that it would flourish, it soon withered away, leaving as one of its legacies a profession yet more irreconcilably divided.

On July 22, 1798, Benjamin Duffield and Caspar Wistar reported two cases of yellow fever to the Board of Health. A month later the fever was epidemic once more. As usual the College recommended evacuating infected areas, as did the Academy of Medicine, which also advised anyone suffering the slightest indiposition to seek medical aid at once. As conditions worsened in September, the Board appealed to public-spirited citizens to prepare a tent city for refugees on the west bank of the Schuylkill and to contribute money for the relief of the sick. Former President Washington sent $200. The Board had nothing else to offer. "We believe that you will think with us," it declared despairingly in an address on September 1, "that the preservation of health is only to be attained by flight."[32] Deaths that summer amounted to 3,446, almost as many as in 1793; in fact, because more had fled the city, the mortality rate was higher.

At the year's end the College issued another review, entitled *Facts and Observations relative to the Nature and Origin of the Pestilential Fever, which prevailed in this City, in 1793, 1797, and 1798.* This in effect complemented the *Proceedings* issued in January, offering a fuller account of the College's actions during the great epidemics and an explanation of its views on the foreign origin of yellow fever and the best ways of preventing and treating it. "Efficient quarantine laws," it affirmed, " . . . are the only effectual means to guard against the future recurrence of a calamity which threatens us with total ruin." From the first appearance of the fever in 1793 to the present time, the statement continued, the College had endeavored to fulfill its obligations by warning the citizens of its appearance, pointing out the means of checking it, and informing the legislature how to prevent its return,

> and although our recommendations have been too little attended to, yet we conceive it to be a duty again thus to publish our opinions on the subject in a more detailed and familiar manner, as well for the information of our fellow citizens at large, as of those who are called to the very important office of legislation.

"In doing this," the College explained, "we have no design of entering into or exciting contention: our sole aim is truth and the public good."[33]

The annual visitation of yellow fever was now accepted as inescapable. There were sporadic cases in 1799, 1800 and 1801. Each year the College met in emergency sessions and called on the authorities to institute the usual precautionary measures. After 1798, however, the Board of Health refused to issue a warning proclamation. "A public notification would perhaps create a terror that might add to the predisposing cause of the sickness, if any such cause exists."[34] Of course, no one knew what caused the disease or how to prevent it. The doctors' treatments varied, and no treatment seemed more effective than another. Every year the same queries were put to the College, and the same answers were returned. The sick were quarantined or hurried into isolation. Many fled to the country. To provide for those who stayed or were too sick to go, the Board of Health ordered that a sufficient number of "Hearses & Bunks" be put in repair.[35]

In response to a question from Governor Thomas McKean in

the late summer of 1799, the College warned of danger to public health from large gatherings of people at the forthcoming local elections. Such an assemblage at the Commissioners' Hall in Southwark in particular would be unsafe, and it was "most adviseable not to hold the Election at the State House." The attorney general, however, declined to recommend postponing the election or moving the voting places, offering as a reason that the College had said only that it was *not advisable,* rather than that it was *dangerous,* to hold the election at the State House. To this, Redman responded tartly, "Had the College supposed it necessary, they would have used this language in their communication—and if you should judge that my explanation is not sufficient we will endeavor to have another meeting."[38]

When the fever broke out in 1802, the Board of Health advised that the sick should be isolated and that others should leave the infected area. Though in some consternation at this, the College endorsed the public proclamation. The result was "a general removal." But every effort by the College and others to strengthen the Board of Health was frustrated. Caught "between the commercial interest and health of the city," the Board was in an awkward position; nevertheless, they proclaimed that the health of the citizens was their paramount consideration, even though this militated against the business interests.[39] Yellow fever took 1,154 lives in 1802.

Inevitably, the successive epidemics attracted the attention of European physicians, who had witnessed epidemics of their own at Marseilles, Cadiz, Malaga, and Leghorn, or had seen yellow fever in the West Indies. But foreign counsel was no more helpful than American. Dr. Bölke of Hamburg, for example, sent the College medicines, which he assured them would cure the fever. (The College wisely took no action.) Johann A. Albers of Bremen was positive the disease was of local origin; John Haygarth of London, that it was imported.[40] Rush pleaded with his friend Lettsom to add his influence to the mounting support for local origins.

> *Do, my friend, give the subject a second investigation.* The evils which flow from a belief in the importation of our American pestilence are incalculable. It has perpetuated the disease in our country. It has demoralized our citizens. . . . It fosters national prejudice and hostility,

> and it consigns thousands every year to the grave who might otherwise have been preserved from it.[41]

In 1806 the College published another pamphlet—*Additional Facts and Observations relative to the Nature and Origin of the Pestilential Fever*—"to prevent any relaxation in quarantine laws."

### *Vaccination*

Not every epidemic proved as unyielding as yellow fever. Just when they were engaged in unremitting battle with yellow fever, the Philadelphia physicians learned of the discovery by a Gloucestershire country doctor Edward Jenner of a defense against a still more destructive and widespread disease—smallpox.

Before vaccination, the only defense against that disease had been inoculation with attenuated virus of the disease itself. Those who were treated successfully in this way received permanent immunity; but the mortality in the treatment was high, and there was always danger that in the process the smallpox would spread in virulent and fatal form to those who had no immunity. Jenner published the results of his observations and experience in 1798 in a slim volume entitled *An Inquiry into the Causes and Effects of the Variolae Vaccinae.* In 1799 Lettsom sent a copy to his friend Benjamin Waterhouse in Boston, and Waterhouse reported on it—'Something Curious in the Medical Line"—in a Boston newspaper. The next year Waterhouse received some "matter" from England, vaccinated his son and other members of his household, and began to supply vaccine to physicians throughout New England. In April 1801 he sent some to Thomas Jefferson.[42]

Jefferson appreciated at once the importance of vaccination and used the vaccine from Waterhouse to vaccinate his Monticello slaves. Not all physicians, however, were so receptive to the new procedure. "Could you believe that not a single case of the cowpox inoculation has yet occurred in Philadelphia?" Waterhouse exclaimed incredulously to Jenner on April 24, 1801. "A young physician applied to me a few days since from that [place] for the infection. It seems that the leading physician there pronounces it too beastly and indelicate for polished society!" Meanwhile, assured of the vaccine's efficacy, Jefferson was providing the matter to physicians in Virginia and the South. At the request of John Vaughan, librarian of the American Philosophical Society, he sent some to John Redman Coxe.

The day the vaccine arrived, November 9, 1801—'A day which I trust will be memorable among the citizens of Philadelphia, from the great benefit connected with it"—Coxe vaccinated himself and four others.[43] In the next few weeks he vaccinated several score more, including children of his friends Benjamin Rush and Charles Willson Peale and his own three-weeks-old son, whom in his enthusiasm for this new therapy he had named Edward Jenner Coxe. Coxe then exposed the child to the natural disease with no ill effects. "This I conceive to be conclusive evidence, not to be overthrown, by cases, problematical, at least . . . ." Coxe was now the principal champion of vaccination in Philadelphia, explaining and defending it in his little book *Practical Observations on Vaccination* (1802), which he dedicated to Jenner, and in the pages of the *Philadelphia Medical Museum,* which he founded in 1804.[44]

Meanwhile the College had received several reports on vaccination. On October 6, 1801, William Currie conveyed to the Fellows a report on the "kine pock" as David Hosack had described it to him in a letter from New York. At the December meeting Lettsom's gift of his *Treatise on the Vaccine Pock* was received. On February 2, 1802, a paper by Thomas Chalkley James on successful cases of vaccination was read; Currie presented a copy of his *Letters on the Kine Pock;* and Jenner and Lettsom were proposed for associate membership. Lettsom was promptly elected, Jenner not—whether because he had no degree in medicine or because his discovery was considered insufficiently tested, or for some other reason, we can only speculate.

Experience with vaccination was conclusive. On March 12, 1802, Rush wrote Jefferson that "the vaccine inoculation is generally adopted in our city and its success has hitherto equaled the best wishes of its most sanguine and zealous friends."[46] At the end of the year the College appointed a committee to consider the health laws of the city, possibly with a view to recommending action on vaccination; but the committee seems not to have reported. In April 1803, forty-nine physicians of Philadelphia, including all the active Fellows of the College except Adam Kuhn, publicly endorsed vaccination as "A CERTAIN PREVENTIVE OF THE

SMALL POX" and recommended it "TO GENERAL USE"[47] In 1809 the Pennsylvania Hospital offered free vaccination to the poor of the city.

### *Meeting Room and Library*

Since 1791 the College had met in the hall of the American Philosophical Society on Fifth Street below Chestnut. Although the interior of the building was not entirely finished, the room was comfortable enough. The Society's custodian was engaged to deliver meeting notices and to attend to other College needs. Charles Willson Peale, who lived in the hall, which also housed his famous natural history museum, provided firewood and swept the chimney. (He also sent the College a description of a newly-invented steam bath, showed it an apparatus for cooking that he had made, and presented a copy of his *Epistle . . . on the Means of Preserving Health.*) But the rent was a burden, and the College repeatedly appealed for a reduction. When the Philosophical Society in 1798 doubled the rent from $40 to $80 a year, the College made a counter-offer—to pay $40 until 1800 and $52 thereafter, and allow the Society to keep its library and apparatus in the College's room. Although this saved the College money, the arrangement was unsatisfactory. The Society frequently encroached upon the College's space. In 1805 it wanted the room for the skeleton of an Indian elephant, and a few years later it proposed that Silvanus Godon be allowed to lecture on mineralogy in the College's room, where the Society's mineral collection was kept, "*if not inconvenient to the College.*"[48]

But the rent remained a burden. In 1800, when it was about to rise to $52 under the agreement of 1798, the College appealed and got the rent restored to $40. To help pay even this amount, the College sublet its room to the Agricultural Society from 1805 to 1812. And still the College complained to its landlord: not only were its funds meager, while the Society's treasury was in a "flourishing state," it pointed out in 1815, but

> The Physicians of this city, as members of the Philosophical Society have not only contributed as much, if not more,

> to the building of the Hall, than any other body according to their numbers, but also by their annual contributions assist in defraying the expences of the Society.[49]

Some of the philosophers were persuaded; their permission to the Athenaeum of Philadelphia and the Agricultural Society to sublet the College's room helped the College in its financial plight.

The College's library, which had begun with a few modest gifts and purchases, grew slowly after 1793.[50] Redman gave the College the works of Boerhaave and Sydenham. Benjamin Moseley of Jamaica presented copies of his treatises on tropical diseases and coffee, and later added copies of subsequent editions. From Thomas Percival in 1803 came a copy of his *Medical Ethics.* Benjamin Smith Barton gave the College two works of Joseph Priestley as well as copies of his own publications. William Currie was particularly generous, on several occasions giving the College copies of his own works on yellow fever and general works by others. Acknowledging his election as an associate fellow, Lettsom sent along a copy of his *Hints designed to Promote Beneficence, Temperance, and Medical Science,* while others presented volumes in hope of obtaining election thereby. From the Medical Society of London came its published *Memoirs.*

Not content with haphazard growth through individual gifts, the College began systematically to order books abroad, appropriating £60 for this purpose in 1794, $120 in 1796, and £28 12s. sterling in 1798. The first of these orders included, among other titles, Alexander Monro's *Description of all the 'bursae mucosae' of the Human Body,* John Howard's *Account of the Principal Lazarettos of Europe,* the works of Senac, the *Mémoires* of the Société royale de Médecine, and "the different periodical Publications on Medicine viz, Reviews, Journals &c which are published on the Continent of Europe, in the Latin or French Languages." Needless to say, not all the titles ordered could be obtained.

Under the direction of the Censors, who were charged with care of the library, the pamphlets were bound and the books numbered and catalogued. In 1796 the College appointed Thomas Chalkley James librarian and in 1797 made a list of books "to be procured from Europe for the use of the College." In 1806 the library was reported to be "in good order," with only two volumes missing—volumes 15 and 27 of the Leipzig *Commentarii de rebus in scientia naturali et medicina gestis.* (They were never found.)

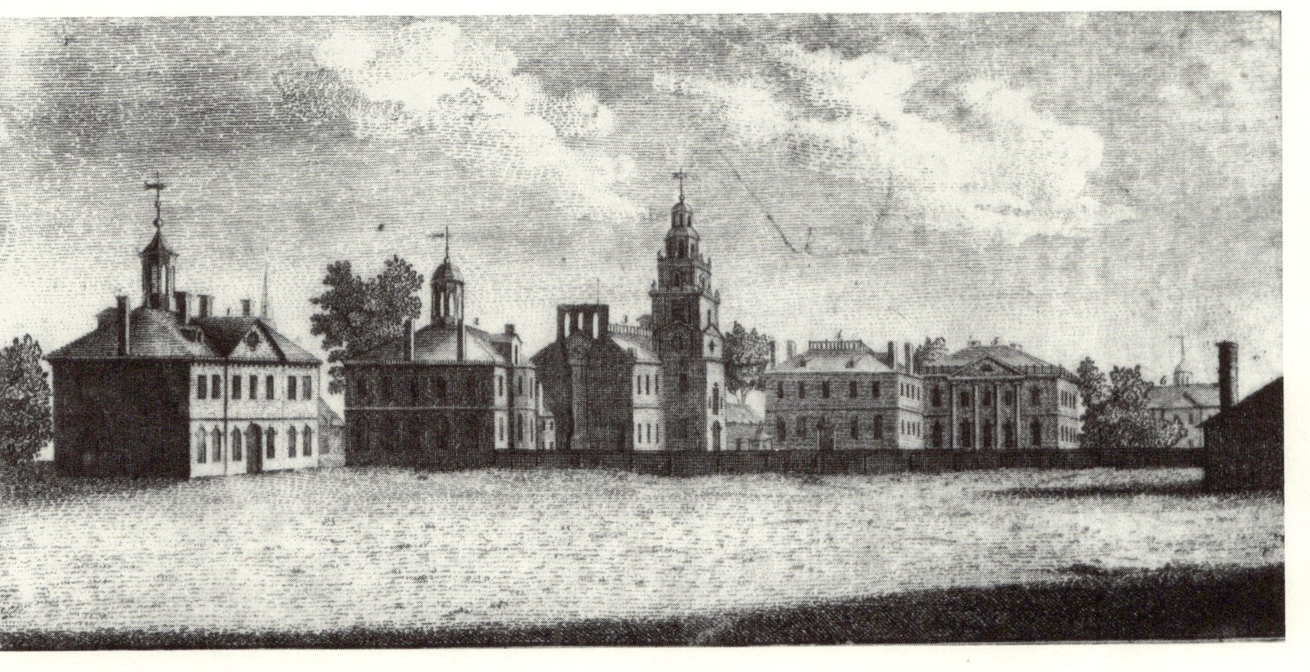

Public Buildings, Philadelphia. Engraving in *Columbian Magazine,* January 1790 *(Library Company of Philadelphia).*

The fourth building from the left, just to the right of the State House (now Independence Hall), is the hall of the American Philosophical Society, where the College met from 1791 to 1845.

A register of borrowings shows that between 1792 and 1810 most of the Fellows took out one or two books, a few as many as six: Thomas Chalkley James twenty-one, Benjamin Smith Barton sixteen, Adam Kuhn eleven, Caspar Wistar, William Shippen, Jr., and Plunkett F. Glentworth six each. John Redman, president of the College, borrowed none.[51]

### *College Business*

During the decade after 1793 yellow fever and related public health measures absorbed much of the attention and energy of the Fellows. An exception occurred in March 1794, when a committee of the legislature asked "the speedy assistance" of the College on a bill it was drafting to regulate the practice of medicine. This was a subject about which the College and its Fellows were always concerned; regulating and improving the practice of medicine had been a reason for establishing the College in the first place. Seeing in the proposed bill a means both of achieving desirable professional and public goals and of raising its own prestige, the College recommended that prospective practitioners, except graduates of the University of Pennsylvania, should be examined in Philadelphia by a board selected by the College from its own membership, and that apothecaries should undergo a similar test. The committee of the Assembly approved this recommendation in principle, but extended the exception to graduates of any college or university, and provided that residents of other counties than Philadelphia should be examined by three physicians appointed by the president judge or any two judges of the county court. However, the bill did not pass.

The withdrawal of Rush did not end contentiousness in meetings. At one meeting, probably in 1795, there was a debate between Benjamin Smith Barton and Charles Caldwell. Caldwell, never loathe to make a good story better, especially if he was its hero, remembered it some years later:

> In the discussion of a subject, in which I took an active part in opposition to him [Barton], having previously made due preparation for the contest, he found himself so entangled by a toil of his own sophistry, that an escape from it by argument was altogether hopeless. He therefore made an

attempt to overwhelm me by an avalanche of authority. But, unfortunately for him as a debater and a lover of truth, his device was a blunder, and his authority a fiction. His reference was spurious; and, to his deep mortification, it was made to a volume which, but half an hour previously, as an act in preparing myself for the occasion, had been taken by me out of the library of the Pennsylvania Hospital, and was then in my pocket. I therefore placed it in his hand, and asked the favor of him to show me the passage alluded to by him; asserting, at the same time, with sufficient firmness, that it was not in the book. With marks of disappointment, embarrassment, and vexation (the latter, perhaps, predominating), he hastily glanced from page to page of the work, and, finding in it nothing to his purpose, acknowledged himself mistaken, said that, through forgetfulness, he had referred to a wrong authority, but that in another publication, which he indiscreetly named, the opinion was contained.

I said to him, with an emphasis on one of my words, 'Are you *sure,* sir, that the sentiment is there?"

"Perfectly sure," was his reply.

The Philadelphia Library being at hand, [across the street from Philosophical Hall], and open, I repaired to it immediately, and returning in a few minutes with the doctor's second book of reference, and, presenting it to him, requested him to turn to the controverted opinion, under a perfect conviction that it was not in the volume, and that he would, therefore, encounter another defeat.

To be thus vanquished a second time, by a young man, who, but a few years previously, had been his pupil, was an event quite too mortifying to be patiently borne by him. After an awkward and unsuccessful attempt therefore to explain and palliate his blunder, and perceiving on the countenances of several members of the college, with whom he was no favorite, a sarcastic smile, indicative of their gratification at his discomfiture and perplexity, he offered as a plea a professional engagement, and left the room under high excitement—not to say, in a paroxysm of anger.[52]

### *Fellows and Officers*

In the quarter century after 1793, twenty-two physicians were elected to the Fellowship of the College, and two other Americans—David Hosack and Samuel Bard of New York—were made Associate Fellows. Of the twenty-two Philadelphia residents, only nine are to be found in Kelly and Burrage's *American Medical Biography* and only five or six achieved much reputation in medicine (Charles Caldwell, Thomas Chalkley James, Thomas T. Hewson, and Nathaniel Chapman) or in one of the sciences (Adam Seybert in geology and William P.C. Barton in botany). The rest, however able and promising they must have seemed when elected, are but names on the membership roll—Hugh Hodge, elected in 1793, John Cumming in 1795, William Annan in 1796, Lewis J. Jardine in 1800, Joseph P. Minnick in 1801, Samuel Stewart and Joseph Woollens in 1814, Samuel Hopkins in 1817. Four of the Americans, it should in fairness be stated, died young or soon after election. Of the twenty-two Fellows only ten are listed in Austin's *Early American Medical Imprints* before 1820, and for six of these ten, the only entry is their graduation dissertation.

Furthermore, this list of Fellows has surprising omissions, which reflect the parochialism and partisanship in the College. This must explain why John Redman Coxe, William P. Dewees, John Syng Dorsey, William E. Horner, James Mease, John C. Otto, Felix Pascalis, and Philip Syng Physick—not a few of them supporters of Rush in the yellow fever controversies—were not then (and only Otto ever) Fellows. The failure of the College to admit these and such as these, or their indifference to membership if in fact they were invited, is evidence both of the decline of the College's reputation, and a reason why it seemed to lack purpose, energy, and drive in these years.

### *Lethargy and Decline*

The fact is that as the College moved into the nineteenth century it was moribund. Only rarely was a meeting enlivened by a scientific paper or other communication. The early promise to issue a volume of *Transactions* from time to time was almost forgotten. Sometimes the Fellows were invited as a body to attend a public function, such as the commencement of the University of Pennsylvania, but at least once the invitation went unanswered because the College lacked a quorum to vote its acceptance.

The decline was chronic. Attendance had fallen steadily since the year of founding—from an average of 12.2 a meeting in 1788 to ten in 1796 to seven in 1804. Redman was absent from eight of the twelve monthly meetings in 1801, from ten in 1802, and after August 1803 he never attended again. On the eve of the annual election in 1804, citing his infirmities and limitations, as he had done for most of the past dozen years, Redman expressed the wish not to be reelected—he was eighty-two—but his colleagues elected him again nonetheless, and let him go only in 1805.

His successor was William Shippen, Jr., vice-president of the College since Jones' death in 1791, one of the original twelve senior Fellows. He had been professor of anatomy and midwifery in the Medical School since its founding. Handsome, elegant, graceful, and gentlemanly in conduct and speech, he had overcome the prejudice against male accoucheurs, lectured regularly to a class of midwives, and was, in the judgment of Thomas Bond, the best obstetrical practitioner he ever knew. However, he had never recovered from the death of a promising son, and by the time he was chosen president, he had largely withdrawn from teaching and practice and from most professional and social life. His election was a tribute to his years, his reputation as a founder and teacher of the Medical School, and to the personal qualities that had made him especially popular among younger people. He had no claim to scientific reputation, and in more than forty years had published only his Edinburgh thesis. In his first year and a half as president of the College, he attended only four of its eighteen meetings.

Shippen died on July 11, 1808. His successor Adam Kuhn, the vice-president, was the last survivor of the first faculty of the Medical School. Son of a physician, he had received his medical education in London and Edinburgh and studied botany for two years in Uppsala, where the great Linnaeus had cherished him "for . . . correct and engaging deportment, . . . unwearied ardor and application in cultivating the sciences, . . . [and] undisguised friendship . . . ." Kuhn was appointed professor of botany and materia medica in the College of Philadelphia and was later named to the chair of theory and practice. He served the Pennsylvania Hospital twenty-three years as a physician, was consulting physician to the Philadelphia Dispensary, and was a physician to the Society for Inoculating the Poor. In the yellow fever epidemic of 1793 he fell ill himself, took refuge in Germantown and so saw few patients, but he strongly opposed the heroic therapeutics of Benjamin Rush. "The most highly and minutely furnished specimen of old-school medical production" one of his students had ever beheld, Kuhn carried a gold-headed cane and a gold snuffbox. Sound but unimaginative, his lectures "mere commonplace," he, like Shippen, wrote nothing during a long professional career: apparently, his only "publication" after leaving Edinburgh was a comment on ulceration of gums following the transplanting of teeth, which he made in a letter to John Coakley Lettsom and which Lettsom quoted in a paper of his in the *Memoirs* of the Medical Society of London.[53]

Kuhn presided at meetings of the College more regularly than his predecessors had; but his example did not reverse the waning interest among the Fellows in its work. Attendance averaged 6.3 Fellows in 1810, 6.6 in 1811, 5.9 in 1812. In 1807 there was no quorum—seven members—at two meetings; none at five in 1808, 1810 and 1811; none at seven in 1812. Sometimes, as the appearance of the minute book suggests, even the secretary failed to appear. By 1813 the College must have seemed dead to any casual observer. In that year there was no quorum at eight meetings, no business done at two others, and at the two remaining meetings nothing but a motion to pay bills. At the annual election only four Fellows appeared, but they went ahead anyway to reelect all the officers and censors. It was much the same in 1815 and 1816. At meeting after meeting, "No business claim'd the attention of the College." When Kuhn died in 1817 the College was at its nadir.

The gap left in Philadelphia medical affairs by the low state of the College was filled by several medical clubs and societies. The oldest, largest, and most influential of these was the Philadelphia Medical Society, founded in 1792 and incorporated three years later.[54] Its weekly meetings, well attended by ambitious students and the more active younger professors, usually included an examination of candidates for admission and a lecture by one of the graduate members, which was followed by lively debate and discussion. After 1814 one of the senior members would report annually on "the state of Medical Science in the United States, & Foreign countries." Some of the papers read to the Society—by, among others, Joseph Hartshorne, Thomas T. Hewson, Thomas C.

James, Joseph Parrish, all Fellows of the College—were printed in Benjamin Smith Barton's *Philadelphia Medical and Physicial Journal,* which began publication in 1804, John Redman Coxe's *Philadelphia Medical Museum,* or after 1811, the *Eclectic Repertory and Analytical Review.* The success of these journals stirred the College to think of reviving its *Transactions.* Although there were enough papers "proper for publication" to fill a volume, the College elected instead to print *Additional Facts and Observations* in support of its view that yellow fever was imported and that the quarantine laws should not be relaxed.

Many physicians obtained such satisfaction and benefit from the Philadelphia Medical Society that they remained active in its work long after they had become Fellows of the College. Its meetings were stimulating, it had a library, and it was more open than the College to new ideas, change, and reform. Some years later, for example, while the College initially opposed creation of the American Medical Association, the Philadelphia Medical Society sent a delegation of twelve to the founding meeting—ironically, all of them also Fellows of the College.

This was the sorry state of the College when William Currie in 1817 called the Fellows to account in a strongly worded, even angry, appeal. One of the original members, Currie had been active in College affairs since 1787, presenting books to its library, reading papers, serving as censor and on the Committee on Publications. Recalling that he had once "fondly hoped" that the College would not only be "the admiration and ornament of this Western World, but would before this time have become more eminent than the most illustrious of the Medical Societies in that portion of the Globe which has been exclusively stiled, 'the Seat of Science and the Nurse of Arts,' " Currie boldly stated that the College had declined in both reputation and usefulness and regretted that it was "of so little use" to the community in general and the profession in particular. Reminding his colleagues of the purposes of their founding, he exhorted them to rescue the institution from "its present state of lifeless apathy." He warned that unless they united

> in emerging from the mists of indolence and indifference, in which they appear to me to have been too long involved for the credit of the Society or the good of the Community, and speedily conclude to do something to rescue the Col-

lege from the opprobrious imputation of being governed by a selfish and illiberal policy, and a culpable indifference to the improvement and extension of useful knowledge, by frequently recording and communicating the results of their own experience, and by inviting Physicians residing in different parts of the Union, by means of circular letters, to communicate such facts as have come into their knowledge relative to the principal objects for which the College was instituted; the College, from present appearances will cease to exist in the course of a very few years, or like the mimic Echo, only live unseen within its airy cell. . . . [55]

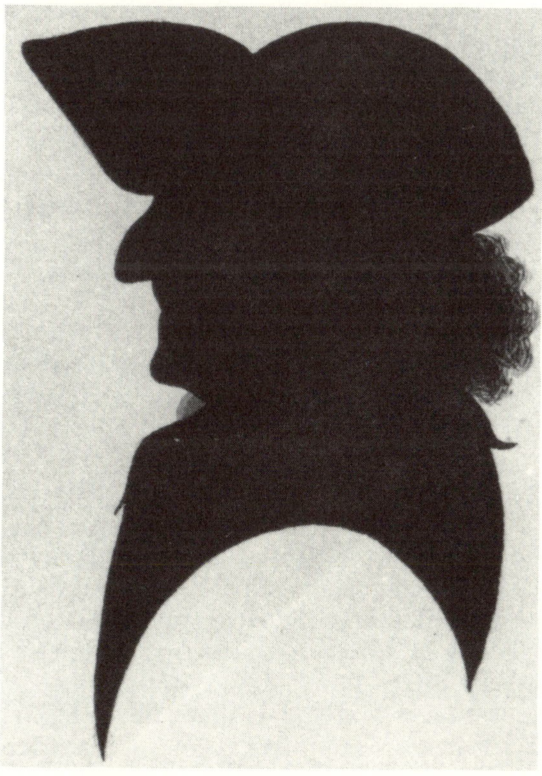

John Redman, (1722–1808). Silhouette by Joseph Sansom, c. 1791.

## CHAPTER III

# *Return to Life*

THE College responded, at least briefly, to Currie's strictures. A revision of the by-laws, under way since 1816, was completed at last and printed in the spring of 1818. The Committee on Library in the same year recommended that "a new catalogue" be prepared, and this was promptly done.[1] Another committee reviewed papers submitted to the College in past years and approved several for publication. Over the next half dozen years, with the example and quiet encouragement of its new president, the College undertook projects for public health and professional control which benefited the profession, the public, and its own reputation.

Thomas Parke, one of the original Fellows of 1787, was elected fourth president of the College on July 7, 1818, in succession to Kuhn, who had died in 1817.[2] The choice was probably more a tribute to Parke's character and years—he was sixty-nine—than to his professional achievements; but it was also a recognition that as vice-president in the preceding years he had provided some leadership to the College.

A native of Chester County and a birthright Friend, Parke had studied medicine with Cadwalader Evans, received the degree of bachelor of medicine from the College of Philadelphia in 1770, and spent two years attending the medical lectures and hospital practice of London and Edinburgh. Since 1777 he had been a physician to the Pennsylvania Hospital and since 1778 a director of the Library Company of Philadelphia. Like many Quakers he took an interest in natural history, acting as agent for Humphry Marshall and other American seedsmen with their English customers; but he published nothing on either medicine or science, and resigned his membership in the American Philosophical Society for lack of interest in its work.

Parke became president when the College was at low ebb. Although conscientious in the performance of obvious duties—until prevented by age and ill health he presided at meetings regularly—he had no clear plan or purpose to offer the Fellows, yet he and some of his colleagues, perhaps stung by Currie's sharp criticism, did respond to professional opportunities. Ten years after his election the College was perceptibly reviving.

### *The Pharmacopoeia*

The first sign of revival was the College's participation in the preparation of a national pharmacopoeia. In his address on the purposes of the College in 1787, Benjamin Rush had named an American dispensatory as one of the first objects of its attention. "The variety in the degrees, and perhaps nature of our diseases," Rush said, "and the many remedies which are peculiar to our country, which have as yet no place in foreign dispensatories, render this undertaking a matter of absolute necessity."[3] The year after Rush spoke, the Fellows voted to prepare such a work "for the use of the College," and, enlarging the plan in 1789, they proposed to "the most respectable Medical Characters in the United States" that a pharmacopoeia be compiled "adapted to the present State of Medicine in America." The response, though favorable, was limited. The College, however, did not give up the project, and in 1797, on recommendation of its Committee on the Pharmacopoeia, resolved

> that an enumeration be made of all such medicinal substances & pharmaceutical processes as shall appear useful and proper to compose the intended Pharmacopoeia—that all the clinical processes be made in a laboratory at the expence of the College, by such members as they may appoint for the purpose—who shall also be directed to compound the different pharmaceutical preparations—and make report thereon to the College.

But this initiative failed; and in the prevailing lassitude in the College in the ensuing decades, it was not renewed.

Meanwhile, John Redman Coxe, a friend of Rush and a follower of his doctrines, but not a Fellow, prepared in 1806 an American edition of Andrew Duncan's *New Edinburgh Dispensa-*

*tory.* Two years later the Massachusetts Medical Society published a pharmacopoeia of its own, and in 1816 the New York Hospital issued a pharmacopoeia for practitioners in New York.

In January 1817 Lyman Spalding laid before the New York County Medical Society a plan for a national pharmacopoeia, to be compiled and issued under the authority of the country's medical societies, colleges, and other institutions, as well as of voluntary associations of physicians and surgeons in states and territories without a general medical society or medical school. Spalding proposed that the country be divided into four geographical districts, that a meeting be held in each prior to a general convention, and that a national convention to approve and adopt a pharmacopoeia be held in Washington on January 1, 1820. This scheme was communicated to other medical institutions by the Medical Society of the State of New York in a circular of May 4, 1818. The response was favorable, and on November 21 a second circular was issued:[4]

> If we advert to the manner in which the first European Pharmacopoeias were formed, we shall find it was by collecting and imbodying the prescriptions and formulae of the most eminent physicians of the time. These recipes have been pruned and polished by the hand of time and experience, until they have approached a state of perfection, as it regards the articles well known in the Eastern Continent, and their application to the particular forms of disease there prevalent. From our native forests and fields we may gather many remedies, and from our practising physicians, original receipts and prescriptions for the cure of the diseases of our country.

The College of Physicians approved the proposal at once, offered its room for the meeting of representatives of the Middle District, and named seven delegates to attend the convention: Parke, Samuel Powel Griffitts, Thomas Tickell Hewson, Thomas C. James, Samuel Stewart, Edward A. Atlee, and Joseph Parrish. On June 1 the representatives of eight institutions, including the College, met in the College's room in Philosophical Hall. They chose Thomas Parke president of the district convention, with Samuel L. Mitchill of New York as vice-president, and Spalding, also of New York, and Samuel Baker of the Medical and Chirurgical Faculty of Maryland as secretaries. The Philadelphia and New York delegations each brought the draft of a pharmacopoeia, from which the delegates fashioned one to present to the general convention at Washington the next winter. Parke and Hewson were two of the ten delegates chosen to represent the Middle District.[5]

Mitchill was elected president of the Washington meeting on January 1, 1820, and Thomas T. Hewson secretary. To their chagrin, the representatives of the Middle District found that the New Englanders had also brought a draft pharmacopoeia. A consolidated version, embodying a major part of the New England proposal, was adopted as the Pharmacopoeia of the United States. In their report to the College of Physicians Parke and Hewson described the convention's work:[6]

> That in addition to the prospectus agreed upon in the Convention of the Middle District, the Delegates from the Northern District presented a regular manuscript Pharmacopoeia. After a mature examination of the list of simples, preparations, and compounds contained in these two plans, the General Convention agreed upon the several articles deemed necessary to be introduced in the work which had been confided to them.
>
> In forming the Materia Medica list some difficulties arose occasioned principally by the multifarious articles presented, whose virtues were not generally known, though, according to the reports made by very respectable authority, they appeared to be well entitled to the attention of the Medical Practitioner.
>
> Wishing not to exclude articles of real value, as yet not introduced into general practice, desirous at the same time of not overloading the catalogue of simples to be kept in the Apothecaries Shops as essential articles of the Materia Medica, the General Convention determined on forming two lists according to the circumstances predicated above.
>
> In the arrangement of the Materia Medica the plan proposed in the Middle District Convention has been departed from. From the variety and confused character of the synonemes [sic] employed to designate particular articles great difficulties presented, to obviate which appeared to be an object of primary importance. By

> selecting the article to be employed in Medicine, and giving it an alphabetical arrangement, according to the most approved nomenclature, in the leading column, and referring in the second column to such authors as had described the sources from which the article was derived, it was believed, that a clear and scientifick list of the Materia Medica would be formed, acceptable to the common Apothecary, at the same time affording that degree of precision required in a work which is to be spread over a wide extent of country, where so many and discordant denominations prevail. In the plan a preference is given to the writers of this country, for the most obvious reason, the desire of rendering the work intelligible to every American.
>
> The list of preparations and compounds is pretty nearly what was agreed on in the Convention of the Middle District. Few additions have been made, and where several preparations of nearly the same character had been introduced, it was deemed advisable to make the selection according to the most approved formula, so that the list has not been increased.

The book was published in Boston in December 1820.

Anticipating the 1830 revision, the College invited its Fellows to list errors and omissions in the first edition and suggest improvements that might be required in existing preparations such as morphia, codeine, and hydrocyanic acid. The Pharmacopoeia Committee, composed now of Hewson, Joseph Hartshorne, and George Bacon Wood, was authorized to hire an assistant (D. B. Smith, president of the Philadelphia College of Pharmacy) to test drugs. The committee held more than one hundred meetings, preparing a draft that Wood and Franklin Bache carried to the Washington meeting on January 1, 1830. The convention judged it "decidedly superior to the original work," and turned it over to a committee of review and publication, headed by Hewson and including Jacob Bigelow and John W. Webster of Boston. In fact, had the College of Physicians not prepared this thorough revision, the convention would have had nothing to discuss. The work was published in 1831 as *The Pharmacopoeia of the United States of America by the Authority of the National Medical Convention.*[7]

It was pronounced by the *North American Medical and Surgical Journal* an "excellent and judicious publication, which will raise our reputation abroad, and give an additional impulse to that spirit of pharmaceutical research which has been awakened, in degree at least, by the influence of the Philadelphia College of Pharmacy."[8]

Meanwhile, another group of physicians had also been at work on a national pharmacopoeia. No New England or New York institution had been represented at the Washington convention. Even Samuel L. Mitchill, who had been elected president of that convention in 1820, failed to appear. Instead, Mitchill inexplicably convened a "General Convention" in New York of representatives of New York and New England institutions. Their production, entitled *The Pharmacopoeia of the United States of America by the Authority of the General Convention for the Formation of the American Pharmacopoeia,* appeared in November 1830, a few months before that of the National Medical Convention.[9] This episode, unnecessary and unexplained, contributed to the ill feeling and suspicion that the Philadelphians bore toward the New Yorkers and Yankees for many years.

Two years after the publication of these two pharmacopoeias, Wood and Bache issued *The Dispensatory of the United States of America.* It was a work of staggering scholarship, the authors explaining that they had consulted but not copied earlier works: "It appears due to our national character, that such a work should be in good faith an American book, newly prepared in all its parts, and not a mere edition of one of the European Dispensatories, with here and there additions and alterations . . . ."[10]

The *Pharmacopeoia of the United States* and Wood and Bache's *Dispensatory* were primarily the work of the College of Physicians and of George Bacon Wood, and for many years both the College and Wood were inseparably associated with them. Wood lived long enough to see the fourteenth edition of the *Dispensatory,* and to know that it would be continued by his nephew Horatio C Wood. As for the Pharmacopoeia, the College and some member of the Wood family of physicians participated in every decennial revision through 1940.[11] The two publications did much to confirm the pre-eminence of Philadelphia in the practice of medicine in the United States.

### *Vaccination Again*

Soon after the College completed its part in the first edition of the national pharmacopoeia, it became concerned with the issue of vaccination and re-vaccination. To protect the poor against smallpox, Philadelphia had created the post of city vaccine agent in 1816. Subsequently, the city was divided into districts and a vaccine agent was appointed for each. In 1822 Joseph Nancrede, with the endorsement of Nathaniel Chapman, Thomas C. James, and Thomas T. Hewson—all Fellows—and of Philip Syng Physick, John Redman Coxe, William Gibson, and some others, opened a vaccine institute, patterned on the national and several state institutes. It offered fresh vaccine matter free to physicians and for $3 to all others.[12] Vaccination had been so widely adopted by this time that one medical journal in 1824 rejoiced in

> the cheering expectation, that Small-Pox will be sooner or later, entirely exterminated, and driven from the face of the globe. We have now arrived at a pretty correct estimate of the powers of vaccination . . . . What though it does not *always* ward off or shield from the attacks of the destroyer! it deadens the blow and renders powerless its efforts—it . . . can do *no* harm, but *much good.* . . . Vaccination . . . if timely, properly, thoroughly and *universally* performed, would in time completely annihilate its deadly foe!—Once dead, it would not easily be revived.[13]

It was just this exception—that vaccination did not "always" provide an impenetrable shield—that created dismay and alarm. Cases were reported of vaccinated persons falling ill with smallpox. When the disease broke out in Philadelphia in 1827, the Philadelphia Medical Society tried to restore confidence in the procedure in the public and among physicians, who were considering resort to inoculation. The College of Physicians followed with its own committee in March 1828—Hartshorne, Hewson, Wood, Moore, and Coates. This committee, which collected information from physicians by questionnaire, asserted that the facts were inconclusive and advised that each Fellow "be left at liberty to act according to the dictates of his own judgment."[14]

From time to time in the ensuing forty years, smallpox reappeared in Philadelphia in alarming proportions, and some of the old questions were raised again. In the wake of the 1840 outbreak, when some physicians re-vaccinated their patients, the College rendered its judgment that re-vaccination, though a desirable precaution in some circumstances, was not generally necessary because vaccination did indeed protect against smallpox. In 1844, in response to a question by William Pepper about the effective life of vaccine virus, the Fellows offered widely varying testimonies. D. Francis Condie reported that in his experience scabs remained active for months, even a year; Henry Bond said up to five years; but Charles D. Meigs would never use any that were more than a few weeks old. Then the discussion veered off onto re-vaccination. On this point Condie cited the Prussian army's successful experience with re-vaccination. Meigs flatly rejected the figures as unreliable, and seemed to question vaccination itself. Re-vaccination, however, won approval. The city authorities gave permission for the College to re-vaccinate school children; and this was done.

Other epidemics in 1855, 1861, and 1864 brought up the old questions as well as some new ones—for example, could vaccination induce other diseases? The College blamed the 1855 outbreak on the Philadelphia authorities, who, amid the problems and confusion of consolidating the city government the year before, had neglected to appoint vaccine physicians. Yet even as late as 1864, a few Fellows, like Squier Littell, denied the efficacy of vaccination, but performed the operation to please their patients, as though it were a placebo.[15]

### *The Zimmerman Case*

In a judicial case of insanity the College called on the knowledge of its Fellows and employed its own prestige. A convicted murderer, John Zimmerman, was awaiting execution in Schuylkill County in 1824. His sanity was in doubt—his mother and two sisters were insane. Joseph Parrish informed the College of the facts, and the Fellows, "believing it a case of such serious moment as to claim their investigation," appealed to Governor Andrew Shulze to postpone the execution until the question could be settled. When a committee of local doctors disagreed whether Zimmerman was insane, the governor asked the College to examine the prisoner. "It is certainly not my wish nor my duty," Shulze told them, "to consign to execution, any person in a state of derangement . . . ."[16] Accordingly Parke, who was then seventy-five years old, with Parrish and J. Wilson Moore, all members of the Pennsylvania Hospital staff and Quakers who shared the Friends' long-standing concern for the mentally ill, travelled to the prison at Orwigsburg. The sheriff was cooperative, for he too doubted Zimmerman's sanity. In four interviews with the prisoner, the committee "entered into a full examination of the state of his mind," read notes made by the judge (who was also cooperative), and unanimously concluded that Zimmerman was insane. Governor Shulze accordingly exercised executive clemency, and the prisoner's life was spared. The trip cost the College $50.25 for the expenses of Parke and his two colleagues.[17]

### *Temperance: Alcohol and Tobacco*

In its earliest years the College had called on both the Pennsylvania legislature and Congress to curtail the excessive consumption of alcohol. Now, thirty years later, in response to a new temperance movement, whose appeal was less to physiology than to morality, the College opened one of its meetings in 1824 to advocates of temperance. The Rev. Mr. Nathaniel Hewitt of Fairfield, Connecticut, an agent of the American Society for the Promotion of Temperance, delivered "an impressive verbal address," after which the College appointed a committee to inquire into the prevalence of intemperance in Philadelphia and to ascertain, as far as practicable, the extent of mortality from overindulgence. Although the College said it "concurred fully" in Hewitt's statement, the Committee made no report. Nonetheless, the movement grew: twenty years later a Philadelphia medical journal ascribed the noticeable "improvement in education and general character" of medical students to the influence of total abstinence societies.[18]

In contrast to its near-silence on alcohol, the College—or at least one of its committees—condemned tobacco in strong terms. A group of young men organized to discourage the use of tobacco, on discovering that they were "railed at" in the newspapers, asked the College for its opinion on tobacco "—whether it be injurious to the human system, or otherwise."[19] John Bell was named chairman of a committee that included John C. Otto, who had been on the temperance committee in 1824. Their "elaborate report" declared:

> Tobacco ranks among the narcotic poisons. When taken internally in the form of powder, infusion or smoke it has caused nausea, vomiting, faintness, great prostration of strength, diminished sensibility, stupor, cold sweats and death, this last sometimes preceded by convulsions.

Tobacco, the committee concluded, was

> in fact doubly dangerous, first on account of the deleterious influences on the animal economy of tobacco itself; secondly, owing to its so affecting the moral nature of man as to throw him open to various untoward influences which in a firmer frame of mind he could readily have resisted.

### *The College Fee Bill*

Yet the interest some Fellows took in the pharmacopoeia, vaccination, or criminal insanity quickly evaporated; it did nothing permanently to revive the College or awaken a sustained concern for its future. Even in 1825 the minutes of five of the twelve stated meetings record "No particular business."

A few of the Fellows, however, determined to change this state of affairs. They were mature, serious, and experienced in the ways of the College. Thomas Chalkley James and Thomas Tickell Hewson had been Fellows for more than a quarter of a century; Henry Neill and Joseph Parrish, for more than fifteen years. John C. Otto was elected in 1819. Joseph Hartshorne, elected in 1824, might be thought a newcomer, but at forty-five was no youthful rebel or visionary. Henry Neill, the youngest, was forty-one.

Their first act—not the most urgent need of the College, one might think—was to propose that the College adopt a fee-bill. Such a list of standard charges, in addition to promising the Fellows obvious financial benefits, would add to the dignity and professionalism of physicians at a time when medicine and its practitioners were not usually highly esteemed. As a result, the following "Table of Charges for Medical Services" was adopted by the College on November 2, 1824.[20]

| | | | |
|---|---|---|---|
| For a single visit & advice in a case | From $1 | to | $10 |
| When detained for each hour | 2 | to | 5 |
| For an ordinary visit | 1 | to | 1½ |
| For a visit at a time appointed by the patient or his friends | | | 2 |
| For verbal advice at the Physician's home | 1 | to | 10 |
| For written advice | 5 | to | 20 |
| For rising at night without leaving the house | 3 | to | 5 |
| For rising at night & visit | 5 | to | 10 |
| For visit in consultation | | | 5 |
| Subsequent visits in the same case | 1 | to | 2 |
| For rising in night and visit in consultation | 5 | to | 15 |
| For a visit in the country: one dollar for each mile beyond the limits of the City in addition to the other customary charges | | | |
| When there are more patients than one in a family, from 25 to 50 cents additional, both for the attending and consulting Physician | | | |
| For vaccination | $5 | | |
| For re-vaccination | $2 | to | 3 |
| For a case of midwifery | 8 | to | 20 |
| For reducing fractures and luxations, exclusive of subsequent attendance | 5 | to | 10 |
| For passing the catheter | 1 | to | 5 |
| For lithotomy, including attendance | 100 | to | 200 |
| For amputation of leg or arm, including attendance | 50 | to | 100 |
| For trepanning | 30 | to | 100 |
| For extirpation of large tumors including attendance | 30 | to | 100 |
| For operation for cataract including attendance | 50 | to | 100 |
| For aneurisms | 100 | to | 200 |
| For hernia | 50 | to | 100 |
| For fistula lachrymalis | 15 | to | 30 |
| For hare lip | 20 | to | 30 |
| For fistula in ano exclusive of attendance | 20 | to | 40 |

> In order that Practitioners of Medicine may exhibit uniformity in their rate of charging, it is proposed that no entry shall ever be made in their account books of lower fees than those contained in the above table. If in any case however the Physician should have reason to believe that his patient cannot pay the full amount without serious inconvenience, a deduction may then be made at the end of the year or at any other time.

The fee-bill was made a part of the College by-laws. From time to time the list of services was revised and extended, and the charges were increased. The exception physicians might make for poor patients was made more explicit in 1840:

> . . . the fee-bill, as at present established by the College, being founded on a just consideration of the important services which its members are called on to perform, it is their duty to conform to it in their charges, whenever the circumstances of their patients are not such as clearly to forbid it.[21]

### *New Members*

Two years after the adoption of the fee-bill, the reformers took a more important step to revivify the College: they encouraged some promising young men to apply for membership. Seven—an unprecedented number—were elected in 1827: John Bell, Benjamin H. Coates, Hugh L. Hodge, René La Roche, Charles D. Meigs, John K. Mitchell, and George B. Wood. Only Meigs had reached the age of thirty-five. All were graduates of the University of Pennsylvania. Meigs, Coates, and La Roche were editors of the *North American Medical and Surgical Journal,* of which Coates was a co-founder. Wood was professor of chemistry in the Philadelphia College of Pharmacy; Mitchell taught chemistry in the Philadelphia Medical Institute; Meigs was a physician to the Philadelphia Dispensary. They were good friends, most of them members of the informal Friday Evening Medical Club, which met weekly over tea and cakes and—sometimes—wine and oysters.[22] All were to have distinguished careers as teachers, authors, and practitioners, and all became active in College affairs. Meigs was elected secretary in 1828 and Wood was chosen president in 1848.

The increase in membership soon brought the College unwonted prosperity. In 1820, with membership dwindling, the College had reduced its fees under the foolish misapprehension that this would make the fellowship more attractive. The next year, when its indebtedness to the American Philosophical Society for rent and service stood at $228.33 and the Society was pressing for payment, the College borrowed $250, which only substituted one creditor for another. In 1829, however, the treasurer reported a balance of $100.82; and four years later, with a surplus of $308.42 on hand, the College purchased four shares of Chesapeake and Delaware Canal stock and created its first endowment.

One of the first acts of James, Hewson, and their collaborators was to get the College to direct that each Fellow in turn should read a paper, "either original or selected," at a stated meeting, on penalty of a one-dollar fine. This practice, they were confident, would provide scientific substance and the basis for profesional discussion, both lacking in College meetings for many years. At the July 1827 meeting President Parke read the first paper on cold and warm baths, and the next month Hewson presented an essay on extra-uterine pregnancy. At other meetings Henry Bond reported on his successful use of the esophagus forceps to remove a needle; Charles D. Meigs read a paper on catalepsy, Hewson on puerperal convulsions, John C. Otto on incontinence of urine. John Bell offered strictures on the usual clothing of young children, and Robert M. Huston spoke severely against the evils of empiricism. On December 28, 1830, in what proved to be a premonitory note, Hugh L. Hodge gave a report on cholera in the East Indies. To encourage and reward the Fellows in their writing, the College authorized publication of some of these reports in the *North American Medical and Surgical Journal.*

### *The Cholera Epidemic, 1832*

On January 31, 1832, a year after Hodge presented his paper, a "conversation" was held at the College on the cholera, which was then moving alarmingly across Europe. Reports of the disease had been coming out of India and Russia for months. Observations by the physician to the British embassy in St. Petersburg on the nature and treatment of cholera in that city, published in London, had been noticed and reviewed in American medical journals.[23] Dr. G. R. B. Horner in a letter to his brother William of Philadelphia had described cases of cholera among the crew of an American warship at Constantinople.[24] By the end of the winter 1831–32, physicians and public health officials were well prepared for the epidemic that they believed was inescapable. "Even the broad expanse of the Atlantic," the *North American Medical and Surgical Journal* had predicted in October 1831, "cannot be considered a certain barrier to its ingress, sooner or later, into the United States."[25] As reports multiplied, the Philadelphia Board of Health, fearing that its own authority and resources were inadequate, expressed the opinion that only state or federal powers could cope with the impending crisis.[26] In April 1832 it called for a meeting of public health officials of the seaboard commercial towns to adopt "some uniform sanitory [sic] measures,"[27] and it requested the College of Physicians and the Philadelphia Medical Society to make "an impartial examination into all the facts in relation to the epidemic cholera" and prepare a report "for the benefit and satisfaction of the unprofessional as well as the Medical part of the community."[28]

It was already known that the disease was not contagious, and that therefore measures of quarantine would not be effective; on the contrary, "an enlightened system of medical police" was required.[29] Cholera found its victims principally among the poor who had insufficient and unwholesome food, lived in filthy, crowded, and ill-ventilated alleys, and drank contaminated water. It was to appear, for example, "in its most malignant and dreadful aspect" in Philadelphia's Almshouse and Arch Street Prison, where overcrowding was "noted and striking."[30] The onset of the disease was sudden: its symptoms were cramps, diarrhoea, and vomiting to dehydration. Death or recovery was swift. Rarely did cholera appear in the large, airy, and cleanly houses of the well-to-do.

The college named a committee of seven Fellows—James, Hewson, Hodge, Meigs, Bell, Coates, and La Roche—to prepare the report the Board of Health had requested. They met with a similar committee of the Philadelphia Medical Society (two of whose seven members were already Fellows; four of the remaining five would become so), but the two groups agreed to issue separate reports. Because cholera had not yet appeared in North America and no physician had treated a case in his own practice, the committees were dependent chiefly on published reports in French, German, and British journals, especially those of British medical officers in India. The College's report, written by John Bell, was presented, discussed, amended, and approved on May 31, and sent to the Board on June 19; next day it was ordered printed.[31]

The Committee reviewed the history of cholera, its predisposing conditions, and the character of its victims; stated firmly that it was not contagious, not transmitted by personal contact, clothing, or merchandise, and that therefore quarantine was not recommended. The "true means of prevention" was sanitation, and the Committee accordingly recommended cleaning the streets; washing, cleaning, and ventilating houses, bedding, and clothing; bathing; and proper diet. Smoked or salted meats should be eaten sparingly, and fat pork not at all. "Lobsters, and the like," the public was warned, "are avowedly pernicious." Persons living in cellars or damp, ill-ventilated, insanitary rooms, especially in the buildings between Front and Water Streets, should be removed; and hospitals should be prepared to receive the sick. The report of the Philadelphia Medical Society was similar, although it contained a greater number of specific suggestions.[32]

In mid-May 1832 two Philadelphia medical students in Paris, Caspar Wistar Pennock and William Wood Gerhard, sent home a report on twenty-three cases of cholera they had observed in the practice of their mentors Pierre-Charles-Alexandre Louis and Gabriel Andral. The paper was published promptly in the *American Journal of the Medical Sciences.*[33] It was useful to physicians treating the disease in Philadelphia; it gave instant reputation to the two young authors; and it was evidence of the opening of a new, more scientific period in Philadelphia medicine and, therefore, in the history of the College.

Meanwhile, on June 8, 1832, cholera, so long fearfully awaited, appeared at Quebec; two days later cases were reported at Montreal; and on June 24 there were cases in New York City. The Philadelphia Board of Health on June 22 sent a commission of three physicians—Charles D. Meigs, a Fellow, Samuel Jackson, and Richard Harlan—to Canada to observe the disease and methods of coping with it.[34] The Board also took steps to handle the expected masses of sick poor. It asked the Secretary of the Navy for use of the Naval Asylum as a temporary hospital, the governor of Pennsylvania for the state arsenal on Juniper Street and for tents and kettles, and the Philadelphia comptroller of public schools for school buildings.[35] When the first case appeared on July 5, the city was reasonably ready. There was little excitement and no panic.[36]

Hugh L. Hodge was in charge of the Almshouse, and each of the other hospitals was in the charge of a physician.[37] Of these sixteen smaller, local hospitals, six were administered by physicians who were or soon afterwards became Fellows of the College. In addition, in cooperation with the publishers Carey, Lea & Blanchard, the doctors issued a weekly news-letter, the *Cholera Gazette,* from July 11 to October 10, with a final double issue on November 21. Factual and dispassionate, without editorializing, the *Gazette* published notes on the history of cholera, reports of outbreaks and public health measures elsewhere, the experience and recommendations of physicians and hospitals in Europe, especially in Paris, and—perhaps most significant—statistics comparing each week's sickness and mortality with those of the weeks before and with the same week in former years. Additional information was provided the public in *All the Material Facts in the History of Epidemic Cholera,* by D. F. Condie and John Bell, which appeared during the summer.

Each day the number of sick and dead rose. Between July 11 and August 10, 984 cases were reported, of whom 393 died. In the hospitals, almshouse, and prison, the mortality exceeded fifty percent, more than twice the rate among private patients. August 9 was proclaimed a day of fasting, humiliation, and prayer. Two weeks later, to the surprise of all, the epidemic was visibly abating. "Is there nothing in prayer?" William Darrach asked, and then dryly answered his own question: "Between prayer & the answer there are many common place events. No Miracle but common human agencies."[39] On September 2 no new cases were reported; by the end of the month the epidemic was over.

Fully engaged during the two months the cholera held the city in its grip, the Fellows had scant opportunity to discuss the disease at stated meetings. After it disappeared, however, several prepared papers on the subject. Samuel Jackson related his "Personal Observations and Experiences," and Isaac Hays reported to the

Philadelphia Medical Society on its pathology.[40] Isaac Parrish read a paper to the College distinguishing malignant cholera from cholera morbus. Although Philadelphia had suffered less than some other cities, the experience of its physicians, including young doctors who had graduated only a few weeks before, was put to use when cholera reappeared, as it did, in subsequent years.

Parke had had no part in the College's discussion of cholera. Citing his "advanced age and declining health," he had resigned the presidency in 1830—he was then eight-one and had given up much of his practice; but the Fellows insisted he withdraw the resignation. On two subsequent occasions he resigned again, and, though he never attended a meeting after August 30, 1831, each time the College sent a committee of old friends to urge him to reconsider. He died on January 9, 1835, and the Fellows chose as his successor Thomas Chalkley James, vice-president since 1826. But James, who was sixty-nine and not in good health, died within three months of his election.

James had studied medicine in London and Edinburgh, where his fellow students included the Philadelphians Isaac Cathrall and John Ruan, both later Fellows of the College, and Philip Syng Physick. In Philadelphia he achieved reputation in obstetrics as one of the physicians of the Pennsylvania Hospital and professor of midwifery in the University of Pennsylvania for a quarter of a century. He was famous for having induced premature labor, which he reported in a paper to the College and printed in the *Eclectic Repertory,* which he founded in 1811. James was "much attached" to the College, to which he was elected in 1795 and which he served almost continuously as librarian, secretary, treasurer, or vice-president. That he was not sympathetic to the changes overtaking the College in the mid-1830s was suggested by his friend Hugh L. Hodge. "Its quiet and dignified course," Hodge wrote, revealing as much of the College in those days as of James,

> well suited the peculiarities of his character. Within its precincts, he was sure to meet with his cotemporaries and personal friends, or with those who were gratified in numbering themselves among his pupils and admirers; and he there never anticipated that rude collision of sentiment, which, although it may occasionally elicit the spark of genius, too frequently generates the fires of envy and passion.[41]

Thomas Tickell Hewson, chosen president on July 7, 1835, was the son of an able English anatomist, William Hewson, who had received the Copley Medal of the Royal Society for his work on the lymphatics, and of Mary Stevenson Hewson, in whose mother's house Benjamin Franklin had rented rooms during his long residence in London as agent of the Pennsylvania Assembly.[42] The friendship that thus developed has remained a warm memory in the Hewson family to the present day. Mary Hewson, after the premature death of her husband, eventually brought her family to Philadelphia. Thomas was graduated from the University of the State of Pennsylvania, spent five years as apprentice to John Foulke before going to London, where he was house surgeon at St. Bartholomew's Hospital, and to Edinburgh, where, however, he did not take a degree. After six years abroad, Hewson returned home and was eventually appointed physician to the Pennsylvania Hospital and professor of comparative anatomy in the University of Pennsylvania. In the College he had succeeded James as secretary, serving ten years, was one of the censors, and took an active and important part in compiling of the national pharmacopoeia.

### *A New Generation*

The renewed activity of the College, amply confirmed during Hewson's presidency, was, of course, owing to new forces at work in medicine and the medical profession generally. In particular, it owed almost everything to the energetic, ambitious men elected in 1827, and especially to the Fellows elected after 1834. In that year Pennock and Gerhard, author of the article on cholera cases they had seen in Paris, were elected; in 1835 Thomas Stewardson, John Marshall Paul, and William Ashmead were admitted. All five were graduates of the University of Pennsylvania, and all had studied medicine in Paris, whose teachers, hospitals, clinics, and medical doctrines had impressed them profoundly. In the next few years, more men with French training were elected—John Rodman Paul and Thomas D. Mütter in 1836, William S. W. Ruschenberger in 1838, George W. Norris, Edward Peace, and William Pepper in 1839; and in the early 1840s Alfred Stillé and his brother Moreton, Meredith Clymer, David Tucker, and Samuel G. Morton.[43] Most of those who nominated these young men for membership had themselves become Fellows only since 1827. Within a few months of their election, Pennock and Gerhard, with two others, proposed their old Paris teacher Louis for election as a foreign Associate Member, and he was accordingly elected on February 3, 1835.[44]

In 1820 most Fellows were graduates of Edinburgh University or had studied under professors who were. But Edinburgh's preeminence as a seat of medical education had passed; and the Paris clinicians and institutions now drew able and ambitious students. In Philadelphia the younger teachers and practitioners were aware of what was being done and published in France. Jason O'B. Lawrance and Benjamin H. Coates repeated in Philadelphia the physiological experiments of Magendie.[45] Chapman's new *Philadelphia Journal of the Medical and Physical Sciences* printed articles, reviews, and notes of French medical achievements and institutions, including an account of Broussais' doctrine of fevers by Joseph G. Nancrede, and a long review by Coates of two reports on the Paris hospitals. John Eberle wrote a review of Johann Ludwig Casper's *Charakteristik der franzosischen medizin* (Leipzig, 1822) for the *Medical Review and Analectic Journal,* which he and George McClellan edited.[46]

Louis, Andral, and their colleagues taught their students the importance of close observation, accurate and full statistics, careful comparison of data, and the drawing of logical inferences from them. The impressions of a busy practitioner were no longer sufficient: one must keep specific and detailed records. From these French teachers the Americans learned, as one of Louis' pupils put it, "not to take authority when I can have facts; not to guess when I can know; not to think a man must take physic because he is sick."[47]

This "numerical system" and all its implications were contrary to what the older men had been taught, had taught their own students, and had lived and practiced by. These French ideas seemed to remove the patient from the center of the doctor's attention, to make him a statistic. Medical "science" was replacing medical practice. In the Philadelphia Medical Society the debates were especially lively, sometimes heated. In the College of Physicians, differences of opinion were no less sharp, but were usually expressed in more muted tones. As an old man Alfred Stillé remembered what the College was like when he joined in 1842:

The College of Physicians at that time was mainly composed of the elders of the profession, who instinctively clung to old and familiar paths, and who resented the intrusion of new ideas as almost impertinent. Age and station then had a much more preponderating influence than at the present day, and the young were as timid in expressing even their well-considered opinions, as the old were prompt to resent and frown down all dissidence and contradiction. There was also a special lack of harmony, if not a positive antipathy and antagonism, between the physicians who had been trained abroad and their pupils, on the one hand, and their elders, on the other hand, who kept to the ancient paths, and were content to plod therein, and who set more value by doctrinal differences and the logomachy of systems, than by the simple, unbiassed observation and comparison of clinical and experimental facts.[48]

As something like this do I recall the aspect of our little province in the medical world, when I first beheld it in 1842, awed, perhaps, by its luminaries, who, however, did not eclipse the greater ones that my eyes had grown accustomed to abroad. At that time, if a Junior Fellow had opened his lips to confirm or to controvert the oracular deliverances of his seniors, he would have been regarded as more presumptuous than wise. It was a day when speculative doctrines were as obstinately maintained and as virulently assailed, as are now the invisible shades of theological dogmas by conflicting religious sects and parties. They gave occasion to a wordy war that filled the air with sound, and which signified nothing, and is as forgotten now as last year's snow. These discussions were often a mere threshing of straw, that raised a blinding dust, and left but scanty grains of truth behind it. . . . Some of these conflicts remain fixed in my memory, in which deep thrusts and hard blows were exchanged by Bond, Bell, Condie, Coates, Jackson, Hodge, Huston, Meigs, La Roche, Morris, Wood, and others. Through the smoke of the conflict I can still distinguish the characteristic fence of the several combatants; the vehemence of some, the placid

> equanimity of others, the fallacies of one's reasoning, and the stern logic of his antagonist. Especially do I recall how George B. Wood was apt to conclude a discussion by one of those convincing statements that issued from his calm, clear mind, as coin from a minting machine. Not less distinctly do I remember the mingled earnestness and conviction with which Charles D. Meigs was wont to plead for a notion that for the time captivated his imagination. Indeed, I shall never forget how, for nearly two hours, he once held the attention of the College while he expounded his most fanciful doctrine of 'The Cholera Squeeze.'

Perhaps it was out of necessity to maintain order in heated debates such as these that the College in 1847 adopted rules on "the right to the floor." No Fellow, they provided, should interrupt another; each should be permitted, "within reasonable license in time, and confining himself to the point," to present his ideas "in the way in which his faculties present them to him."

The year 1834 saw constitutional changes which reflected and strengthened the scientific ideas and professional ideals of the younger Fellows. Although the College had altered some of its practices by resolutions, the by-laws had not been revised since 1818. After some months of consideration, a revision was approved. The most obvious of the changes was the elimination of the "Constitution" from the governing documents of the College. Henceforth, instead of three documents—charter, constitution, and by-laws—there would be only two—the charter and the by-laws.[49]

Other changes in the 1834 by-laws were more important. Instead of applying in writing for membership, prospective Fellows were to be nominated by three Fellows and approved by three-quarters of those present. The old rule requiring approval by three-quarters of the whole membership had made it nearly impossible to elect anyone. Another change extended the residence requirements beyond the narrow limits of the city, Northern Liberties, and borough of Southwark to include all the "incorporated districts" of Philadelphia. The "Regulations to Promote Order," now renamed "Rules of Professional Conduct," were amended and extended to incorporate the College fee-bill that had first been adopted in 1824.

But the most important change in the by-laws was the creation of standing committees in each of seven specialties—theory and practice, surgery, midwifery, diseases of children, materia medica and pharmacy, meteorology and epidemics, and public hygiene. The committees were required to report annually on "interesting facts and doctrines," and were composed principally of the younger, more active Fellows: of thirty-one persons who served on these committees, twenty-three had been elected since 1827.

### *Public Health and Pediatrics*

Especially noteworthy in this list of standing committees is the recognition of "diseases of children" and "public health." Concern for public health, to be sure, was rooted in the original College purpose and the activities of forty years; it arose also inescapably from conditions of health and sanitation in rapidly growing Philadelphia. As for separating the diseases of children from the more common comprehensive designation of "diseases of women and children," the College was responding to the practical experience and studies of some of its younger Fellows: three of the four first members of the committee had been Fellows for less than five years.

The Committee on Public Hygiene presented its first report within six months of its appointment. This promptitude was owing principally to the commitment of its chairman, John Bell. Born in Ireland but reared in Virginia, Bell was a graduate of the University of Pennsylvania, where he was noticed by Nathaniel Chapman, who habitually encouraged fellow Virginians. He contributed frequently to Chapman's *Journal,* edited the *Select Medical Library and Eclectic Journal,* and wrote on mineral springs, the rearing of children, and bathing and personal hygiene. He was president of the Phrenological Society, belonged to the American Colonization Society, was an active member of the literary Athenian Institute. Throughout his life he strongly opposed alcoholic beverages, which he denounced as "a poison, a constant source of disease, of strife, and of turmoil, of personal misery, and social disorder." As a professor of the institutes of medicine at the Pennsylvania Medical Institute, he was said to attend "more to the matter than to the manner" of his lectures. He was a member of the National Medical Convention in 1846 which led to the creation of the American Medical Association the next year. In the College of Physicians, Bell was a member of the Library Committee after 1841 and headed the Committee on Public Health during its entire existence from 1834 to 1851.[50]

In his committee's first report on November 4, 1834, Bell offered several general recommendations for improving the sanitary conditions of the city—cemeteries, for example, should be "tastefully enclosed & planted with trees"—and urged that all existing laws and ordinances concerning public health be enforced. But the committee's recommendation, he knew, would avail little without the enlightened concern of the citizens. His suggestions were unexceptionable, but they were made in full awareness that any legislation for public health involved substantial economic interests. Nothing was said in this report about conditions in the city's prisons, almshouse, hospitals, schools, and other public institutions; nor was any particular factory named as a public nuisance and source of pollution.

No consideration of the public health of Philadelphia could long overlook the Schuylkill River, principal source of its water supply. Here the College put itself ahead of its committee. Calling itself "a guardian of the Health of the Inhabitants of the Community," the College directed Bell's committee to investigate discharges by manufacturing plants into the pool from which water was drawn into the reservoir atop Fair Mount. The College also offered to provide the City Councils with information on public hygiene and to give assistance "in perpetuating to our Citizens all the intended benefit of a great and noble enterprize which by its completion has justly confered [sic] on Philada. a character beyond her Sister Cities for the purity and salubrity of the water, with which she is abundantly supplied." For its part the Board of Health consulted the College about draining and filling the city's ubiquitous ponds of stagnant water.

As "a guardian of the Health of the Inhabitants," the College took other actions. It petitioned the legislature to provide for parks and shaded walks in newly incorporated districts of the city; and in 1841 it began urging the Councils to purchase Lemon Hill to protect the city's drinking water.

The creation of a standing committee on diseases of children in 1841 was a recognition of pediatrics years before that specialty was generally acknowledged elsewhere. Not until 1860, for example, was an effort made to establish a section on pediatrics in the

New York Academy of Medicine; it failed; and the section was not organized until 1887. The section on pediatrics in the American Medical Association was not created until 1880 and the American Pediatric Society was organized only in 1888.[51] Meanwhile, the Children's Hospital of Philadelphia had been founded in 1855.

D. Francis Condie, appointed to the Committee on Diseases of Children in 1841, immediately became its leading figure, and was the author of its annual reports for ten years. A graduate of the University of Pennsylvania in 1836, he was elected a Fellow of the College in 1838, and for more than thirty years was active in its affairs. He was secretary of the College from 1843 to 1854, served on the standing committees on publications and public hygiene, was a delegate to the National Quarantine and Sanitary Convention in 1857 and 1858, and often represented the College at the annual meetings of the American Medical Association. Condie was also an active member of the County Medical Society and in 1859 was president of the Medical Society of Pennsylvania. He was never a medical teacher, but had a large, though probably ill-paying, practice in South Philadelphia. His *Practical Treatise on the Diseases of Children,* published in 1844, went through six editions and was said, to be "one of the best, if not the best, in the language." Conscientious, conservative, a bit old-fashioned in opinions and manners, he always made visits on foot, holding, as he declared contemptuously, that "those who rode in one-horse carriages were physically deficient; those who rode in two-horse carriages were mentally deficient."[52]

Condie's annual reports were principally reviews and discussions of recent publications by French, German, and British physicians. In 1845, for example, he warmly recommended the recently published treatise on diseases of children by Frédéric Rilliet and Antoine-Charles-Ernest Barthez, warning, however, that as their cases were taken almost entirely from among children of the poor, their conclusions might not be applicable in private practice and to children of the better-to-do. Some diseases and chronic conditions were subjects of comment in almost every one of Condie's reports—cyanosis, meningitis, diphtheria (with special reference to tracheotomy), rectal polyps, tuberculosis, measles, and a spectrum of intestinal disorders often lumped together as "softening of the stomach." Not content simply to report, Condie sometimes offered a sharp judgment of his own. On the subject of milk for babies, he wrote in 1846, "We have no hesitation in stating, that all which has hitherto been said and written on the subject, so far at least as regards the peculiar qualities of milk in relation to the nourishment of infants, is absolutely valueless."[53]

### *Unethical Conduct*

As Fellows of the College became more confident in their scientific knowledge and more aware of their professional status, they also became more sensitive to professional ethics, as the case of Joseph Togno showed. A graduate of the University of Pennsylvania in 1829, who, while still a student, had translated Bichat's *Pathological Anatomy* and other French works for a Philadelphia publisher, Togno seemed just the sort of able, industrious, and ambitious young physician the College wanted to elect to its fellowship in the 1830s. His application for membership was endorsed by Thomas C. James, Joseph Parrish, and John C. Otto, and he was elected in 1830. He contributed articles to the *American Journal of the Medical Sciences* and read at least one paper to the College. When standing committees were created under the bylaws of 1834, he was put on those for surgery and public hygiene. Then or soon afterwards, he opened an Infirmary for the Cure of Deafness and wrote *A Popular Essay on the Laws of Acoustics, and on the Anatomy and Physiology of the Ear* that included an account of seventy-seven cures of deafness. In the Infirmary's annual report for 1834–35 Togno also claimed to have restored hearing to the deaf. This elicited in the *Boston Medical and Surgical Journal* a slashing attack on Togno's "specious pretensions" and a hint that the honor of the College was involved because Togno identified himself as a Fellow on his title-page.[54] The review was brought to the attention of the College.

Although they disapproved the content and tone of Togno's pamphlet as "not in accordance with . . . strict professional propriety," the Censors found insufficient grounds for action. This satisfied neither Togno nor all the Fellows. Had he accepted the Censors' judgment, Togno might have retained his membership. But he defended his conduct aggressively, charged another Fellow, Reynell Coates, medical editor and author and brother of Benjamin H. Coates, with a malevolent determination to drive him out, and demanded that this statement be recorded in the minutes. When the demand was rejected, Togno sued Coates in the civil courts.[55] The issue had now escalated beyond the question of the cure of the deaf; and Togno was dropped from the fellowship.

### *Library and Publications*

The authors of the revised by-laws of 1834 anticipated the revival of the College library. Like other College activities, the library had been neglected for many years, for it had no constituency and the resources of the College were not adequate even for elementary College needs. The by-laws provided for a committee to "attend to the increase and preservation of the Library," and directed that the College should appropriate annually to the library "such a sum as may be deemed compatible with its funds." The first Library Committee was composed of J. Wilson Moore, William S. Coxe, and Simon A. Wickes. Wickes died in 1835 and Coxe in 1837, and they were replaced by Henry Bond and Squier Littell. The committee's first report in 1835 pronounced the library "in a bad condition and going to decay." A few months later, however, they contrived to get money enough to rebind "certain folio volumes;" and their energy and dedication were recognized when the College voted to place its records in their keeping. A second annual report, on June 7, 1836, showed that the collection contained 291 volumes and a number of unbound pamphlets, that during the past year not a single volume had been called for, and that only one or two books had been added to the collection. Nothing changed over the next few years: the library contained principally ancient and out-of-date books of scant use to practicing physicians. The Library Committee in 1836 presented the situation in the best light it could:

> They are in fact to be regarded as a mere foundation, although a valuable one for a medical library; and your committee trust that whenever a place of deposit shall be obtained, at the same time safe and easily accessible, funds for adding to their number will be appropriated more frequently and more abundantly, so that the collection may become an object of greater interest, and may better correspond with the dignity of so ancient and so honor-

> able a literary body as the College of Physicians of Philadelphia.

In 1839 the library was reported still to be "but little used." A proposal the next year that the committee inquire into the possibility of acquiring, by purchase or deposit, the splendid and extensive library of John Redman Coxe came to nothing.

No less important than the revival of the library was the reestablishment of the *Transactions.* This, too, took several years to effect. That regular publication of papers presented to the College was a desirable object, even an essential obligation, most Fellows would heartily have agreed. From time to time in the preceding thirty years, the question had been raised in the College, but without result. The new by-laws directed, but no more than that, that papers intended for publication should be turned over to the Library Committee. But the College had no funds for publication. In 1839, however, at the instance of J. Wilson Moore, the papers were given to the Censors to review for publication. The Censors, finding no "convenient vehicle for their publication at the command of the College," returned them to the Library Committee.

Two years later D. Francis Condie moved that the College consider the "propriety and expediency" of publishing a bulletin of College proceedings. The motion passed; and Condie, Benjamin H. Coates, Isaac Parrish, Henry Bond, William Pepper, and J. Wilson Moore were appointed to make a recommendation. They lost no time in doing so, proposing the next month that a quarterly bulletin be issued containing papers, abstracts of papers and oral communications, and such reports of College business as the membership and profession at large might find instructive. The publication was to be called *Quarterly Summary of the Transactions of the College of Physicians of Philadelphia.* Condie, Parrish, and John Bell were named the publication committee.

The first issue of the *Quarterly Summary,* reporting on the meetings of November 1841 to February 1842, appeared in February 1842. "It is hoped that the result of adopting this course," the editors declared in the brief preface to the first number,

> will be to revive that spirit, which actuated the college in its earliest years—to encourage the number and value of

> the communications of the fellows—to promote a more punctual attendance, and to ensure to the institution, by more fully deserving it, that prominent place in the public respect and confidence to which it has heretofore been deemed to be entitled.[56]

The reviewer in the *American Journal of the Medical Sciences* hailed the appearance of the *Transactions* as evidence that the College had "at last awakened, for from its respectability and postion, it might, by well directed efforts, exert a wholesome influence over the profession, and contribute largely to the advancement of our science."[57]

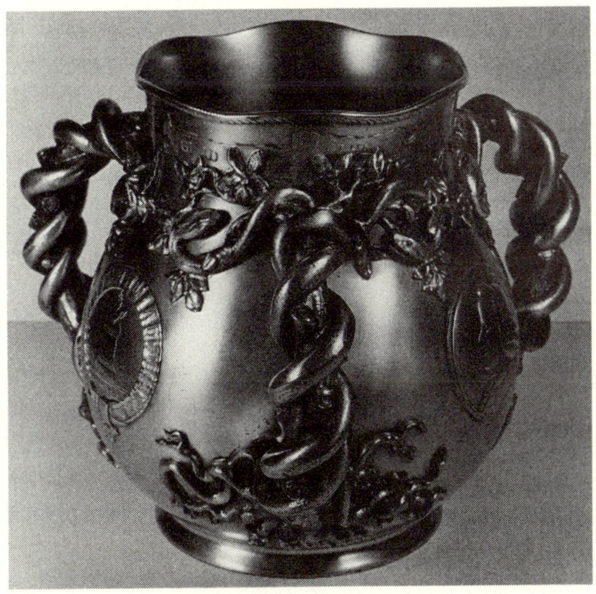

College Loving Cup.

CHAPTER IV

# *Into a Wider World*

No single event or date signalizes the emergence of the College of Physicians from its long years of inactivity. On the contrary, decisions were taken and practices inaugurated—not every one wise or fruitful—which together gave the institution a new spirit of confidence, purpose, and institutional pride. This spirit was clearly recognizable in the early 1840s. Membership was growing, and attendance at the regular monthly meetings was large enough for stimulating exchanges of information and opinion. After nearly half a century, publication of the *Transactions* was resumed. The library began to grow. A pathological museum was established. A new form of membership certificate was adopted; a seal was purchased for official letters; and, with surplus funds in hand, in 1847 the College invested $300 in municipal bonds. In 1845 the College moved to more spacious and convenient rooms, and the Fellows, who had often wanted to reduce their dues, now cheerfully raised them to pay the increased rent and even to erect a building of their own. Thanks to these reforms and the reawakening they signified and to the reputation of such individual Fellows as the authors of the *Dispensatory,* the fame of the College spread. A Boston medical journal, reviewing a publication of the New York Academy of Medicine in 1849, reminded its readers that no one could ignore "the brilliant and eminently successful medical institutions of Philadelphia."[1]

On the other hand, the College of Physicians was increasingly less representative of the Philadelphia medical profession as a whole. Without exception, the Fellows were men of education and wide experience; they were the professors in the medical schools, the attending physicians of the oldest and largest hospitals, the authors of standard textbooks; they were men who exemplified the highest ideals of their profession. Their practice was varied and extensive, but it was different from that of neighborhood doctors in Kensington, Moyamensing, and West Philadelphia. The number of physicians in the city increased as the general population rose, but the fellowship of the College remained limited.

Elections, which had totalled forty-nine in the decade 1831–40 (up from eighteen in the preceding ten years, two-thirds of whom were elected in 1827–29 alone), increased to fifty-nine in 1841–50 (an average of nearly six a year), and to sixty-four in 1851–60. The total active resident membership rose from thirty-one in 1834 to sixty-four in 1840, to 102 in 1851, and to 136 in 1864. Most of the new members soon achieved, if they had not already attained, distinction in their profession and took active parts in College business. Of the Fellows elected in 1842, for example, Henry H. Smith became president of the County and State Medical Societies; Caspar Wister was treasurer of the American Medical Association from 1854 to 1877; and Alfred Stillé was president of that Association in 1871. Several of the new members were professors in local medical schools, while Meredith Clymer became professor of practice in the medical school of New York University. Robert Bridges was president of the Academy of Natural Sciences of Philadelphia, and Paul Beck Goddard was president of the city's Board of Health. In the College, Bridges served thirteen years as librarian; he, Goddard, Wister, Stillé, and John D. Griscom were also delegates to annual meetings of the American Medical Association; and Stillé, after holding a variety of elective and appointive offices, was elected president of the College in 1883.

The regular monthly meetings in the 1840s were filled principally with papers and case reports. The subjects ranged widely from fractures to fevers; and there might also be remarks on the deleterious effects of tobacco, on quackery, or the importance of physical education of women. John K. Mitchell in 1842 read a paper on mesmerism, which took up two meetings and provoked a long discussion in a third. Remarks by Franklin Bache illustrated how even a casual episode might contain a useful lesson. While walking in the street one day,

> he was called into a store to see a child who, it was said, had swallowed a portion of tin. The child was crying vio-

> lently, had some slight difficulty of breathing, and had discharged a portion of bloody sputa. On examining the throat, he [Bache] had at first some doubts as to the presence of any foreign body, but on introducing his finger far back into the fauces, detected the edge of the piece of tin at the upper part of the oesophagus. Having with him no appropriate instrument to extract it, he curved, by means of a common vise, the point of a straight dressing forceps, and placing one of the wooden pins used to attach clothes, when drying, to the line, between the teeth of the child, succeeded in seizing and bringing away a disc of tin of about an inch in diameter. The patient experienced no unpleasant symptoms, and was soon able to play as usual. The Doctor did not relate this case as one possessing any peculiar features, or any novelty in its management, but to show how readily suitable instruments may be extemporaneously devised upon any emergency.[2]

Under the by-laws of 1834, committees presented annual reports on recent advances in the principal medical specialties. These reports proved less productive than expected; and in 1840 responsibility for the annual surveys was given to individual Fellows. Several, like Charles D. Meigs for midwifery and Joseph Pancoast for surgery, offered no reports for several years running; and, when pressed, resigned the responsibility, and were replaced. Some reports were merely anecdotal: J. Wilson Moore for meteorology and epidemics told the College in 1845 that on the preceding May 9 "fire-flies were seen, like little stars, moving over the surface of the ground," and that during the last week of June "the cheering and active scenes of mowing, reaping, and cradling were observed" in eastern Pennsylvania.[3] On the other hand, D. Francis Condie regularly presented detailed and informative reports on the diseases of children, as Wilson Jewell did on meteorology and epidemics, and Isaac Parrish on surgery. These men abstracted significant articles and notes in medical journals of France, Germany, and Russia, as well as of England and the United States, offered critical assessments of treatments and procedures, and sometimes warned against hasty acceptance of statements that were based on unsubstantial evidence or conflicted with reason and common sense. Parrish in 1844 gave a full account of the injuries sustained by rioters and bystanders in the Nativist "tumults" in Kensington and Southwark earlier that year.[4]

### *Puerperal Fever*

At the conclusion of the regular meeting of May 3, 1842, Condie spoke informally about a disease "of a peculiarly insidious and malignant character," which was then prevailing chiefly in the southern sections of the city: puerperal fever. Nearly every case that had come under his observation or that he had learned about from colleagues, had ended fatally. "In the practice of one gentleman, extensively engaged as an obstetrician [David Rutter, a Fellow]," he continued, "nearly every female he had attended in confinement, during several weeks past, within the above limits, had been attacked by the fever."[5]

Many of the Fellows were well acquainted with it. Robert M. Huston was seeing the fever currently at Blockley Hospital, where he was on the obstetrical staff.[6] Thomas Stewardson recalled an epidemic at the Pennsylvania Hospital in 1830, and Henry H. Smith gave an account of puerperal fever and erysipelas in the wards of a Paris hospital when he was a student there.

Condie also described the symptoms of the fever, its usual progress, and the treatments he and others followed. As he reflected on the cases, one question irresistibly presented itself: "Is it, namely, capable of being propagated by contagion, and is a physician who has been in attendance upon a case of the disease, warranted in continuing, without interruption, his practice as an obstetrician?" Although he could not accept contagion as a universal explanation in cases of puerperal fever, Condie admitted he had

> nevertheless become convinced by the facts that have fallen under his notice, that the puerperal fever now prevailing, is capable of being communicated by contagion. How otherwise can be explained, the very curious circumstances of the disease, in one district, being exclusively confined to the practice of a single physician, a Fellow of this College, extensively engaged in obstetrical practice—

> while no instance of the disease has occurred in the patients under the care of any other accoucheur practising within the same district; scarcely a female that has been delivered by this gentleman for weeks past has escaped an attack?

Condie was questioned by a number of the Fellows present, including Huston and David Rutter, who offered their own testimony.[7] Through Francis West, Samuel Jackson (of Northumberland), for example, gave facts from his practice to prove the contagiousness of puerperal fever. Not a few practitioners had long recognized or suspected a connection between childbed fever and the physicians, midwives, and nurses who attended women in labor; and, like Jackson, they acted on this premise. Not everyone, of course, accepted this conclusion. William P. Dewees, professor of midwifery in the University of Pennsylvania, flatly denied that puerperal fever was contagious. Hugh L. Hodge, professor of obstetrics in the University, and Charles D. Meigs, professor of midwifery and diseases of women and children at Jefferson Medical College, had they been present to hear Condie's report to the College, would also have strongly opposed the idea. The report, with the accompanying discussion, was printed in the *Summary of the Transactions* of the College and reprinted in the *American Journal of the Medical Sciences.*[8]

The College resumed its discussion of childbed fever on July 5. Further discussion inside and outside the College was stimulated by Condie's review of Meigs' *The History, Pathology, and Treatment of Puerperal Fever,* which firmly rejected Meigs' recommendation of bleeding as "neither a certain, essential nor proper remedy." Meigs, however, was not without supporters. Rutter espoused bleeding, and in return Meigs warmly praised the "brilliant example" of his well merited successes: of some seventy cases in Rutter's practice, "only some fourteen or fifteen proved fatal."[10]

Meanwhile, puerperal fever was discussed by the Boston Society for Medical Improvement in June and October 1842 and at subsequent meetings. In December Oliver Wendell Holmes began a careful review of the relevant literature. He read Condie's report and quoted from it in an eloquent and persuasive paper to the Boston Society in February 1843. By statistics and careful reasoning, Holmes showed that childbed fever was contagious, and that obstetricians were the carriers. He called it "a private pestilence." "The Contagiousness of Puerperal Fever" was published in the short-lived *New England Quarterly Journal of Medicine and Surgery* in April, and reached a national audience through a two-page abstract that was printed in the *American Journal of the Medical Sciences* of Philadelphia in July.[11]

For some years, however, the question of the contagiousness of puerperal fever remained unsettled. The idea was opposed in Boston by Walter Channing and in Philadelphia by Hodge and Meigs. The College minutes of June 1, 1852, for example, record that Dr. Meigs made some remarks on the causes and pathology of childbed fever, "principally with a view to disprove the contagiousness of the disease." The discussion, if any, was not recorded, nor were Meigs' remarks printed in the *Summary of Transactions.*[12] Two years later, in his work *On the Nature, Signs and Treatment of Childbed Fever,* Meigs asserted unequivocally that there was not "the least reason to suppose I have ever conveyed the disease from place to place, in any single instance," and he dismissed the arguments for contagion as

> the jejeune and fizenless [sic] dreamings of sophomore writers, who thunder forth denunciations, and would mark, if they might, with a black and ineffaceable spot, the hard-won reputation of every physician, who, in the Providence of God, is called upon to contend with the rage of one of the most destructive of epidemics . . . .[13]

In this overblown rhetoric Meigs displayed not only his uncompromising opinion that contagion was not the cause of childbed fever, but also a sense of personal hurt that his care of lying-in women should be branded as harmful. Meigs, Hodge, and their supporters and disciples were well-trained and widely experienced; they had delivered hundreds of women, bringing most of them successfully through even the most threatening complications. They were often selfless, even courageous, in the face of terrifying epidemics like the cholera, having only the welfare of their patients in mind. Meigs could not believe that doctors like himself, high-minded and able, as, without immodesty, he knew himself to be, could bring a fatal infection to his patients. "Medicine," he wrote, "is Doctors, not physic."[14]

Born in Bermuda in 1792, the son of a Connecticut Yankee

temporarily resident there, Meigs was graduated from the University of Georgia, of which his father was president, studied and practiced medicine in Georgia, and then entered the University of Pennsylvania Medical School, from which he was graduated in 1817.[15] In Philadelphia he acquired a large practice as an accoucheur, was elected to the staff of the Pennsylvania Hospital, wrote an authoritative standard textbook, *The Philadelphia Practice of Midwifery,* and enjoyed both scientific and social reputation. In Jefferson Medical College, to whose faculty he was elected in 1841, he was a graceful and effective lecturer and teacher. His description of Adam's reactions on finding Eve in labor was long remembered. His students extended his influence throughout the country. Toward mothers fearful of the dangers attendant on childbirth, he showed an understanding tenderness, throwing an atmosphere of romance and sentiment about them. But on the cause of childbed fever he was, even on the basis of the facts available to him, wrong. Perhaps he almost admitted this to himself before he died, for, his son tells us, he became depressed about 1855 and often complained of fatigue. It is at least worth noting that the son made no mention of puerperal fever in his obituary memoir of his father. Modern scientific knowledge would soften the harsh judgment of Meigs by his contemporaries.

The persistence of Hodge and Meigs in rejecting contagion and the offensive tone of Meigs' treatment of Holmes' arguments roused Holmes to republish his essay with a long introduction rebutting "the two Professors in the great Schools of Philadelphia." Forcefully refuting Meigs point by point, Holmes in conclusion appealed to his readers:

> If I am wrong, let me be put down by such a rebuke as no rash declaimer has received since there has been a public opinion in the medical profession of America; if I am right, let doctrines which lead to professional homicide be no longer taught from the chairs of those two great Institutions. Indifference will not do here; our Journalists and Committtees have no right to take up their pages with minute anatomy and tediously detailed cases, while it is a question whether or not the 'black-death' of child-bed is to be scattered broadcast by the agency of the mother's friend and adviser. Let the men who mould opinions look

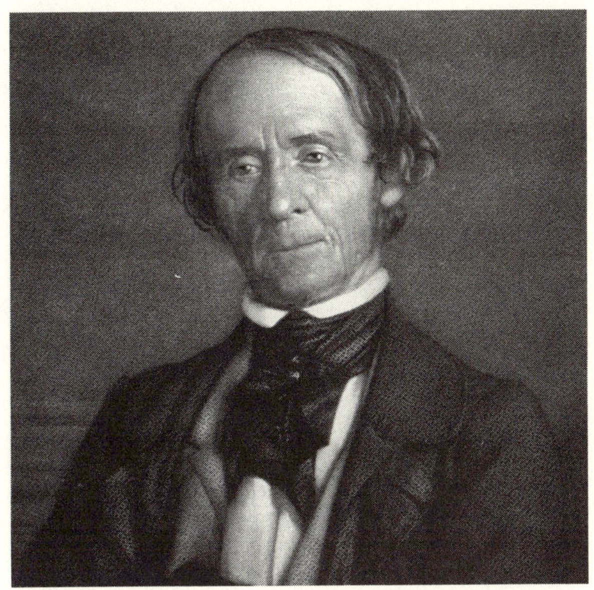

Charles D. Meigs, (1792–1869). Engraving by Welch & Walter, Philadelphia, from a daguerreotype by M. P. Simons.

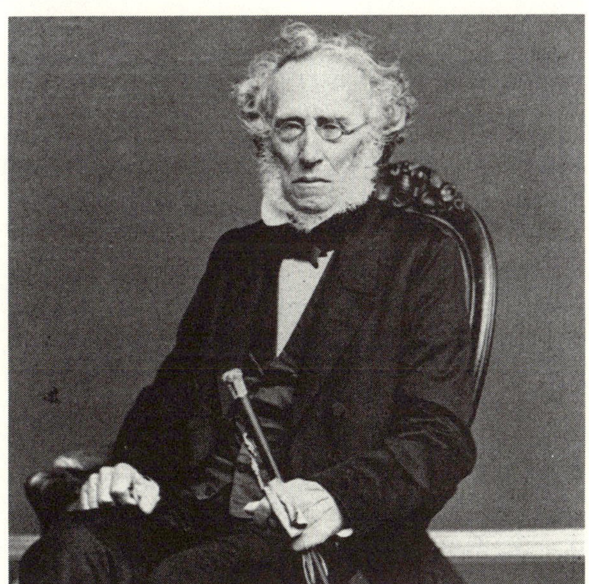

Hugh L. Hodge, (1796–1873). Photograph by F. Gutenkunst, Philadelphia.

> to it; if there is any voluntary blindness, any interested oversights, any culpable negligence, even, in such a matter, and the facts shall reach the public ear; the pestilence-carrier of the lying-in chamber must look to God for pardon, for man will never forgive him.[16]

These differences over the transmission of puerperal fever, which descended so close to personalities, fed the rivalry of Philadelphia and Boston. They strengthened the sense of superiority with which each regarded the other, barred mutual respect and confidence, and prevented the free exchange of information from which the physicians of both cities might have benefited. Philadelphia's reception—rejection rather—of surgical anesthesia was another illustration of this rivalry.

### *Anesthesia*

"Dr. Parrish," the College minutes of December 1, 1846, record,

> read a paper containing an account of the experiments performed by Dr. Bigelow and others, with an etherial preparation, proposed by Drs. Jackson and Morton, of Boston, Mass., as a means of preventing pain during surgical operations, detailed in the Boston Medical and Surgical Journal; with some animadversions on the conduct of Drs. Jackson and Morton in keeping the composition of the etherial preparation a secret from the profession, and in attempting to secure the use of it to themselves and their agents by a patent.
>
> The paper gave rise to a discussion in which several of the Fellows participated.[17]

Parrish's report was made just six weeks after the day—October 16, 1846—when Dr. John Collins Warren, the respected senior surgeon of the Massachusetts General Hospital, removed a tumor from a patient's neck. The operation was not unusual; the preparation and reaction of the patient, however, were unprecedented. At the surgeon's request Dr. William T. G. Morton, a Boston dentist, had anesthetized the patient, as he had been doing recently for tooth extractions in his own practice, and the patient had experienced no pain. The next day Dr. George S. Hayward, with Morton again as anesthetist, successfully removed a fatty tumor from the shoulder of another patient. Dr. Henry J. Bigelow, who was present on both occasions, reported briefly on the operations to the American Academy of Arts and Sciences on November 3, and in detail to the Boston Society of Medical Improvement on November 9. A few days later Bigelow's full report, which now included additional cases, was printed in the November 18 issue of the *Boston Medical and Surgical Journal* under the title "Insensibility during Surgical Operations produced by Inhalation."[18]

News of this astounding discovery spread rapidly. Extracts from Bigelow's report were printed in Philadelphia in *Medical News and Library* within two or three weeks of its appearance in Boston.[19] Isaac Parrish, surgeon of the Wills Eye Hospital, read Bigelow's and other reports with "a thrill of delight and gratitude," and at the first opportunity—the regular meeting on December 1—as a member of the Committee on Surgery, gave the College a short account of the "experiments" at Boston.

A member of an ancient and famous Quaker family, educated in Friends' schools, and himself "a strenuous Friend in his manners, customs, and doctrines," Parrish had studied medicine with his father Joseph (a Fellow since 1810) and received the M.D. degree from the University of Pennsylvania in 1832. His dissertation, on spinal irritation, based on data collected as a pupil in Blockley Hospital, was published in the *American Journal of the Medical Sciences.* During the cholera epidemic of 1832 he had assisted his father in one of the hospitals, and in 1834 was named to the staff of the new Wills Hospital, where his associates included Isaac Hays, George Fox, and Squier Littell. There Parrish took a lead in opening the wards to students, and in 1839–40 offered the first course of lectures on ophthalmology. In the College of Physicians, to which he was elected in 1836, he played a conspicuous part, "clear, precise, and forcible in debate, always winning the attention and respect of the house." In addition to being on the Committee on Surgery, he served on the Committee on Publications from 1841, was a benefactor of the library, and was the first to propose that the College establish a museum, to which he gave his father's collection of specimens and models.[20]

In his account of anesthesia at Boston, Parrish reviewed

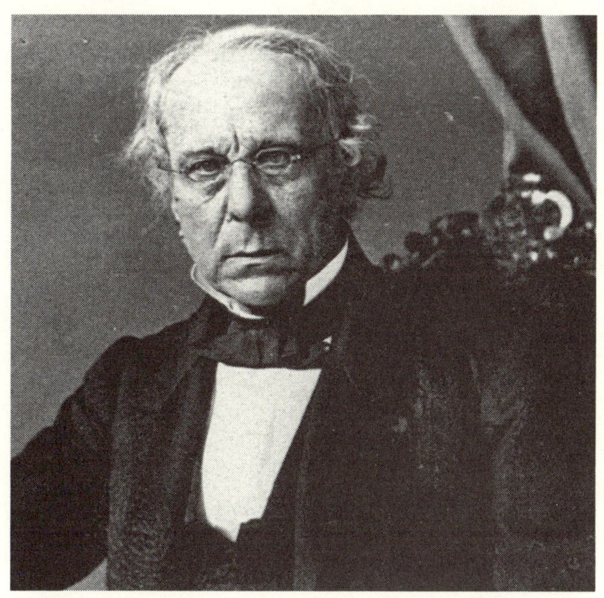

D. Francis Condie, (1796–1875). Photograph by M.P. Simons, Philadelphia.

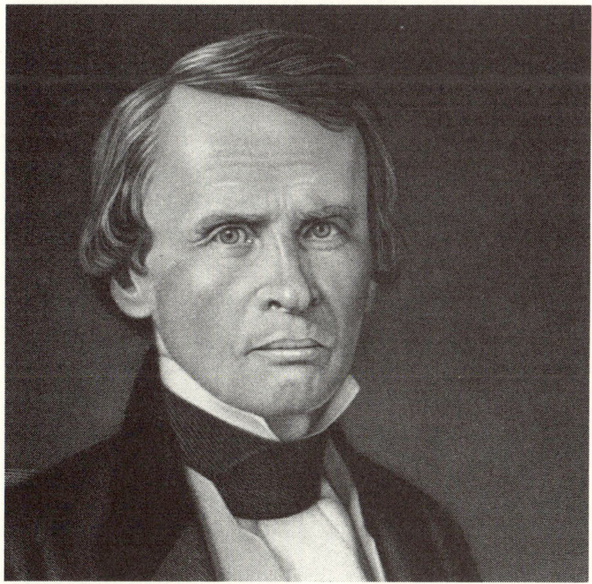

Isaac Parrish, (1811–1852). Engraving by A.B. Walter, Philadelphia, from a daguerreotype by Frederick DeB. Richards.

Bigelow's article at length and reported on subsequent operations and on the successful use of anesthetics by two Philadelphia dentists. "If the favorable accounts received . . . should be confirmed by subsequent experience," he concluded, "and if no serious effects should be found to follow its application, it may justly be considered as an important medical discovery." He urged that etherization be tested "by repeated and well directed experiments." But he strongly deprecated as contrary to principles of the medical profession and of humanity the decision of Morton and his colleague Dr. Charles T. Jackson to patent and "merchandize" their formula and keep it secret. The College at first took no action on Parrish's report; a month later, however, as the significance of ether anesthesia became inescapably clear, it voted to print the report in the *Transactions,* but without the Fellows' comments.

Many of those comments must have been skeptical at best. To some Philadelphians, strongly prejudiced against other sections of the country, anesthesia was just another "Yankee notion," another example of New England sharp practice, of a piece with Connecticut's wooden nutmegs. Surgeons who had worked successfully all their lives in "the old regime of shouting and twisting under the inflictions of the knife," could not believe that anything could—or should—suppress all sensation in a patient.[21] Indeed some believed that pain had its uses—the patient's cries told the surgeon when he had gone too far—and that it had therapeutic or moral benefit. Cautious practitioners understandably feared a powerful and mysterious agent, which might have alarming, dangerous, even fatal effects. But whatever their feelings about the "etherial preparation" (which was quickly identified as sulphuric ether), the Fellows were unanimous in denouncing Morton for patenting his vapor, which he called "Letheon." In their view Morton and Jackson were clearly quacks and "Letheon" another "secret" quack remedy. It meant little that Bigelow had acquiesced in Morton's action and defended it, while assuring medical colleagues that Morton would act generously toward the Massachusetts General Hospital and the profession. "We are persuaded that the surgeons of Philadelphia," wrote Robert M. Huston, editor of the *Medical Examiner and Record of Medical Science,* "will not be seduced from the high professional path of duty, into the quagmire of quackery by this will-o'-the-wisp . . . ." If a patient should die under anesthesia, he asked,

> what would be the effect upon their conscience, their reputation and business, and how [would] the practice . . . be likely to be viewed by a Philadelphia court and jury? . . . If such things are to be sanctioned by the profession, there is little need of reform conventions, or any other efforts to elevate the professional character—physicians and quacks will soon constitute one fraternity.[22]

How strong and widespread the resentment was against Morton for patenting his discovery was illustrated by the concern of an outstanding New York surgeon: Valentine Mott. One of those who had just issued the call to found a New York Academy of Medicine, Mott feared that he might not be allowed to sign its constitution because he had used "Letheon" in his practice.[23]

Reports multiplied of the successful use of sulphuric ether in Boston, New York, and Europe. By March 1, 211 operations had been performed in the hospitals of Paris.[24] From Vienna Moreton Stillé, younger brother of Alfred Stillé and soon to be elected a Fellow himself, wrote that he had witnessed two operations under anesthesia and had heard of no "untoward consequences" of its use in any of the Viennese hospitals.[25] In the late spring of 1847, some Philadelphia surgeons cautiously introduced the anesthetic into their practice. William Gibson, professor of surgery in the University of Pennsylvania, amputated the finger of a medical student in May; a few days later William E. Horner, also of the University, removed a cancerous breast. Neither Gibson nor Horner was a Fellow of the College. At Jefferson Medical College operations under anesthesia were performed by three Fellows: John K. Mitchell, who visited Boston to learn the procedure from surgeons there, Joseph Pancoast, and especially Thomas D. Mütter, who performed forty-five operations under anesthesia in his clinic between July 19, 1847, and February 26, 1848. Mütter assured a committee of the American Medical Association that in two hundred cases "no instance of a fatal event or even of serious mischief in any way attributable to the ether, has come to our knowledge."[26]

In the report on surgery that he made to the College in November 1847, Parrish reviewed the experience and testimonies of the year since Warren's first operation in Boston. "With the exercise of a sound discretion," he concluded, "we can see no reason . . . why etherization should not now be considered as a safe preparatory process to be instituted before the most important operations in surgery." He paid particular attention to sentiment in Philadelphia, warning his colleagues against "nurturing an overweening conservatism and incredulity, and shutting our eyes to . . . a great Truth."[27]

In Edinburgh meanwhile, Dr. James Y. Simpson had discovered the anesthetic properties of chloroform. By January 1848 chloroform had largely replaced ether in Britain, as Simpson explained in a letter to Charles D. Meigs. But, as Meigs' reaction to the idea of the contagiousness of childbed fever had shown, he was inclined to make hasty judgments, which pride and confidence in his practical experience kept him from modifying. He acted like this again on the subject of anesthesia.

In a stiffly worded letter on February 18, 1848, Meigs replied to Simpson. He had never "yielded," he stated proudly, to even the strongest appeals to administer ether or chloroform to women in labor. His reasons were moral and philosophical, not statistical and pragmatic:

> . . . notwithstanding I have seen so many women in the throes of labour, I have always regarded a labour-pain as a most desirable, salutary, and conservative manifestation of life-force. I have found that women, provided they were sustained by cheering counsels and promises, and carefully freed from the distressing element of terror, could in general be made to endure without great complaint, those labour-pains which the friends of the anaesthesia desire so earnestly to abolish and nullify for all the fair daughters of Eve.

Meigs admitted that ether and chloroform had been safely administered to thousands, but there had been "alarming accidents," however rare. "In all cases of chloroform anaesthesia," he wrote, "there remains but one irrevocable step more to the grave," and then he asked, a question for which neither Simpson nor any other had a ready and conclusive answer:

> should I exhibit the remedy for pain to a thousand patients in labour, merely to prevent the physiological pain, and for no other motive—and if I should in consequence destroy only one of them, I should feel disposed

> to clothe me in sack-cloth, and cast ashes on my head for the remainder of my days. What sufficient motive have I to risk the life or the death of one in a thousand, in a questionable attempt to abrogate one of the general conditions of man?[28]

The Simpson-Meigs exchange was reprinted and often quoted. Meigs sent the College of Physicians a copy of the journal in which it appeared.[29]

Some Philadelphia doctors, like Washington L. Atlee, W. Kent Gilbert, and Joseph Parrish, now began to use chloroform in their obstetrical practices; but others, citing Meigs' authority and their own reservations, rejected it. At the Pennsylvania Hospital the surgeons refused to use anesthetics in any case. Henry S. Patterson, a Fellow who had originally opposed anesthesia, spoke with the impatient scorn of the converted against the "unreasonable" conservatism in which some of his colleagues took a perverse pride: "Why should we in Philadelphia alone," he demanded, "occupy this position of dogged resistance and refuse to receive them [anesthetics]?" Since anesthesia was sure to be adopted soon everywhere, the most the Philadelphia profession could achieve was "the merit of having been the drag on the wheel that prevented a too rapid attainment of the goal."[30]

From time to time in the early 1850s, the College received papers on the use of anesthetics. John D. Griscom's report on midwifery in January 1849 elicited a lively discussion of the use of ether and chloroform in cases of labor.[31] The fullest discussion, however, took place at two sessions of the Philadelphia County Medical Society in March and April 1852. All those whose remarks were recorded were Fellows of the College. Time and experience had by now confirmed the efficacy of anesthesia; most of the objections had been successfully rebutted; and even opponents of the procedure used it in certain conditions. But reservations continued to be voiced. The pediatrician D. Francis Condie opened the discussion in the County Society with an unequivocal personal statement: "I feel no hesitation in announcing myself as one entirely opposed to their [anesthetics] employment when this is done for no other object than merely to prevent or assuage pain." Until ether and chloroform were proved to be absolutely safe, with never a serious or fatal issue, he could not accept them. In a strong reply, in which he admitted that ether had taken one life and chloroform eighteen, Isaac Parrish cited the record of five years, including cases in his own practice. Rejecting the notion that relief of pain was "a mere luxury," he asserted firmly that anesthesia was "a positive remedial agent of great power and utility." William Darrach, who had been a pupil of the great Philip Syng Physick, supported Parrish, rejoicing that the surgeon was no longer "the butcher-knife-man." Similar testimony came from another of Physick's pupils, Gouverneur Emerson. But Condie repeated the argument Meigs had offered Simpson four years before: "The life of one patient in 10,000 ought not to be sacrificed to obtain for the remaining 9999, relief from what is, in fact, in most cases, a very short period of suffering."[32]

By this time, of course, opposition had softened; it was soon abandoned altogether as its most eloquent spokesmen died, retired, or, like Charles Evans and John Wiltbank, changed their minds.[33] Whatever its scientific limitations and moral burdens were thought to be, anesthesia was universally adopted. Ether was finally admitted into the Pennsylvania Hospital in the summer of 1853; after 1863 all amputations there were performed under anesthesia.

### *Public Health*

Unlike anesthesia, which occupied the Fellows' attention for only six to eight years, public health remained a frequent, even constant, concern of the College. Every observant practitioner was aware of the insanitary conditions prevailing throughout Philadelphia in the middle of the nineteenth century; every doctor knew what overcrowding, intemperance, impure food and water meant to the health of the inhabitants, especially the poor. These matters were also a concern of the American Medical Association. In Isaac Parrish the Association found an ardent champion of medicine as an instrument of urban improvement. He was named to the Committee on Public Hygiene that the Association appointed at its second annual meeting in 1848, and wrote the report on public health in Philadelphia.

Parrish described sanitary conditions in the city in clear and forceful terms. Philadelphia had not kept William Penn's generous street plan. The squares had been divided and subdivided by alleys and courts, into which ever more people were crowded together. The tenements in these narrow streets and alleys had no yards. No current of air ever swept through them. Water was supplied from hydrants at the ends of rows of houses; the common privies were often built nearby—though sometimes they were placed in cellars, "which is still worse." Filth and offal accumulated, to be rooted through by roaming hogs from the city's piggeries, or blown about on dry days, or watered down into a sodden mess when the sprinkling carts came through. Unpaved streets were never cleaned; drains were open sewers; and the sewers were often clogged and overflowing. The old city was overbuilt, and new sections like Spring Garden were being developed with little thought to their residents' health.

Parrish argued that the city should require that water be supplied to every house, not simply for drinking and cooking, but also for bathing, a practice as yet "confined to a relatively small number," although most new houses, especially along the main streets, were being equipped with "conveniences" for bathing, a bath room being considered "indispensable to domestic comfort." There were only five public bath houses within the city limits and one in Spring Garden, and their general use was restricted by an admission charge. Parrish also urged cities to adopt a building code and a zoning ordinance:

> It is the opinion of the writer, as well as that of the committee with which he is associated, that the construction of dwellings should be, to some extent, under legal control; so far, at least, as to prevent the building up of confined courts and alleys, or of houses without provision for privies, hydrants, and a certain amount of open space in their rear. Surely, the protection of human life is one of the highest and noblest ends of government; and if a sordid self-interest interferes with the public good, by depriving any portion of the honest and industrious poor, of those natural elements, essential to the preservation of health, it should be within the province of the State to interpose its authority to prevent it. This principle is recognized in the powers given to Boards of Health, and other municipal bodies, to remove nuisances, &., and should, we think, be extended much farther than is now generally regarded as essential. . . . If, therefore, the municipal authorities do not move in this matter, it is greatly to be feared that the large

> and flourishing cities, which are now rapidly rising up in different sections of the Union . . . will be permanently defaced, and their facilities for diffusing health and comfort for ever impaired, for want of such timely interference. For while taste and elegance may adorn the mansions of the rich, and increasing splendour may mark the structures which public munificence or private enterprise rears to charity and science; yet, if the dwellings of the poor are neglected, if the light and air of heaven are shut out from their abodes, and avarice is allowed to feed and fatten upon their helplessness, we shall fail in establishing cities worthy of that high destiny to which our country aspires. It is the boast of the Republic to regard with an equal eye the happiness and interests of all classes, and especially to throw the aegis of its protection around those who, from adverse circumstances, may be exposed to privation and suffering, at the hands of their more favoured fellow-citizens; let our legislators, then, be inspired with the genius of our institutions, and act upon this principle, and the work which we advocate would be speedily accomplished.[35]

In support of projects for the public health in the College of Physicians, Parrish joined Condie, John Bell, Wilson Jewell, Gouverneur Emerson, and Henry Gibbons (who was to have a distinguished career in public health in California). They urged the College to call on the Philadelphia Board of Health to pay attention to the streets. There was much to criticize in the Board's actions and inactivity, but it had less authority and power than it might seem to have (it had no control over the contractors engaged to clean the streets); and, as some of the Fellows were members of the Board—Jewell and Paul Beck Goddard were presidents in the 1850s and 1860s—the College's views were already presented there as fully as it could hope.

In 1843 the College again warmly endorsed the proposal that the city acquire the Lemon Hill estate to protect the purity of the Schuylkill water supply; the memorial was particularly mentioned by the City Councils' joint committee on the purchase.[36] The Fellows called on the state legislature to reserve squares in the growing cities and larger towns of Pennsylvania as a means of ensuring the purity of the air and affording opportunities for physical exercise. When the Philadelphia City Councils sent out queries concerning burials and burial grounds within the city limits, Condie, Emerson, Robley Dunglison, Mütter, and other Fellows replied at once, although their attention at that time was focussed principally on the cholera epidemic sweeping through the city.[37] In 1862 the Select Council asked the College whether salting railroad tracks to prevent their freezing in winter was deleterious to health, as the Common Council believed. The College had one of its Fellows Robert E. Rogers, professor of chemistry in the University of Pennsylvania, make some experiments; he concluded that the practice was safe. Among those testifying in support of Rogers' conclusion was young Robert S. Kenderdine of the staff of Episcopal Hospital: salting icy streets, he remarked dryly, harmed only physicians, who would earn fewer fees for setting fractured limbs.[38]

Less apparent aspects of public health were also presented to the College in the 1840s and 50s. J. Wilson Moore questioned the discipline of the public schools; he considered one long session of four to five hours, with no opportunity for outdoor exercise, harmful to children.[39] Parrish offered statistics that showed that Pennsylvania's cherished prison system of solitary confinement produced mental illness and insanity. As a result, the system was eventually changed.[40] Insanity in the civil population was also a concern. Pointing out that insane persons were sometimes confined in prisons and that sane persons were sometimes committed to asylums, John Bell recommended that medical schools pay attention to this and related matters of medical jurisprudence.[41] Charles Evans, one of the attending physicians of the Friends Asylum for the Insane, agreed: lunacy hearings in Pennsylvania, he thought, were "a perfect farce." The subject of insanity came up in the College several times. Discussions tended to be anecdotal, and there was no agreement on treatment. Nor was there agreement whether insane persons should always be institutionalized. Evans, for one, had no doubt

> that it was a common error that, in all cases, the recovery of the patient is rendered more speedy and certain the earlier he is removed to an asylum, and surrounded with strangers, after indications of insanity present themselves. Dr. Evans was convinced that there are a large number of

> cases that are rendered worse by such removal, and that a disordered condition of the intellect, which could have been better treated and readily controlled in the patient's own home, has not unfrequently been aggravated by his removal.[42]

### *Transactions*

Some of these reports, as well as scientific papers and discussions, were printed in the *Quarterly Summary of the Transactions* of the College. Each issue included also a brief abstract of College business of general interest, such as committee reports, the record of elections, and memoirs of deceased Fellows. Of 250 copies printed, 150 were reserved for the Fellows and for editors of medical journals, and 100 were retained for sale. Although the appearance of the *Summary* had been hailed by the medical press, and a Hamburg physician prepared an "Analysis" of it through 1844,[43] there were few subscriptions and no sales of individual numbers. With such limited circulation, the journal offered no inducement to Fellows to contribute the results of their observations and experiments; it did little to enhance the reputations of the authors or the College, little to promote or spread medical knowledge. Thus, the principal reasons for issuing the *Transactions,* which cost the College $300 a year, were unrealized.

In 1851 Fellows considered how they might increase circulation of the periodical without increasing cost, "and in a mode not to impair its dignity or character." Rejecting the suggestion of Isaac Parrish that the papers be published in the *American Journal of the Medical Sciences,* the College contracted with the local publisher Lippincott, Grambo & Co. to print five hundred copies, of which half would go to the College and half be retained by the publisher for subscriptions and sale. The cost to the College would be less than when it printed the *Transactions* itself. Under this arrangement a "New Series" was begun.[44]

This new arrangement, however, produced no more sales and income than the previous one. The fault was not the publisher's. The Committee on Publications could not provide copy enough to fill the scheduled issues: only three numbers appeared in 1855, only two in 1856 and 1857. Nor was the committee entirely to blame. Philadelphia was the principal medical publishing center in the country. The *Transactions* had to compete with such powerful, well-edited, and widely-distributed periodicals as the *American Journal of the Medical Sciences,* the *American Medical Intelligencer* (continued as *Medical News and Library* ), and the *Medical Examiner.* It did not help the Committee in getting manuscripts that each of these journals was edited by a Fellow of the College.

The condition of the *Transactions* remained a subject of concern. In 1857 it was decided that it should contain only papers and reports of cases actually presented at meetings.[45] The next year, still searching for some way to publish the *Transactions* "at less cost to the College and so as to secure a more extended circulation," the College ended its contract with Lippincott, Grambo & Co., and accepted an offer from the *American Journal of the Medical Sciences* to publish papers and abstracts of papers quarterly in its pages at no cost except for steel and copperplate engravings and expensive woodcuts. The *Journal* would provide 250 reprints separately and consecutively paged and with new headings, so that the several issues might be gathered and bound as a single volume.[46] This form of publication lasted for fifteen years.

### *Cholera Again*

Improvements in public hygiene came slowly and epidemic diseases were not entirely banished from Philadelphia before the twentieth century. None of the epidemics, however, had consequences for the city and the College like those of the yellow fever visitations in the 1790s. Physicians and laymen alike had profited from their experience in the earlier crises. Professional collegiality and civility, not to say a resort to objective facts, tempered differences of opinion; and there were no public quarrels and angry resignations as in 1793.

On June 1, 1849, two cases of cholera were reported in the city, and on June 2 another. The count rose steadily through June and July—twenty cases on June 26, forty-three on June 27, forty-eight on June 29, eighty-one new cases on July 13—and then fell off in August. The Board of Health solicited the views of the physicians and, recalling the experience of 1832 and at the prompting of the College, set about erecting hospitals. One of these was "in full readiness" only nine hours after the decision to build was made, with physicians, attendants, nurses, medicine, and kitchen equipment all on hand.[47]

In the emergency the College met weekly. At one of the first sessions, Charles D. Meigs reviewed the history of the disease and its treatment, and offered his own explanation—that "cholera consists of an exaggerated intensity of the motor force, produced by the poisoning cause of the disease," and recommended bleeding. He summed up this murky idea as "a cholera squeeze" (a term which Oliver Wendell Holmes was to deride). More helpful was Henry H. Smith, who reviewed points on the pathology of cholera made by William E. Horner in 1835, and presented some morbid specimens for examination. Varying opinions on post-mortem appearances continued to be offered until Professor Samuel Jackson moved that a committee should examine lesions of the intestinal mucuous membrane microscopically:

> The disease is now amongst us; let us examine it systematically and thoroughly, without prejudice, and unbiassed by the authority of names or systems. What are the anatomical lesions in cholera . . . . Let us investigate the subject for ourselves . . . .[48]

This appeal to facts, not authority or doctrine, indicates how far medicine and the Fellows of the College had come since the days of yellow fever and Benjamin Rush.

The College was involved in a different way in an outbreak of cholera in 1854 in Columbia, Pennsylvania, a Susquehanna River town some seventy-five miles west of Philadelphia. The disease first appeared in the first days of September among some German immigrants. It spread rapidly, and on Saturday, September 9, thirty persons, including one of the town's six doctors, died. Panic seized the place; half the population of 4,500 fled to the surrounding farms and villages; and late that Saturday night a hastily-formed Sanitary Committee sent the College an urgent appeal for help. Its messenger arrived in Philadelphia at four o'clock Sunday morning. Two Philadelphia physicians—apparently one was Henry Hartshorne—went to Columbia that day. On Monday, September 11, the College held an emergency meeting, after which Wilson Jewell, Caspar Morris, and René LaRoche also travelled out to Columbia. They met the local doctors, found nothing unusual in the outbreak, drafted and published some sanitary regulations, and arranged for the delivery of medical and other supplies.[49] After these three returned to Philadelphia and made their report, the College assured the Columbia authorities

> that they will hold themselves in readiness to aid you with advice or with their personal assistance if required: being willing to repair to Columbia to help you bear the fatiguing labours of your service if the Epidemic should unhappily become still more prevalent in your town.[50]

Fortunately the disease vanished as rapidly as it had appeared, though leaving 127 dead. The Columbia people sent the College their warmest thanks for its "prompt and God-like aid . . . in the dark hour of their calamity." But, as one of the volunteer physicians had submitted a bill for $300 for his services, the local committee also asked what compensation would be appropriate for the College Fellows, who had "sacrificed their business and perilled their lives" to save the lives of their fellow-citizens.[51] The College replied that its members had acted "entirely without expectation of any pecuniary reward," and that the doctor who had billed the town for his services was not a Fellow.[52]

CHAPTER V

# *A Hall of Its Own*

THE revival of the College in the 1840s was an episode in the advance of medical knowledge and the medical profession in the United States and Europe. The increase of scientific knowledge and the growing professional confidence that flowed from it were reflected in medical practice and institutions everywhere. In the United States they led to the founding of local, state, and national societies, which, in turn, initiated and supported additional scientific inquiries and professional reforms. As the College pursued its particular objectives more vigorously, many of its Fellows were also involved in the formation of the American, Pennsylvania, and Philadelphia County Medical Societies.

### *Professional Societies*

The first step toward founding the American Medical Association was taken by the New York State Medical Society. In 1845 the Society called for a national convention to adopt measures to raise the standard of medical education. The initial response of the College (and of other medical institutions in Philadelphia) was cool, for the Philadelphians resented the implied slur on their professional qualifications and suspected that the New Yorkers' real motive was to promote their own medical schools and the reputation of New York as a medical center.[1] After all, the Philadelphians were the most famous medical teachers, authors of the most widely-used medical textbooks, and heirs to the oldest medical tradition in the nation, which their achievements strengthened daily; and they were sure that in the College of Physicians and the Philadelphia Medical Society they had instruments sufficient to any professional purpose. Under pressure from some of its younger and active members, however, the Philadelphia Medical Society reversed its decision not to attend the New York meeting. All but one of its delegation of twelve were also Fellows of the College. John Bell was elected one of the vice-presidents of the convention and Alfred Stillé one of the secretaries. The presence of these and other Philadelphians proclaimed the national character of the convention and assured its success.

In a move calculated in part to confirm this support, the delegates voted to hold their next meeting, which would form a national medical society, in Philadelphia in May 1847. Other Fellows, either as individuals or as members of the Philadelphia Medical Society, also supported the call for a national organization; and the College of Physicians now joined in the movement. It named sixteen Fellows to represent it at the organizing convention in 1847. The officers chosen at the first meeting of the American Medical Association included Nathaniel Chapman as president, Stillé as one of the two secretaries, and Isaac Hays as treasurer—all three Fellows of the College.[2] In the 1848 convention the Philadelphia institutions were represented by forty delegates, of whom thirty-three were Fellows of the College.[3] Stillé and Hays were returned to their offices, and Professor Samuel Jackson, another Fellow, was elected one of the four vice-presidents. The chairman and two other members of the important standing committees on practice, medical literature, and publications were also Fellows. The College sent delegates to each annual meeting thereafter for nearly thirty years until 1874, when the Association restricted representation to formally organized county and state societies affiliated with the national body.

One of those representing the College at the Association meeting in 1849 was George Bacon Wood. He entered in his journal an impatient judgment of its limitations and probable future usefulness:

> The heavy reports from Standing Committees . . . are of no other earthly use, as a general rule, than to enable the chairmen of the Committees to gain a brief notoriety. They are mere abstracts of what may be found in the journals, and repetitions of similar abstracts now published in various periodicals. Indeed, I do not think the

> Association can do much directly towards the promotion of Medical Science. If it do good, it must be indirectly, by elevating the standards of professional attainment & character, and by promoting a professional spirit among its members & others. In the arrangement of the committees for next year, I declined taking a place.[4]

The formation of the American Medical Association was followed quickly by the establishment in 1848 of the Medical Society of the State of Pennsylvania. The first calls for such a state-wide organization came from the Chester and Lancaster county societies. The College sent ten representatives to the founding meeting, which elected Professor Samuel Jackson as president.[5] The new state society invited the College to affiliate with it as one of three local societies allowed to the city and county of Philadelphia; but the College declined, unwilling to lose its independence.[6]

At the same time Fellows of the College and other physicians formed the County Society. The College had ten delegates at the first meeting in 1849, as did the Philadelphia Medical Society, all of whom were also Fellows of the College. Of the forty-seven men who were the first subscribers of the County Society's constitution, twenty-nine were Fellows. All the first officers except the treasurer were also Fellows, as were three of the five censors. In fact, of the first twenty-four presidents, who served from 1849 through 1875, twenty-one were Fellows of the College at the time of their election, and one became a Fellow afterwards. After 1856 the County Society met in the College's rooms.[7]

This broad overlap in membership between the two Philadelphia medical societies was a reason why they pursued their several aims so amicably. On many issues of public and professional concern, such as registration of births, deaths, and marriages, the College and County Society spoke with one voice. Thus, the two societies were not rivals, but complemented each other. The Fellows of the College appreciated that the County Society was more widely representative of the physicians of the city, with fewer professors and consultants and more general practitioners in the neighborhoods. The County Society more eagerly concerned itself with matters of public health and relations with the public, and was better organized and suited to approaching City Councils and the legislature, a task which officers of the more conservative College often found distasteful. On the other hand, the College could approach public bodies with a prestige and tradition, such a concentration of ability, reputation, and influence as no other Philadelphia medical institution could match.

Still, this overlapping membership does not mean that the County Society was only a lesser, imitative College. Many men gave their first loyalty to the County Society. Its younger members were sometimes restless, even resentful, at what they perceived as domination by the older members, many of whom were also Fellows of the College. The County Society was thus in their view more conservative than it might have been otherwise. In an expression of this spirit of independence, as early as 1850 the County Society called on the American Medical Association to limit representation to organized state and local societies. To include medical colleges, hospitals and asylums, and independent organizations like the College of Physicians, it was argued, unfairly favored the profession in large cities, diminished the importance of county societies, "and thereby discourages the formation of medical societies in rural districts."[8]

### *Reform of Medical Education*

Improvement of professional standards—in Benjamin Rush's phrase, the introduction of "order and dignity" into medical practice—was one of the purposes of the founders of the College of Physicians. It was always mentioned when physicians discussed the state of their profession in the United States. Such reflections addressed particularly the quality of education, the prevalence of quacks and quackery, and the conduct doctors observed toward one another and their patients. The American Medical Association also sought to raise educational standards. Leading physicians charged that the profession was crowded with illiterate, unqualified, and incompetent doctors; and the public, which also saw this, held both physicians and medicine in low regard. What Hugh L. Hodge had said in 1823 was even more true twenty years later:

> . . . it is the low opinion entertained of medical talent, which has inundated our profession with the refuse of schools and colleges; which has degraded it in the eyes of the world; which has given character to every ignorant

> pretender, to every undaunted, impudent empyric, and brought even the utility of the science into serious question and disrepute.[9]

To make matters worse, just as medical science was beginning to advance after 1820, the quality of medical education and practice fell as medical schools proliferated, especially in the United States. In Pennsylvania, for example, as the Committee on Medical Education of the American Medical Association reported in 1849, "there have never been any laws regulating the practice of medicine and surgery; any one may engage in practice, and recover his fees."[10]

Although the College deprecated the legislature's willingness to charter unneeded medical schools, "all clothed with the power of granting the degree of Doctor in Medicine," as a body it seemed less concerned with the problem than were many of its Fellows as individuals. This reflected the confidence the College as an institution felt in the adequacy and superiority of Philadelphia's medical schools. In any case, the College judged it best to allow the city's medical teachers and their schools to deal with standards of education and training.

However, individual Fellows spoke out strongly for reform and through their efforts acquired a national reputation. In 1847 the University of Pennsylvania inaugurated a six-month term of study in medicine, and in the same year the Philadelphia College of Medicine advised students to follow a logical sequence of courses from pre-clinical to clinical subjects.[12] The American Medical Association, as part of its effort to raise professional standards, also endorsed lengthening the regular terms of instruction. The Harvard medical professors, however, clung to the old pattern, arguing the merits of the traditional apprenticeship system and claiming that students could not absorb more material than could be presented to them in a four-month course. Lest there be any misunderstanding about where the national medical association stood, George Bacon Wood called on it to go on record as favoring the longer term; and Professor Samuel Jackson, Alfred Stillé, and John L. Atlee, appointed for the purpose, drafted a strongly-worded report.[13]

The committee asserted unequivocally that the public no longer respected the medical profession. The reason was simply want of proper education, which led to incompetence and invited not only the ignorant and gullible, but also the educated and intelligent, to tolerate and accept "absurd, fallacious, and dangerous doctrines." The medical profession, the report argued,

> had ceased to be a highly educated class. In its ranks were found those not only devoid of all pretensions to general science, but many who were absolutely illiterate. He must have occupied a low station, indeed, who could not produce the evidence of a diploma. The parchment refused in one quarter could be procured from another.[14]

The dispute, the committee declared, was more than the matter of a couple of months; it involved the whole rapidly increasing body of medical knowledge and the relations of the profession and the laity. Two four-month terms—even two six-month terms—were simply not enough to master the essential body of available medical knowledge. Medical students and their teachers owed more to the profession, the public, and the whole body of medical science. "It is an improvement in the quality, that the public good now requires," asserted the Committee, rejecting the Harvard professors' arguments and presenting their own reasons for advocating longer terms.

The profession, the committee's report went on, must look to the medical schools to raise standards by lengthening the course of study, adding new branches to the curriculum, raising graduation requirements, and requiring appropriate pre-medical education: "It is absurd to suppose that any effectual improvement can be made in the education of our schools, bringing their instruction up to the present elevation of medical science, while the four-month courses are retained."

But these arguments and appeals made scant impression. Dependent on students, who did not realize they were being cheated, the teachers and their institutions were unwilling to initiate practices that might lose them fees. Furthermore, the democratic temper of the time, allowing all sorts of sectarian cults to flourish, thwarted every effort to establish higher standards. The efforts of the American Medical Association came to nought. Even the University of Pennsylvania professors abandoned their lengthened curriculum in discouragement after six years in 1853.

***Professional Ethics***

Proper conduct among colleagues in the profession was always a concern of leading physicians. It is worth noting that within four months after it was added to the College library in 1803, Percival's *Medical Ethics* was taken out by five Fellows. Almost as urgently as education, professional ethics concerned the College and the American Medical Association at mid-century.

Through the first quarter of the nineteenth century written rules of conduct had not seemed necessary in the College. The faculty was dominated in general by men of integrity and manners, whose example in a still-aristocratic age was likely to be followed. The College by-laws of 1790 made no provision for bringing or hearing charges of misconduct. But the large increase in the number of doctors after 1820 changed this. The sense of common feelings and interests that had characterized the profession in the time of Redman and Parke weakened. Competition for "business"—patients and profits—became keen, and the temptation to self-promotion stronger. As late as 1855 one Philadelphia medical editor, citing specific cases, deplored the "pugnacity" and "disposition to quarrel" which, he said, pervaded much of the profession in Philadelphia.[16]

In this situation the College in 1839 took cognizance of "the present condition of the medical profession" in the city, and named a committee to examine why doctors were held in low esteem. The committee listed a dozen "evils" which in its view explained why the profession fell "below the standard . . . contemplated in the chartered constitution of the College."[17] A number of the charges were familiar: too many students and physicians with inadequate general education and of questionable moral character; deficient instruction in medical schools; advertisements and endorsements of medical wares by physicians. Several complaints went to the pocket-book: the fee-bill was not universally honored; some doctors waived fees for services "to richly endowed charitable institutions." Several reasons, of particular interest, reflected the unsettled state of medical science:

> 4th. The inattention of the College to the revision of papers and works published by its members & the doctrines taught by them as public lecturers . . . .
> 8th. The want of unity in the medical profession in refer-

> ence to modes of practice . . . .
> 12th. The want of legislative authority delegated to this College or other corporate medical body for the regulation of the important concerns of the profession in its community interests with the public.

The complaints were a miscellaneous lot, and some of the "evils" might more properly have been regarded as consequences than causes of the low rank of the profession. Nonetheless, the report called for issuing "a full & comprehensive code of medical ethics" under the sanction of the College.

While the College committee was preparing this report on the condition of the profession, the Pennsylvania legislature chartered the Medical College of Philadelphia, which was given power to confer medical degrees on any candidate who took its examination, without reference to where he had studied. By this act the legislature hoped to check the proliferation of medical schools and to separate licensing from teaching. Needless to say, the faculties of the established institutions were not ready to surrender their prerogative, and the Medical College of Philadelphia proved to be no different from other institutions.[18]

In 1842, at the instance of Benjamin H. Coates, the College, responding to its report of three years before, drafted a set of rules of conduct which Fellows should observe towards their colleagues and patients. (At the same time the Philadelphia Medical Society also prepared rules for its members.) During the twelve months that the College discussed the proposed rules, suggestions also came from outside. For example, the *Medical Examiner,* while skeptical whether any rules would do much good without power to enforce them, sharply criticized draft provisions concerning educational qualifications and free attendance on clergymen. Both these provisions were dropped.[19] The revised rules were adopted on December 5, 1843, and were printed in the by-laws, with a revised fee bill, in 1844.

The rules set forth in general terms the ideals that should govern physicians in their relations to other physicians, their patients, and the public. But the most important rule in the minds of the Fellows was that which read as follows:

> No person who gives his support to any system of practice, which is sustained by efforts to weaken or dimin-

> ish public confidence in the science of medicine, or in the medical profession, or who, by advertisement, announces his claim to superior qualifications in the treatment of diseases, or of a particular disease; or who holds a patent, or a part of a patent for a surgical instrument; or gives a prescription to any apothecary, which he refuses to give to other apothecaries; or who deals in secret medicines, or publicly recommends them, shall be considered eligible as a Fellow or Associate of the College. And, any Fellow or Associate who may be hereafter so engaged, shall forfeit his right to membership, on the fact being reported by the Censors. But an appeal from the decision of the Censors is permitted, as in other cases.

This provision, the Fellows said, had "necessarily the force of law;" all the others were "merely recommendatory."

No set of rules, however, could anticipate all conditions and every problem. In the next few years a dozen questions were presented to the College and its Censors: Had physicians the right to charge for making post-mortem examinations at the behest of coroners? Should a physician charge for attendance on servants in families whose medical adviser he was? How should a physician respond to an invitation to attend an operation or practice of an empiric or irregular practitioner? Was a physician called to attend the patient of a brother physician ever entitled to receive a fee for his attendance? (He was, a committee decided, "provided that this rule shall not be understood to interfere with a friendly reciprocal exchange of services between physicians.")[20] Although many, long-standing precedents and practices on patents seemed clear, there was room here for argument, if not for doubt: "Why shall a man be allowed the advantages of patent right [i.e., copyright] for a book he may write, but be disgraced among his professional brothers, if he claim a share of the profits arising from an extensively useful instrument of his own invention?"[21]

Some responsibility for answering such puzzling questions was taken out of the College's hands in 1847, when the American Medical Association as one of its first acts adopted a code of ethics for the profession. Large parts of the College's rules were translated into the national code; what was new in it the College incorporated into its own by-laws. For example, there were few substantial changes or additions to the College's statement of physicians' obligations to patients; but a section on patients' obligations to physicians, adopted by the national association, was added by the College to its by-laws. The extended rules were printed in the 1848 edition of the *Ordinances and By-Laws of the College.*

Towards their patients physicians were enjoined to observe "the strictest temperance." They "should minister to the sick with due impressions of the importance of their office," uniting tenderness with steadiness, and condescension with authority. A physician "should not be forward to make gloomy prognostications, because they savour of empiricism," but he should rather appear as "the minister of hope and comfort to the sick." And at the close of every important case he should scrupulously review all the steps in treatment for the benefit of future cases.

Other regulations dealt at length with physicians' relations to other physicians, especially the etiquette of consultations, and with fees. Then came a paragraph headed "Esprit du Corps"—something akin to Rush's notion of "collegiality:"

> The Esprit du Corps is a principle of action founded in human nature, and, when duly regulated, is both rational and laudable. Every man who enters into a fraternity, engages, by a tacit compact, not only to submit to the laws, but to promote the honor and interest of the association, so far as they are consistent with morality, and the general good of mankind. A physician, therefore, should cautiously guard against whatever may injure the general respectability of his profession; and should avoid all contumelious representations of the faculty at large, all general charges against their selfishness or improbity, and the indulgence of an affected or jocular scepticism, concerning the efficacy and utility of the healing art.

### *George Bacon Wood*

Before President Hewson died in 1848, the College had become active again, with reasonably defined objectives, attainable hopes, and practical means. Though an older man, born and educated in the eighteenth century, Hewson had taken a large part in preparing the national pharmacopoeia and in performing a variety of services for the public health. He had gently encouraged and supported the changes that brought the College into the middle of the nineteenth century. In the years of his successor, George Bacon Wood, whose presidency of thirty-one years was the longest in its history, the College erected a permanent physical home in Philadelphia and acquired reputation and influence throughout the nation.[22]

A graduate of the University of Pennsylvania in 1818, Wood linked the age of Wistar, Chapman, and the eighteenth century with that of Gerhard, Stillé, Mitchell, and the mid-nineteenth. If he retained something of the thought and practice of the earlier time, Wood was also willing to study and adopt current ideas and methods. When the stethoscope was introduced, for example, he learned how to use it, even asking his younger colleague William Wood Gerhard to instruct him. Wood's contemporaries had confidence in his ability, wisdom, and personal integrity and in "his reserve force," and he was for more than thirty years the single most influential figure in the profession in Philadelphia, and one of the most influential physicians in the nation.

Born in Greenwich, New Jersey, of a Quaker family, a student of Joseph Parrish, who invited him to join the faculty of his private school (later named the Association for Medical Instruction), Wood was professor of chemistry and then of materia medica in the newly-established Philadelphia College of Pharmacy from 1822 to 1835. In the latter year he was elected to the staff of the Pennsylvania Hospital and was named professor of materia medica in the University of Pennsylvania, where he succeeded Chapman as professor of theory and practice in 1850. Wood was also president of the American Philosophical Society for twenty years until his death and of the American Medical Association in 1855–56.

His carefully prepared lectures were enriched by copious illustrative materials. To show his students articles of the materia medica, he grew as many plants as possible in his own garden and greenhouse, employing a Scots gardener to tend them. "It is my intention to introduce in time into the garden & hot houses," he wrote in 1836, "all the medicinal plants which can be procured from all parts of the world—at least so far as the limits of my grounds will allow."[23] What he could not grow, he imported, and, when living specimens were unobtainable, he used drawings and paintings. Upon his appointment as professor of theory and practice, he visited the medical schools, hospitals, and famous teachers of Europe, and is said to have spent $20,000 for diagrams, casts, and models for his teaching. Gross recalled that Wood once spread seventeen stethoscopes on a tray before him when he lectured on the normal sounds of the lungs.[24] "Everything," said a friend, "was done to give the class all possible experimental knowledge of the subject."

The private income that enabled Wood to do these things also allowed him to live in ease far above that of any of his colleagues. "Elegant" was the adjective often applied to his manner of living. He had "a beautiful & complete establishment," remarked Sidney George Fisher approvingly.[25] Wood's style in travels to the West, Niagara Falls, Saratoga Springs, even to his Jersey farm suggested the progress of an English milord—a handsome private carriage drawn by four horses, sometimes with liveried servants atop and behind. No matter how remote his destination or how tired he might be, he would never take a public conveyance. "When I ride," he told his nephew, "I ride in my own carriage."[26] Tall, dignified, formal, and distant, he always dressed faultlessly in black, and wore a black wig that was increasingly incongruous as he grew older.

After the early years, Wood's practice was principally of a consulting kind. In addition to his regular teaching, he had many private pupils, who respected, admired, and feared him.[27] A tireless worker, he was the principal author of several editions of the *Pharmacopoeia;* he presided at the National Conventions of 1850 and 1860 to revise it. With his friend Franklin Bache he compiled the *Dispensatory* in 1833 and revised or supervised fourteen editions before he died. His *Practice of Medicine,* published in 1847, was famous, went through six editions in his lifetime, and was used as a text in Edinburgh University. It is said to have sold 50,000 copies and, like the *Dispensatory,* brought him a handsome income.

Between 1848, when Wood became president, and 1863, when the College moved into its own hall, 105 men were elected Fellows. In only five of those sixteen years were more than seven chosen, in eight years four or fewer. Only one Fellow was elected in 1861, which may reflect wartime dislocation. The average number elected each year for the period was 6.5. These 105 included several men of great distinction who, however, took little part in College business: Joseph Leidy (1851), almost the last person who took all natural history as his field of study, and Philadelphia's two

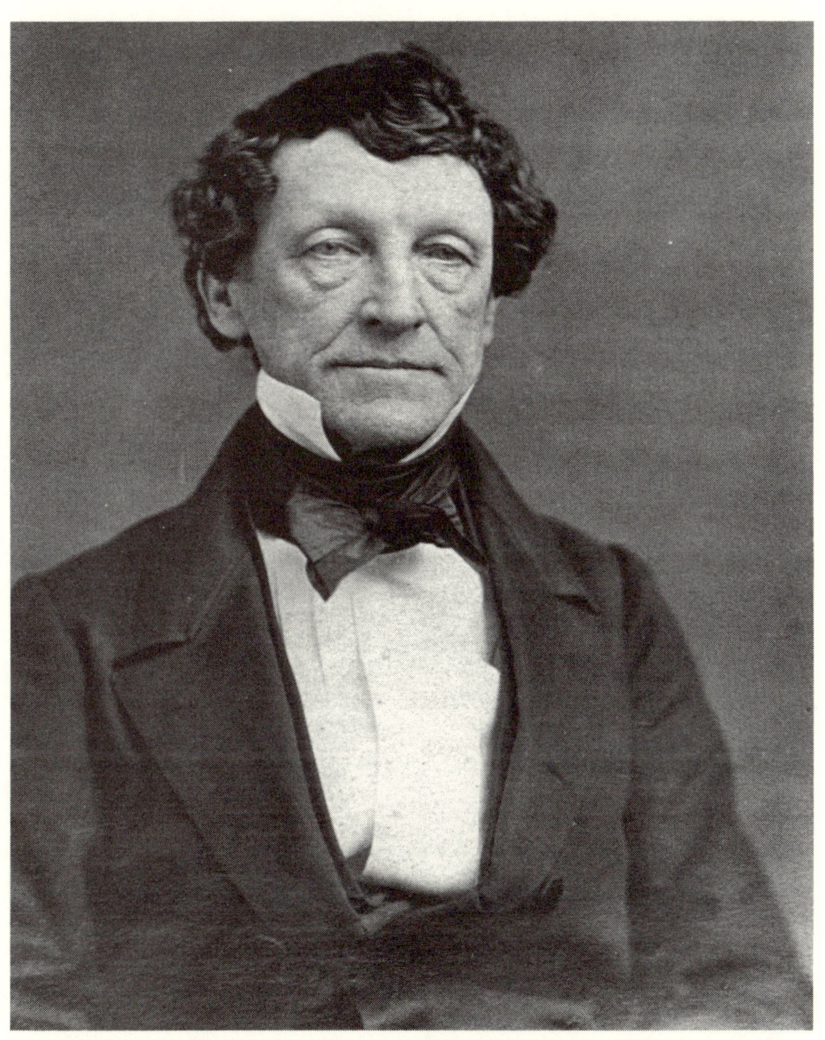

George Bacon Wood, (1797–1879). Photograph.

great surgeons, Samuel D. Gross (1857) and D. Hayes Agnew (1859). Among the rest were a score who became leaders in College affairs, presenting papers, serving on committees, holding office. They included D. Paul Lajus (1849), Henry Hartshorne (1851), Wilson Jewell (1851), who reported annually for some years on climate and disease, T. Hewson Bache (1852), who served many years first as librarian, then as curator of the Mütter Museum, J. Aitken Meigs (1856), and John H. Packard (1858), subsequently secretary and vice-president, and the first Mütter lecturer. In December 1855 the name of S. Weir Mitchell was proposed by John Bell, John Rodman Paul, Alfred Stillé, and Lajus; and he was elected a Fellow the next month.

What the meetings were like then, a combination of formality and passion, Mitchell recalled thirty years later:

> The debate used to be sharp in those days. There was Wood in the chair, most courteous of men, gently formal, and of ever-ready kindness to younger physicians; a peacemaking presence when the too-positive Condie was raging in debate, and Charles Meigs, with his poetic nature and talk of singular freshness, was spurred to sharp reply, and [Hugh L.] Hodge grew graver and yet more sedate, and [Franklin] Bache sat ready to drop with deliberate slowness of contradiction on the inaccurate. As I write, the visage of [William Wood] Gerhard returns to me with its grim humor. A man quick of speech and as quick to regret, an unbalanced nature, but a keen and subtle observer. There is stout George Fox, and the slight, delicate form of [René] La Roche beside our great surgeon [Joseph] Pancoast, sturdy, earnest, kindly, and original, a curious physical contrast to his colleague Mütter, small, exquisitely neat in person, and courtly in manner.[28]

When Wood died in 1879 the Fellows attended his funeral in a body. In resolutions on the occasion Squier Littell, his colleague in the College for more than forty years, wrote:

> His mental characteristic was not genius properly so called; but he possessed capacity of a high order, and had a methodical and mathematical mind, a striking feature of which was its strong, masculine common sense. With this

was united the greatest, perhaps, of all talents, steady and unwearied application.[29]

Wood made many gifts and performed many services for the College in his half-century as a Fellow. Perhaps his most important and influential service was helping to procure a permanent meeting place.

### *Library, Museum, and Hall*

Although the regular meetings of the College after the early 1840s were instructive and well-attended, and the *Transactions* were appearing quarterly, no one paid much attention to the library. It was, the chairman of the Library Committee reported in 1842, "but little used, and there has been but the addition of one volume during the last year."[30] The books were kept on a stair-landing in Philosophical Hall, in a case, painted black, through whose glazed doors, Alfred Stillé remembered, a few hundred volumes "could be dimly seen . . . all by their musty and dingy bindings proclaiming their long disuse." This "ancient receptacle," Stillé continued, "irresistibly suggested the chamber of an Egyptian tomb."[31]

In 1844, however, the Fellows took an action that was to have far-reaching consequences for the library and for the College. John C. Otto, vice-president of the College, who was about to leave the city in search of rest and health, put his library up for sale. It was reported to be "a valuable collection of works on the medical and collateral sciences, all of which are in a good state of preservation." Acting with unusual speed, the College bought it for $200. Because there was no more space on the stair-landing, the books were stored in a room over Hugh L. Hodge's office at Ninth and Walnut Streets, where they were safe but virtually inaccessible.[32] Accordingly, the College on May 7, 1844, directed the Library Committee to present plans at the next meeting "for rendering the Library more useful and accessible to the Fellows, and to ensure its permanent increase in size and value."

Although entirely in sympathy with these objectives, the committee was annoyed that it had been so long ignored and that now, when its advice was sought at last, it was given scant time to prepare a considered reply. Nonetheless, its suggestions were practicable: the collections should be catalogued; the library should receive an annual appropriation; a librarian should be named, and the library opened at least two hours a month; and a more convenient place should be found for the books. This last suggestion, which was to be repeated in ever-stronger terms almost annually for the next fifteen years, was a principal reason why the College moved twice to larger quarters and finally built a hall of its own in 1863.

There were, of course, other reasons why the Fellows were increasingly dissatisfied with the small, crowded room they rented in Philosophical Hall. The Philosophical Society repeatedly asked to use the College's space; there was no security for the minute books, ledgers, correspondence, and other archives; and, though the Society had not raised the rent for years, the Fellows constantly complained about what they were charged. From time to time someone would suggest that they move, but no better accommodation at so convenient an address for such low rent was ever found.[33]

The College was not the only medical society looking for permanent quarters commensurate with its "influence and respectability." In 1840 a joint committee of three of these societies—the College, the Philadelphia Medical Society, and the Medical College of Philadelphia—proposed to acquire or construct a building in which each might hold its meetings. The central feature, in addition to a meeting room, would be a library and a museum. Since the estimated cost of $15,000 was more than the societies, either separately or jointly, could contemplate, it was recommended that a stock company of individual shareholders be formed to erect the building. The corporation would be called the Medical Hall Association of Philadelphia. Although this proposal had the support of Henry Neill of the College and of Henry Bond, also a Fellow, who represented the Medical College, the College of Physicians judged it premature and inexpedient.[34]

The new building of the Mercantile Library, rising on Fifth Street across from Philosophical Hall, offered a practical, if temporary, solution; and the College rented space there. The room was large enough to allow all the books to be shelved and even to provide for expansion; it had its own street entrance; and the library could be open as many hours daily as the College wished, thus in some measure answering the requirements of a medical athenaeum. A subscription was taken up to pay for the necessary furnishings—"1 Presidential chair," ten ball back settees, thirteen arm chairs, carpeting, and four spittoons, for a total cost of $280.42 1/2.[35] The first meeting in the new quarters was held on August 5, 1845; thereafter, the secretary headed his minutes, not "Philosophical Hall," as he had done for so many years, but "Hall of the College." To meet the rent of $175 a year the College increased its entrance fee to $15 and the annual dues to $5. On October 7 the Committee on College Room reported proudly that most of the medical journals published in the United States and one in Canada were being received in exchange for the *Summary of Transactions* "and are placed on the table, agreeably to the design of the College, for the use of the Fellows who may visit the Chamber during the hours it is daily open."

As the College flourished, there was growing recognition of the library's benefits. Now that there was ample space for the collection, Fellows were moved to donate books and periodicals. On September 2, 1845, a month after the College moved into its new quarters in the Mercantile Library building, Isaac Parrish presented seven volumes and gave three more in October. In November Henry Bond gave sixty-six volumes, and in December George Bacon Wood gave seventeen titles and D. Francis Condie twenty-three.[36] John Bell got a publisher to present some books; and from Isaac Hays came the first of many gifts of books, journals, and pamphlets received by the *American Journal of the Medical Sciences,* which he edited. A subscription was entered for publications of the Sydenham Society; thereafter each volume was reported to the Fellows as it was received. By July 1846 the books were all labelled and numbered and a catalogue was prepared, the first since 1818. Almost for the first time, the Library Committee could report that the library was "in good condition." At the end of 1846 the Philadelphia Medical Society deposited its library in the College.[37] But each year, usually on the motion of D. Francis Condie, who was always sensitive to financial limitations, the College "dispensed with" its annual appropriation for the library.

Meanwhile, in 1849 Isaac Parrish proposed that the College establish a museum of pathology. The idea was appealing, and the Fellows quickly approved it, appropriating $50 to construct cases and prepare the specimens. As curator they named the thirty-year-old John Neill, who had been a physician in one of the city cholera hospitals that summer. Parrish gave the College the large collection his father Joseph Parrish had assembled for his teaching.

Benjamin H. Coates presented a microscope. Other Fellows came forward with gallstones, monsters, and plaster casts of one condition or another. Isaac Hays presented "a horn-like substance" more than four inches long, which had been given him by a gentleman who knew no more about it than that he had received it from another, who claimed it was "a horny excrescence taken from the knee of a negro man." But the initial enthusiasm for the museum waned. In 1853–54 there were no accessions, and in 1861, when John H. Packard became curator, the specimens were suffering neglect. There were then ninety-two exhibits in all—forty-nine wet preparations, three wax casts, six bone specimens, twelve injected specimens (dried), and seventeen injected specimens (wet).

Before long the steadily growing library, the new museum, not to mention the regular meetings, which were now usually attended by forty or fifty Fellows, required more room. The Library Committee in 1852 took the opportunity of its annual report "for pressing the necessity of additional room for the accommodation of the library upon the attention of the Fellows, as a strong inducement . . . for the collection of a fund adequate to the erection of a hall suitable for the use of the College."[38] Even outsiders urged the College to move. The city's medical societies, remarked the *Philadelphia Medical and Surgical Journal* in 1854, were "entirely destitute of a permanent place in which to hold their meetings, wandering about, begging or hiring rooms," and it urged them—the College, the County Society, the Northern and Southern Medical Associations—to erect "a splendid brown stone hall . . . in the middle of the city (somewhere near the Schuylkill river), at once . . . ."[39]

But the College could not afford to build a hall, and so in 1854 it rented the "Picture House" of the Pennsylvania Hospital on Spruce Street between Eighth and Ninth; here Benjamin West's painting "Christ Healing the Sick" had until recently been displayed. The building was described as "comparatively elegant and commodious," with one large room for meetings and a smaller one for the library. The College met there on July 4, 1854. The rent was $250 annually, but that burden was lightened when the College allowed the County Medical Society to meet in its rooms for $125 a year.

In 1855 the College, whose secretary had discharged the duties of librarian for some years, elected a librarian again after many years. Thomas Hewson Bache, son of Franklin Bache, a graduate of Jefferson Medical College in 1850, was never a leader of the profession or even of the College; but he was a sound and useful practitioner. As librarian for eight years and curator of the Mütter Museum for seventeen, he enriched two of the College's principal functions on many occasions.

Bache's guiding principle, he once explained, was to keep the library before the Fellows constantly.[40] In his first report, made a month after he was named, Bache revealed that hardly any run of periodicals was complete: the College did not even possess a complete set of its own *Transactions.* He organized the collection, filled incomplete files of journals and had them bound, sold duplicates, acquired more books, and eventually persuaded the College to put the library in its annual budget. In that same report he announced a gift of fifty volumes from Samuel Lewis, the first donation by the man who was to become the library's greatest benefactor.

In addition to hundreds of modern, useful texts and monographs, the library received some rare and curious titles. Among twenty-five volumes given by Paul Lajus were editions of William Harvey's *De Motu Cordis* and *De Generatione Animalium;* Theophilus E. Beesley gave six volumes of a student's notes of Alexander Monro's lectures at Edinburgh; and from Caspar Morris came a volume he had acquired thirty years before when, as a young doctor on a merchant vessel, he had visited India: *Qanoonchen: or, A Treatise on the Theory and Practice of Physic* by Ahmud-bin Muhmood Chughmeenee (Calcutta, 1827), with a commentary in Persian and brief notes in English.[41] With 1,700 volumes on the shelves in 1855, the Library Committee now regarded the library "more encouragingly" than in former years; but the College once again dispensed with the "special annual appropriation," as it had done for so many years.

Interest and pride in the library, however, were growing among the Fellows, several of whom paid to have a bookplate made for the College in 1855. Finally, in 1856 Bache succeeded in winning $125 for the library (though Condie tried to reduce the amount to $50), and in the next year he blandly asked for a renewal of what he now called the "usual" appropriation, which was approved.[42] Shortly afterwards, the sum was raised to $150 per annum, and in 1862 Condie himself put the motion for that amount.

A large addition to the library came from Thomas F. Betton, a Fellow of the College who had recently been president of the County Medical Society. In 1856 he offered the College his library and that of his father—an estimated two thousand volumes of "the best editions of the best authors, all in perfect order, some of the books very rare." The conditions attached to the gift were, however, unacceptable. President Wood and Alfred Stillé were asked to visit Betton to explain why. But Wood, who at the moment was incapacitated by an injury, asked Betton to see *him* at his convenience. Betton refused, replied that he would still gladly meet Wood and Stillé at *his* house, broke off communication, and resigned his fellowship. Matters were soon patched up. Betton withdrew his resignation, dropped his unreasonable stipulations, and donated the books as a memorial to his father. They were added to the library in 1857–58.[43] With 3,560 volumes now crowding the shelves, the Library Committee reminded the Fellows once more that "additional accommodations for the books has [sic] become absolutely necessary."[44] In fact, such accommodations were about to be provided.

The College was hardly settled in the "Picture House" in 1855 when it became clear—and not only to the friends of the library—that still larger quarters were required. Not only was the library growing at an accelerating rate, but the new museum was sure to expand, and the regular meetings were more fully attended than ever before. Furthermore, the proposal that the city's medical societies should join in erecting a hall for their own uses, though not approved, had awakened hopes and expectations. As one of the city's oldest and more prestigious institutions, the College was thought by its Fellows to deserve a home of its own, like the Library Company, the Philosophical Society, and the Academy of Natural Sciences. What was needed, the president of the College reckoned, was a building fund; with this in mind Wood privately resolved to donate $1,000 "as a nest-egg for such a fund," and he persuaded one of the Fellows, George Fox, to present the matter to the College.[45]

### *George Fox*

In 1849 Fox was one of the physicians of the Pennsylvania Hospital, a member of the Board of Managers and visiting surgeon of Wills Hospital, a vice-president of the Philadelphia County Medical Society, and the treasurer of the Medical Society of the State of Pennsylvania. As a young resident in the Pennsylvania Hospital he had invented an apparatus for the treatment of fractures of the clavicle; and, though not a major writer, he contributed several papers to the *American Journal of the Medical Sciences.* Practical, unpretentious, concerned for his patients' welfare, he was in the words of a contemporary "an accomplished general practitioner." In the College, to which he was elected in 1831, Fox served several years on the committees on surgery and on materia medica and pharmacy; and he was one of the College's delegates to the national convention that formed the American Medical Association in 1847.[46]

Fox retired from active practice and from his hospital appointments in 1854 and eventually moved to Torresdale, north of the city. His attention to the College funds, however, was unflagging. For nearly a quarter of a century he gave unstinting advice and support to every step toward his and the other Fellows' dreams of a hall. "He had able and zealous coadjutors throughout the work," wrote his friend W. S. W. Ruschenberger of the significance of his service,

> but it is generally conceded that, from first to last, his tact in affairs, financial sagacity, and alert prudence as well as persistence exercised a guiding and helping influence, essential to the accomplishment of the project, which strengthened the foundation of the College and accelerated the growth of its means of utility.[47]

When the proposal for a Medical Hall Association was abandoned, Fox had called on the College at once to get an estimate of the cost of erecting a building for itself. However, the committee—composed of himself, D. Francis Condie, and John Rodman Paul—seems not to have made a report. But Fox's interest did not wane; he responded enthusiastically to Wood's suggestion and renewed his motion for a building committee. Fox insisted, the committee recommended, and the College voted, that monies collected for a hall should be placed in a trust, so that donors could be assured that their gifts would not be used for other purposes. On January 15, 1850, Fox, Wood, and Paul were named trustees of the fund; and Fox was put on the committee to solicit funds, along with Condie, Moreton Stillé, Francis West, and George W. Norris. Other Fellows promptly followed Wood's example, and within six months the building fund amounted to $4,085. The College assigned annual surpluses and its Chesapeake and Delaware and other securities to the fund. Almost every year Wood added another $1,000.

### *Mütter Museum*

Meanwhile, Thomas D. Mütter, retiring in 1856 from the chair of surgery at Jefferson Medical College because of ill health, indicated his intention to donate his collection of pathological specimens to the College—nearly 1,600 bones, wet preparations, casts, oil paintings, and water colors. The College responded promptly. Mütter's travels abroad in search of health delayed execution of the deed of gift until the winter of 1858–59. By its terms the College would receive the specimens if, within five years, it erected a fireproof building to house them. Mütter's gift would include an endowment of $30,000 to support and extend the collection, pay a curator, and provide a lectureship. The offer was accepted by the College on January 8, 1859, two months before Mütter died.[48] The collection, on which he is said to have spent $20,000, was the largest single gift the College received in the nineteenth century. With its own endowment, the Mütter Museum for many years was used for teaching purposes. Presidents in their annual reports invariably spoke of it with pride.

Thomas Mütter was a native of Virginia. Orphaned at the age of eight, he was reared by a kinsman Robert Carter of Sabine Hall, attended Hampden-Sydney College, and was graduated in medicine from the University of Pennsylvania in 1831. He spent a year in Paris, and used thereafter, rather pretentiously, to refer to the great clinicians there—Dupuytren, Lisfranc, Velpeau, Louis, Roux, Chomel, and Baron Larrey—as his "friends." Eager for approbation and personal influence and position, he was, in fact, inclined to puff himself. His friends excused this trait, for he was friendly, able, honorable, and wealthy. He lived in a style almost as grand as George Bacon Wood, dispensing an "elegant hospitality" in a large house, richly furnished. He taught in the Philadelphia Medical Institute, and in 1841 was elected professor of surgery in Jefferson Medical College. He made plastic surgery a specialty, operated successfully for club-foot, wrote little, but was, as we have seen, one of the first in Philadelphia to appreciate and use ether anesthesia.[49]

Mütter's gift forced the College to take action about a hall. By 1859 the Building Fund amounted to $21,545. This was the figure the College had set as the Fund's goal, but as the amount was still insufficient for a building, the College renewed the trust for five years, expressing its thanks for the committee's "skill and industry" in bringing the fund "to so brilliant and useful a result."[50] Then, on Fox's motion on March 2, the committee took its first action, purchasing a lot on the northeast corner of Locust and Thirteenth Streets for $10,500. Two years later, for $3,500 a small adjoining property was acquired, which gave an area 60 by 110 feet to build on.

## *Hall of the College*

Under the terms of the agreement with Mütter, a modern fireproof building had to be erected within five years, that is, by January 1864. To do this, the Building Fund had to be increased substantially. Accordingly, when the purchase of the Locust Street property was authorized, a committee of Seven was named to solicit additional contributions. The committee was headed by Francis West and included T. Hewson Bache, Edward Hartshorne, and S. Weir Mitchell, in whose office at 1226 Walnut Street it usually met. This solicitation brought in only $3,065, of which $1,000 was another gift from Wood. The suggestion that "well-to-do laymen" also be approached was initially rejected because "the older fellows" thought it improper. Even a warm recommendation of the College and its campaign in one of the local newspapers embarrassed them.[51] There was no response to Samuel D. Gross' suggestion that Fellows deliver lectures around the city to help increase the Building Fund.

At the beginning of 1860 approximately $13,500 was available for a building, $10,500 having been spent for the Locust Street lot. This was about half of what it was estimated the hall would cost. About to depart on a two-year tour of Europe, Wood offered to give $5,000 when the College had $25,000 in hand. Further donations by the Fellows (including Wood, who gave another $1,000 in March 1861),[52] as well as improved financial conditions in the na-

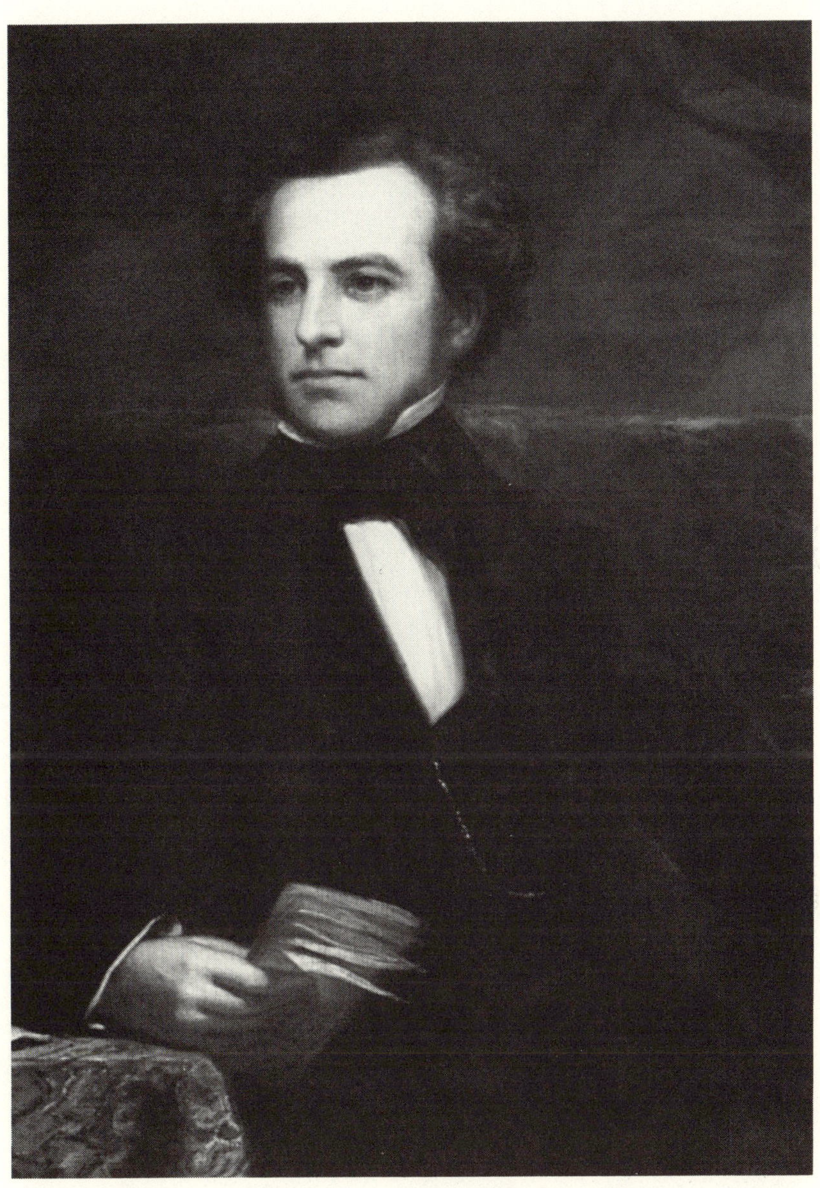

Thomas D. Mütter, (1811–1859). Portrait by Daniel Huntington.

tion, gave the College confidence: it directed a committee, headed by Isaac Hays and including Fox, to make plans and obtain estimates. These were submitted in May 1861. There was, however, still some hesitation: Ought the College to commit itself for more money than it had in hand? Could any estimate made in wartime be relied on? "It is a serious thing to build in these times," Franklin Bache reflected in a letter to Wood, then in Italy, "and it is to incur a serious risk to postpone building."[53] Even the Committee on Plans was not strongly committed, and "after a warm discussion," the plans were tabled. John H. Packard, who was also keeping Wood informed, thought that only "a proper degree of energy" was needed to "carry us completely through all the difficulties apprehended by the opposers of the building."[54] Wood replied with exhortations to action.

Despite these doubts and delays, however, support for the building was mounting rapidly. At last, at an adjourned meeting on December 18, 1861, the Fellows voted unanimously to invite proposals for the hall.[55] Isaac Hays, Edward Hartshorne, George W. Norris, and Franklin Bache, together with the trustees of the Building Fund—Fox, Wood, and Paul—were appointed the Building Committee. One last effort was made to postpone action, ironically by George Fox, who, perhaps the best informed about financial realities, was apprehensive because the market value of the College securities had declined. His motion was tabled; and on February 19, 1862, at another adjourned meeting, the newly-appointed Building Committee was authorized to prepare a contract for a sum not to exceed $13,700. "I have seldom seen a more unanimous action in the College, upon a question of policy," John H. Packard wrote Wood a few weeks later, "when there was not only so much room for doubt, but opinions had varied as much at different times." Well pleased with the outcome, Wood promised to give another $1,000 on his return home from Europe.[56]

James H. Windrim, who was to design the Masonic Temple on North Broad Street ten years later, was engaged as architect, and Michael Errickson, "well known as a very experienced, trustworthy & responsible builder," as general contractor. At first the College decided to build only so much as the Mütter Museum and College library required; then they decided to build over the entire lot, leaving a portion of the interior unfinished; but finally they confidently directed that the entire building be completed inside and out.[57] In addition to a museum, library, and lecture hall, it would contain rooms for the librarian, curator, and janitor, and a retiring room for lecturers. There was no cellar, but the building was designed to permit the addition of a third floor.

Except for some library furnishings and lecture room fittings, the building was completed in the late winter of 1863, and the first meeting in the building, with fifty-two Fellows in attendance, was held on March 4, 1863. Isaac Hays presented the final report of his Building Committee. The total cost, including land and interior furnishings, was $40,858; this was several hundred dollars under the revised estimate. All but $2,500, the Building Committee reported with satisfaction, had been contributed by members of "our hard worked and inadequately compensated profession."[58]

With the completion of this building the College became visible, an institution with a permanent home and a certain address, no longer a loose association wandering about the city looking for cheap lodging. Presiding over a meeting of the State Medical Society in the hall a few months later, Wilson Jewell, who was also a Fellow of the College, hailed the opening of the building "as constituting a new epoch in American medical history."[59]

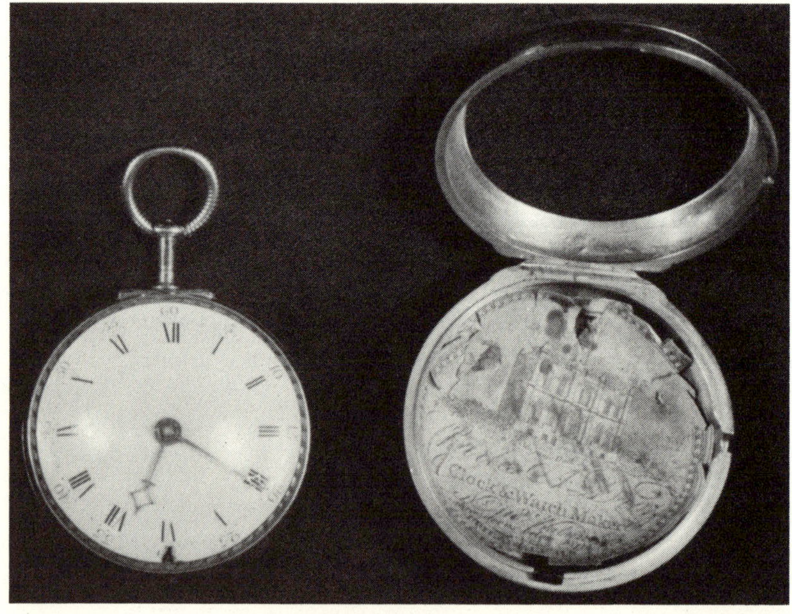

Benjamin Rush's Watch *(Abbe Collection, College of Physicians).*

CHAPTER VI

# *Professional Concerns*

NOW in possession of a hall of its own, the College of Physicians was not only the most visible of Philadelphia's medical societies, but its hall was a central location for their meetings. The County Medical Society and the Philadelphia and Rush Medical Book Clubs met there. The Pathological and Obstetrical Societies also held their meetings at Thirteenth and Locust Streets, paying in 1867 a rent of $40 a year—raised fifteen years later to $60 and $50 respectively. Scientific associations holding conventions in Philadelphia were sometimes offered the use of the hall. The usual charges for the lecture room in 1882 were $6 for its use during the day, $10 for an evening.

Income was not the only benefit the College received from its hall. The Committee on Hall spelled out the more lasting returns the College might expect:

> . . . the library-rooms might be not only used for the meetings of the College, but might be lighted up on stated evenings, for conversation meetings. This it is believed would promote the social intercourse of the Fellows, tend to preserve harmony among them, render the Library more accessible & useful, be a point of attention to strangers, members of our profession, who may visit our city, & in various other ways greatly advance the objects & extend the usefulness of the College.[1]

As president George Bacon Wood took special pleasure in decorating the hall. He had copies made of portraits of Redman, Shippen, Parke, and James; and he persuaded his friends to give paintings of their fathers and grandfathers. Mrs. Mifflin Wistar, for example, donated a picture of her father-in-law Caspar Wistar, and John Lambert Cadwalader presented a painting of Thomas Cadwalader, a leader of the medical profession in the generation before the founding of the College. Through the years other similar donations followed. Mrs. S. Weir Mitchell and a friend paid for a painting of Rembrandt's School of Anatomy "by the best copyist in Holland." On January 2, 1878, Mitchell himself delivered to the vice-president of the College a sealed envelope with the solemn, mystifying injunction that it was not to be opened until after his death. The enclosed note, it turned out, bequeathed to the College Mitchell's own portraits of Harvey and John Hunter, copied from originals in the Royal College of Surgeons.[2]

The obligations and expenses of the hall, the expanding membership of the College—136 resident members in 1864—a greater variety of College activities, the Mütter museum and lectureship supported by income paid out by an independent trustee, all created problems which leaders of the College recognized could not be handled properly at the stated monthly meetings. Those meetings were often poorly attended; still less were those attending likely to be adequately informed on financial or legal matters. Their votes were unpredictable, their decisions liable to postponement and delay. What was needed was a smaller body, possessed of full knowledge of the facts and issues and able to advise informedly or act swiftly. New by-laws enacted in 1863, in addition to codifying the rules and practices about officers, meetings, committees, rules of order and the like, also created a council. It was composed of the elected officers, including the four censors, and six Fellows chosen by the whole membership for three-year terms. The new by-laws provided:

> The Council shall exercise a general supervision over the affairs of the College, carefully consider all questions that may be referred to it, and report to the College in writing its decisions thereon, and from time to time submit to the College, for its approval or rejection, such measures as it shall believe to be adapted to further the objects for which the College was organized and to promote its interest generally.[3]

In particular, all nominations for election of Fellows or Associate Fellows were to be referred to the Council, which, after full inquiry into the candidate's character, professional standing, and other matters of eligibility, would certify the result to the College.

At first the Council had little to do: it met only four times a year; at some meetings there was no quorum, at others no business. After 1882, however, it met regularly before each monthly meeting of the College. The Council gave College activities direction and consistency, but it could also lengthen the period of deliberation. A question might be addressed to the president or secretary of the College. If the matter was judged to involve policy, the Fellows would refer it to the Council; the Council, after consideration (which could mean asking for further information), might then return it to the College for action. Each of these steps required at least a month, sometimes more. The system ensured that the College would not act precipitately and unwisely; it also risked not acting at all.

Among those elected under the new procedure in the next four or five years, were Harrison Allen, professor of comparative anatomy in the University of Pennsylvania; William Goodell, physician-in-charge of the maternity hospital Preston Retreat; William W. Keen, of the Philadelphia School of Anatomy; William Pepper, pathologist and curator of the Pennsylvania Hospital and lecturer on morbid anatomy at the University of Pennsylvania; William H. Pancoast, demonstrator in anatomy in Jefferson Medical College; and Horatio C Wood, who was soon to be elected a professor in the University of Pennsylvania Medical School. One of those chosen in 1866 was William Fisher Norris, who, after studying in Vienna, made diseases of the eye his specialty. Such specialization was regarded unsympathetically by Philadelphia doctors, who took pride in being able to treat the complete spectrum of medical and surgical conditions. Specialization, especially on the eye, recalled to their minds a procession of quacks.[4] Norris' demonstrated competence and his unassailable social position, however, silenced, if they could not entirely overcome, the prejudice; and he was invited to lecture on ophthalmology at the University of Pennsylvania.

More remarkable than the admission of specialists to the College fellowship was the election after 1865 of several men who, though possessing the degree of doctor of medicine, were not primarily practitioners. Theodore G. Wormley, named professor of chemistry and toxicology at the University of Pennsylvania in 1877 after a distinguished career in Ohio, was elected a Fellow, but only with the strong support of Stillé and Ruschenberger. Rush

Shippen Huidekoper, an M.D. of the University, was elected a Fellow in 1881, perhaps fortunately, for he soon afterwards began the study of veterinary medicine and became the first dean of the School of Veterinary Medicine of the University of Pennsylvania. But a suggestion that the College might consider electing an M.D. engaged primarily in dentistry, was summarily tabled.

### *Civil War*

Most of these new Fellows, many older members of the College, and other physicians of Philadelphia served as military surgeons in the Civil War, some in the field at Antietam and Gettysburg, most in the great general hospitals in Philadelphia, Washington, and other places. They remembered the experience to the end of their lives.

An intimation of what the war might mean to the profession occurred in the last months of 1859, when two hundred Southern students, reacting to the raid on Harper's Ferry and Northern sympathy for John Brown, withdrew from the local medical schools to continue their studies in the politically more congenial atmosphere of Richmond and other Southern cities. As tensions increased, old friends and acquaintances no longer found pleasure in one another's company. Some members of the Philadelphia Club, for example, withdrew and formed the Union Club as a "refuge for loyalty." The Wistar Association, the city's most congenial social-cultural gathering, stopped meeting. Even the American Philosophical Society was torn by the expulsion, not easily accomplished, of the distinguished oceanographer Matthew Fontaine Maury, who had resigned his commission in the United States Navy and joined the Confederacy. Although no Fellows seceded from the College of Physicians, personal relations among them probably cooled, reflecting divided opinions elsewhere.

On the Sunday morning in April 1861 when news of the fall of Fort Sumter reached Philadelphia, John Neill, a Fellow of the College, who had been on the staff of the Pennsylvania Hospital and a professor of surgery in Pennsylvania Medical College, made a tour of the city. Believing that the war just opening would be long and that Philadelphia would become a center for the care of sick and wounded soldiers, he made note of the halls and public buildings that might be adapted to hospital purposes. Moyamens-

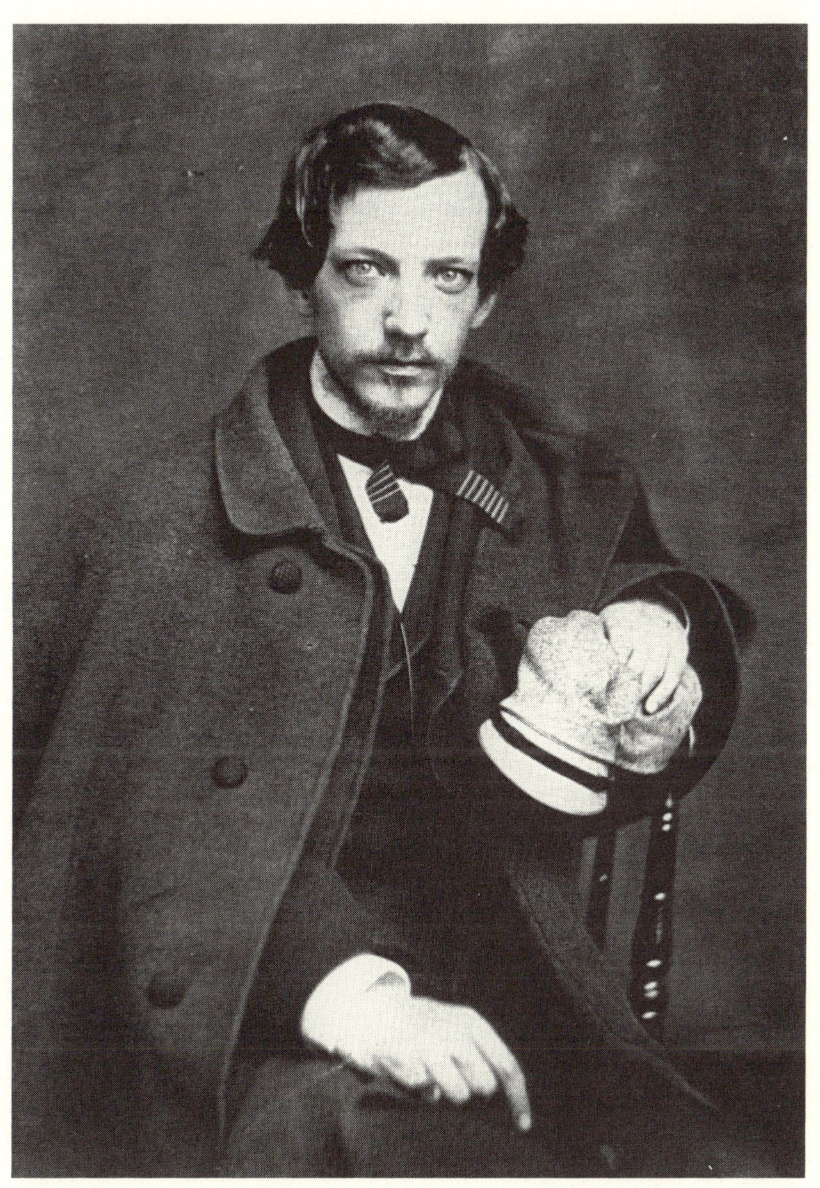

S. Weir Mitchell, (1829–1914). Photograph, 1859.

ing Hall in South Philadelphia, formerly the seat of the borough government, seemed especially suitable. Neill obtained permission to take possession, received orders from the Surgeon-General of the Army to organize a military hospital, appointed a staff and collected supplies, and within a few weeks had all in readiness. The first patient was received on May 6. In the next few weeks, Neill was called on to select other suitable buildings. Under his direction they were remodeled, equipped, and staffed. "With him," a friend wrote of Neill's accomplishments, "to think was to act."

> Thus, on one occasion, he received a telegraphic order from the Secretary of War to be in readiness for some hundreds of sick and wounded—nine hundred, I think—then actually upon their way. The hospitals were all full to overflowing, but he at once secured a large storehouse, had it swept and arranged, necessaries supplied, and in a very few hours was ready to receive this large number of patients, with soup, coffee, bread, beds, medical stores and medical aid all at hand.[5]

During this time Neill had no other authority than that of a contract surgeon paid $80 a month. In the fall of 1862, however, he was commissioned a surgeon of Volunteers and put in charge of the 650-bed receiving hospital at Broad and Cherry Streets, where patients were classified before being sent to special hospitals. In 1863, on the eve of Lee's invasion of Pennsylvania, Neill was made medical director of Pennsylvania hospitals.

Other physicians also joined military units activated in the summer of 1861. Some served short terms in the field, especially during the Gettysburg campaign, when Philadelphia seemed in danger from the enemy. Others were assigned to the military hospitals in Philadelphia. One of the two largest of these was the West Philadelphia (later Satterlee) General Hospital. It was erected in seven weeks in the late spring of 1862, organized and directed by I. I. Hayes, who had learned about the war only in October 1861, when his ship put in at Halifax on its return from an expedition in the Arctic. Satterlee's visiting surgeons constituted a roll of the ablest physicians of Philadelphia: D. Hayes Agnew, Walter F. Atlee, Jacob M. Da Costa, William S. Halsey, Hugh Lenox Hodge, James B. Hutchinson, Francis W. Lewis, John H.

Packard, Richard A. F. Penrose, Edward A. Smith, Thomas Stewardson, Alfred Stillé, Francis West, and Caspar Wister. Before the end of the war, Satterlee General Hospital had 3,500 beds. Mower General Hospital in Chestnut Hill, which opened in January 1863, was even larger, with more than four thousand beds. Its director was Joseph Hopkinson; its executive officer, John H. B. McClellan; and among its assistant surgeons were Robert Bolling, Horace Y. Evans, Isaac Norris, Jr., and William M. Welch.[6] All these men on the staffs of the two hospitals were then, or soon became, Fellows of the College.[7]

Many of the other military hospitals in the city—at one time there were twenty-four—were also directed and staffed by Fellows. James Darrach was in charge of Cuyler General Hospital in Germantown; his executive officer John Ashhurst, Jr., later gave the College photographs of it. The Fifth Street Hospital was established under the direction of Thomas G. Morton, surgeon to Wills Eye Hospital, who was later surgeon-in-charge at the Twelfth Street Hospital and a consulting surgeon at Mower General Hospital. D. Hayes Agnew was director of the 172-bed hospital at Hestonville; and Lewis Taylor headed the McClellan Hospital with four hundred beds. At Turner's Lane Hospital S. Weir Mitchell, William W. Keen, and George R. Morehouse, who had been together in the Christian Street Hospital, made those observations and experiments which they reported in their classic monograph *Gunshot Wounds and Other Injuries of the Nerves.*

As surgeon-general of Pennsylvania, the modest Henry Hollingsworth Smith, professor of surgery in the University of Pennsylvania (who had resigned his Fellowship in January 1861 in protest against measures the College had adopted to collect unpaid dues), displayed unusual administrative talents in organizing the evacuation of casualties from the Virginia battlefields. John H. Brinton, lecturer in operative surgery at Jefferson Medical College, commissioned as a brigade surgeon on August 3, 1861, was medical director of Grant's army in the campaign that captured Forts Henry and Donelson in the spring of 1862. Then, assigned to the War Department in Washington, he planned the great *Medical and Surgical History of the War of the Rebellion* and laid the foundation of the Army Medical Museum.[8] From all these experiences the doctors obtained more, and more varied, knowledge of medicine and surgery than they had hitherto; and although the practice of medicine in military hospitals was not of the highest order, doctors came to understand the fundamental importance of sanitation and to appreciate what women nurses and volunteers might do for patients and for hospital discipline and efficiency. The lessons learned in 1861–65 they applied in civil practice in the next three decades.

The wartime achievements of military surgeons, Weir Mitchell wrote afterwards, raised both the reputation of the medical profession and the doctors' own self-esteem. The change from national indifference to general respect was owing not simply to advances in medical science and practice, however impressive they may have been, but even more to the remarkable organizing abilities that the physicians displayed. The construction, organization, and administration of more than a score of hospitals, which, with a total bed capacity of 14,000 or 15,000, received and treated some 157,000 patients during four years of war, was an impressive feat. These hospitals, Mitchell wrote in his novel *In War Time,*

> were planned and admirably built, without the advice of architects, by physicians, who had to learn as they went along the special constructive needs of different climates, and to settle novel and frequent hygienic questions as they arose. In and near the locality of my tale, the hospitals numbered twenty-five thousand beds for the sick and wounded; and these huge villages, now drawn on by the war, now refilled by its constant strife, were managed with a skill which justified the American test of hotel-keeping as a gauge of ability. A surgeon taken abruptly from civil life, a country physician, a retired naval surgeon, were fair specimens of the class on which fell these enormous responsibilities.[9]

On the College of Physicians as an institution, however, the effect of the war was less noticeable. Attendance at meetings dropped, of course. But there was, after all, little that the College, apart from its individual Fellows, could do. From time to time a member read a report of cases of amputation, gunshot wounds, or paraplegia.[10] One of the more interesting reports was Henry Hartshorne's account of what he called "cardiac Muscular exhaustion."

The humane and practical judgment of this Quaker physician was that soldiers suffering from this condition were

> entirely unfit for ordinary field service in the army. They would soon be broken down by the 'double quick,' or even by the knapsack and musket alone. It would, therefore, be not cruelty, but false economy, to compel them to undertake duty of which they are really incapable. No doubt many, perhaps most of them, would be quite able to do light service in various ways; but I am well satisfied that it would be cheaper and wiser, as well as more just, to discharge them, than to return them to regimental duty before the exhausted heart has had time for full recuperation.[11]

No one who served in the field or in hospitals behind the lines ever forgot the frightful scenes he witnessed. "Only too sharply do we remember the dreadful things that we did," wrote William W. Keen, "and the good things that we did not dare to do."[12] The memories were the more harrowing and ineffaceable because the surgeons knew what an adequate supply of drugs, medicine, instruments, above all of anesthetics, would have meant. Keen reckoned there were not half a dozen hypodermic needles or half a dozen clinical thermometers in the whole Army of the Potomac. Antisepsis was unknown. Healing "by first intention" was so rare that the surgeons marvelled and boasted when it happened. Erysipelas, pyaemia, and "hospital gangrene" were universal; and the death rate was appalling.[13]

After the war surgeons sometimes recounted their experiences in non-professional writings. Weir Mitchell used them in his novels and short stories. He and Keen made several reminiscent addresses to the College,[14] and two former Confederate surgeons were invited to speak on their experiences.[15] It was Mitchell's hope during many years that the College would erect a tablet in its hall honoring those Fellows who served in the Civil War; and it was through his influence that the Surgeon-General of the Army and the Gettysburg Park Commission decided, on the fiftieth anniversary of the battle of Gettysburg, to mark the positions of the Union and Confederate hospitals there.[16]

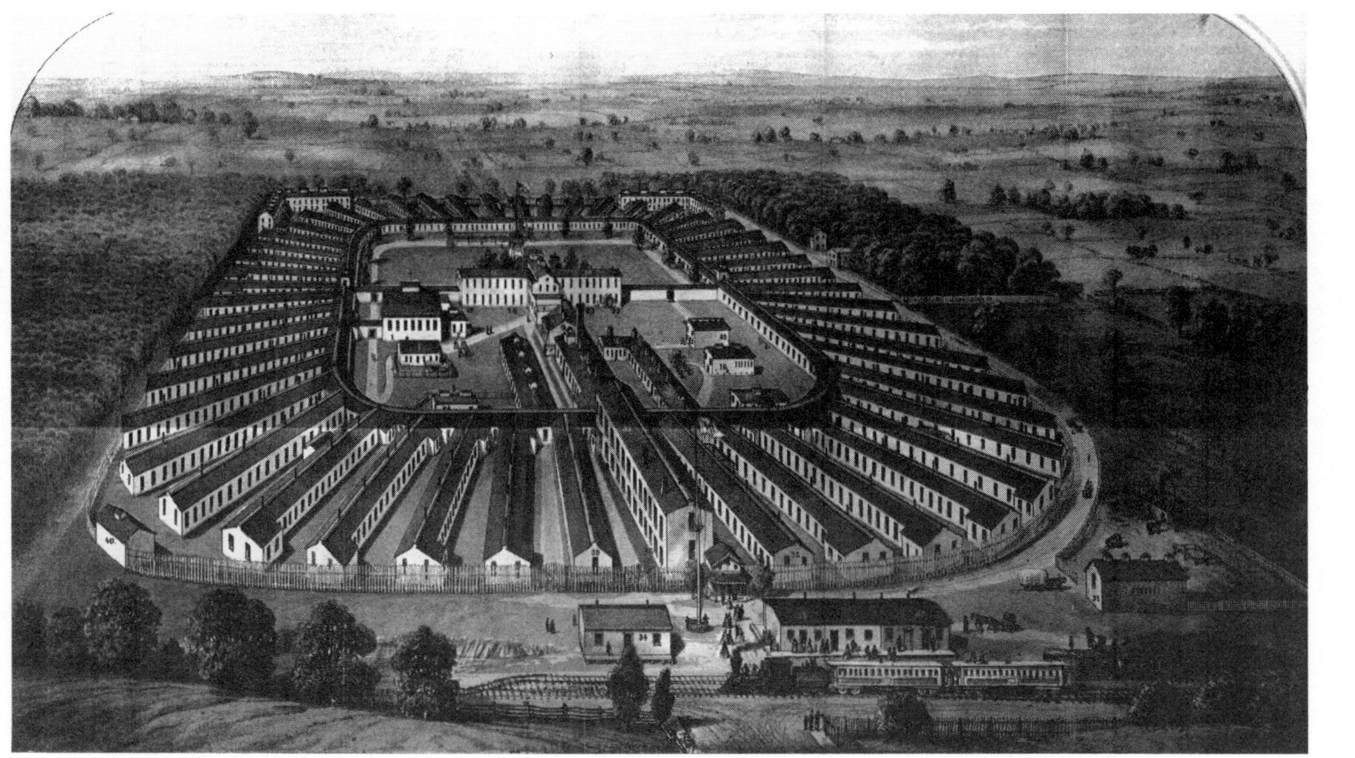

Mower General Hospital, Philadelphia. By James Queen; lithograph by P.S. Duval & Son, Philadelphia, c. 1863. *(Library Company of Philadelphia).*

Mower General Hospital, with a capacity for 4,000 patients, was the largest military hospital in Philadelphia.

### *Scientific Papers*

The release of energies from wartime concentration and the surge in medical knowledge and techniques were reflected in the confidence with which the College turned to its work after the war ended in 1865. The regular monthly meetings, some Fellows believed, allowed too little time for scientific papers, and so the College in 1869 instituted a second monthly meeting exclusively for reading such papers. The papers varied in content, quality, and significance. Many were records from the practice of observant and thoughtful physicians, and a few were reports of a general kind, like William W. Keen's notes on medicine in Japan made on a visit there in 1877.[17] Reports on meteorology and epidemics, which had been presented annually by Wilson Jewell for eight years until 1863, were made by William Lehman Wells from 1864 to 1873, and by Richard A. Cleeman from 1874 through 1880. The committee was abolished in 1882 after existing for ninety-five years.[18] An increased number of papers on surgical procedures reflected the striking advances made in surgery in the two decades after the Civil War. For example, John Ashhurst, Jr., professor of clinical surgery at the University of Pennsylvania, read several papers on amputations and excision of the knee joint, operations often required by railroad accidents.[19] A curious after-effect of amputations was the continued sensation of a phantom limb, which had intrigued S. Weir Mitchell ever since his work at Turner's Lane Hospital, and it intrigued the Fellows when he reported on the phenomenon in 1871.[20] And while no one any longer doubted the efficacy of anesthesia, physicians continued to search for better anesthetics. Horatio C Wood reported to the College on acetic ether, on which he had been experimenting; and John B. Roberts' account of his use of cocaine in an operation for cataract in 1884 elicited a lively discussion, which called forth other papers on cocaine.[21]

At least two cases reported in the 1860s and 1870s had improbable features. Both were, in a sense, reports of industrial accidents, like Ashhurst's railway amputations. Elisha B. Shapleigh, a surgeon in the Coroner's Office, invited to read a paper soon after his election as a Fellow in 1868, told about a patient, "an intelligent German," who kept rattlesnakes as pets in his beer saloon. Bitten once, the saloon-keeper had recovered, thanks to applications of whisky and caustic. However, bitten a second time by a newly-arrived, large, young, and active specimen, he died within forty minutes.[22] One of Ashhurst's patients also pushed his luck too far. The man, an animal tamer with a travelling menagerie, thrust his head into a lion's mouth to demonstrate something or other about the beast; the lion closed its jaws, and the spectators had to beat it about the head to make it release the man. Angered and mortified by the animal's behavior, the keeper once more entered the cage and advanced upon the beast "with a mad determination to obtain the mastery." He failed to do so. The lion tore away part of his thigh, and he died within forty-eight hours. Ashhurst characterized the accident correctly, if understatedly, as one of "unusual character . . . (in this country at least)."[23]

New instruments and procedures were also described or demonstrated at the stated meetings. The obstetrician Albert H. Smith showed the Fellows a compact portable obstetric case. John H. Packard described a splint he devised for resection of the knee. Addinell Hewson showed how the electric light might be used in diagnosis (this was in 1884, less than five years after Edison's successful invention); and Morris J. Lewis, a few months after he was admitted to the College, was asked to demonstrate the ophthalmoscope "as an aid to medical diagnosis." Several papers were illustrated with photographs and some with the patients present. Foreshadowing the increased interest in public health, including nutrition, the College invited Professor Albert R. Leeds of the Stevens Institute of Technology, to address them in 1883 and 1884 on infants' food and human milk. In 1884 Nathaniel Archer Randolph, a newly elected Fellow, a lecturer on physiology in the University of Pennsylvania, recommended that "branny foods" be included in everyone's diet.[24]

Despite their wide experience and general medical knowledge, the Fellows seem not to have produced enough papers for College meetings, much less for publication in the *Transactions.* The explanation, of course, is that those who wrote articles preferred to publish them in one of the monthly medical journals published in Philadelphia. Although newly-elected Fellows seemed a likely a source of papers, this had limits. In consequence, the College dropped the semi-monthly scientific meetings in 1873; and ten years later, recognizing the fact of summer vacations, it dropped the regular July and August meetings. At the same time John B. Roberts tried to persuade the College to impose a twenty-minute limit on papers, but his motion was tabled.[25] The same motion made in later years met the same fate—or, if approved, was unobserved and unenforced.

### *The Siamese Twins*

No scientific meetings in the two decades after the Civil War excited as much attention as those at which reports were given of the autopsy on the bodies of the original Siamese Twins. In addition to the anatomical information provided, the event had important consequences for the publication of the College *Transactions.*

Chang and Eng, joined from birth by a band extending from the junction of the thoracic and abdominal cavities, were brought from Bangkok to Boston in 1829 at the age of eighteen. In the next few years they were exhibited throughout this country and in Britain and Europe.[26] Everywhere they were both a popular sensation and an object of serious medical inquiry. They were examined in Boston by John C. Warren,[27] in New York by Samuel Latham Mitchill, and in London by Sir Astley Cooper. Becoming naturalized American citizens in 1839 under the names of Chang and Eng Bunker, they married sisters and settled as planters near Mount Airy, near Greensboro, North Carolina, but returned occasionally to touring. Several times they consulted surgeons about the feasibility of separation, but apparently seriously considered the operation only once. For more than forty years they remained a focus of interest and curiosity by anatomists and psychologists.[28] On their last trip to Europe in 1869, they were carefully examined by Sir James Simpson.

The twins died on January 17, 1874—Eng a few hours after Chang. When the news reached the newspapers, physicians everywhere hoped that at last the mystery of their union would be discovered. One of those interested was William H. Pancoast of Jefferson Medical College, about to be elected professor of anatomy there in succession to his father. Encouraged by Samuel D. Gross, Pancoast prevailed upon Mayor Stokely of Philadelphia to telegraph the mayor of Greensboro to ask whether a post-mortem examination had been made, and, if not, whether Pancoast might be permitted to make one, either at Jefferson or in Mount Airy. The mayor of Greensboro disclaimed both knowledge and influence in the matter. Meanwhile, Dr. Joseph Hollingsworth, brother of the twins' physician, learned of Pancoast's inquiry, and notified him that he would be in Philadelphia on January 23. That evening and in the next two days, Pancoast and Hollingsworth consulted with other surgeons and anatomists in the city. On January 26 they met with Joseph Leidy, W. S. W. Ruschenberger, vice-president of the College, and John Neill, professor of clinical surgery in the University of Pennsylvania (the only physician who responded to an invitation to meet). These men agreed to form themselves into a commission, that Pancoast and Harrison Allen, professor of comparative anatomy in the University, should go to North Carolina at once, and that the commission should report its findings to the College of Physicians. Although all the participants in the undertaking were Fellows, the College up to this time had no part in their decision.

Pancoast and Allen set out on January 29, taking with them Thomas H. Andrews, demonstrator in anatomy at Jefferson. The party reached Mount Airy on January 31. The Bunker widows and their legal adviser gave permission to embalm the bodies and perform the autopsy. But there were no proper facilities for a thorough examination, and Pancoast asked to take the bodies to Philadelphia. "Without their active co-operation," he wrote afterwards of the Hollingsworths and the Bunkers' lawyer, "we should have failed in our effort." The commission's team returned to Philadelphia on February 4, and completed the autopsy in the Mütter museum of the College.

A special meeting was called for February 8; 101 Fellows attended.[29] After considerable discussion the College, on Leidy's motion, adopted the commmission as its own, agreed to pay its expenses, and, on a motion by S. Weir Mitchell, authorized an expenditure of $350 for photographs, drawings, and casts to illustrate Pancoast's report. Although this was not a public meeting, someone reported it to the newspapers. The result was that attendance at the next special meeting, on February 18, was also large—some eighty Fellows and a number of visitors, including the well-known New York pediatrician Abraham Jacobi. Pancoast and Allen reported orally on their findings, illustrating their observations and conclusions on the bodies of the twins with drawings and casts.[30] Their written reports were presented at later meetings.[31]

After giving the full history of Chang and Eng and reviewing other cases of joined twins, Pancoast answered the question that

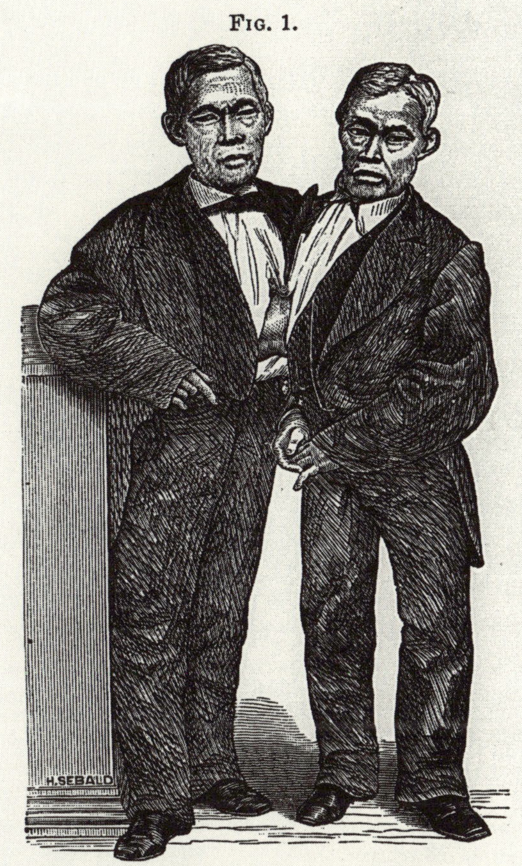


Fig. 1. The twins in the acquired position (E. R., C. L.). From a photograph taken in St. Petersburg, 1870.

Eng and Chang, The Siamese twins. Woodcut by H. Sebald in College of Physicians, *Transactions,* Third series, VIII (1875), facing p. 3.

every anatomist and layman was asking: "No operation . . . for the purpose of separating the twins in adult life," he wrote, "could have been performed and their lives preserved." However, Pancoast continued, to have attempted to separate Eng from Chang when the latter died, would have been "judicious surgery." As for separating the twins in childhood, it was "problematical" whether the operation would have succeeded, "but . . . it would have been the part of wisdom and humanity to have made the effort . . . ."

To satisfy the "anxiety" of the medical profession for the report of the post-mortem examination, the College directed that a stenographic record of the proceedings of February 18 be made, and that extracts from this record be given to the *Philadelphia Medical Times.* The report was printed in that journal the next day.[32]

To Isaac Hays, editor of the *American Journal of the Medical Sciences,* which had printed the *Transactions* of the College in its pages for fifteen years, this was a breach of contract. Not only had the College given a rival publication a timely story of the widest professional and public interest, but it proposed to publish the full report of the Pancoast-Allen commission in an illustrated pamphlet of 1,500 copies. The College rejected Hays' protest, insisting that it had the right to publish what it would; and, after several exchanges of letters, the arrangement between the College and the *American Journal* was terminated.[33]

## *Transactions, Third Series*

This left the College with no vehicle of publication. Horatio C Wood would have had the Committee on Publication ask the Smithsonian Institution to publish the report on the Siamese Twins. But at the end of the year it was decided that the *Transactions* should appear, one volume a year, under College auspices. Abstracts of papers would be provided to the medical press immediately after delivery in order to secure early and wide dissemination of important facts and observations, and reprints would be supplied the authors. The cost to the College, it was estimated, should amount to only $100–150 more than the total costs under the contract with Hays' *Journal.* Among the benefits of the new arrangement would be one for the College library—separate volumes of the *Transactions,* sent to other societies and to medical journals for review, would bring their publications in exchange, to be added to the library's holdings.[34]

The first volume of the third series of *Transactions* appeared in 1875. It was well designed, printed, and bound. In addition to the report on the Siamese Twins, it contained articles by the most prestigious Fellows—John Ashhurst, Jr., William S. Forbes, William W. Keen, S. Weir Mitchell, and Jacob M. DaCosta—as well as the roll of Fellows, officers, and standing committees; but it included no record of College business. The *Boston Medical and Surgical Journal,* welcoming the volume, judged it "elegant" in appearance, its contents "certainly highly creditable to the college," and its style as "much superior to that customary in this country."[35] The Fellows understandably were proud of it.

### *Public Health*

As the Fellows' confidence in medical science grew, so did their inclination to speak out on matters of public concern. Public health questions had, of course, engaged their attention in the past, if only intermittently. But such questions pressed more insistently upon them after the Civil War, when Philadelphia, no longer the "greene countrie towne" Penn envisioned, became an industrial city with all the overcrowding, crime, and grime that characterized such places. Most physicians were aware of the links between public hygiene and private health: after mid-century physicians became more sensitive to the conditions of the growing city and sought means of coping with them.

No one could ignore the filth in the streets. In 1868 the College unanimously sent "an earnest but respectful appeal" to the mayor, councils, and Board of Health to attend promptly to cleaning the streets, alleys, and gutters. Calls to pave the streets were repeatedly issued by independent civic groups, for unless the streets were decently paved, they could not be properly cleaned.[36] But the doctors were not in charge of municipal contracts. "At present," one Philadelphia medical editor remarked wryly, "Philadelphia, unlike a warmer place, is not even paved with good intentions."[37]

Cleaning the surfaces of the streets was, however, primarily a matter of aesthetics. A hint of their true condition is contained in the suggestions of the College to the Philadelphia Fountain Society in 1874 that the Society place urinals "in places of daily resort," and to the City Councils a few years later that the city require "sanitary fixtures" in houses constructed hereafter.[38] William Pepper drew the connection between defective drainage and diseases, and the College endorsed his plea in 1878 that the municipal authorities engage a competent engineer to study the matter and report how other cities dealt with the problem. "It is believed," the College said, "that with such information at hand it will be more easy for those entrusted with the duty of determining upon the changes to be made in our present system to adopt such as will be well adapted to the peculiar needs of this city." Later that year the motion was renewed in stronger terms. William V. Keating, who had been professor of midwifery and diseases of children at Jefferson Medical College, described the connection between defective drainage and typhoid fever, and moved that a sanitary engineer or medical expert be employed to report. Colonel William Ludlow, chief engineer of the Philadelphia Water Department, which he had reorganized and reanimated, was invited to address the College on the water supply of cities.[39]

The water department, however, was infiltrated with politics and corruption; and despite the earnest representations of the physicians and the best efforts of reformers, little was done for years. James Bryce in *The American Commonwealth* cited Philadelphia's water supply as evidence of the bad government of American cities. He quoted a memorial that the citizens sent to the Pennsylvania legislature in 1883:

> . . . the streets of the city have been allowed to fall into such a state as to be a reproach and a disgrace. Philadelphia is now recognized as the worst-paved and worst-cleaned city in the civilized world.
>
> The water supply is so bad that during many weeks of the last winter it was not only distastesful and unwholesome for drinking, but offensive for bathing purposes.
>
> The effort to clean the streets was abandoned for months, and no attempt was made to that end until some public-spirited citizens, at their own expense, cleaned a number of the principal thorough-fares . . . .
>
> Inefficiency, waste, badly-paved and filthy streets, un-

> wholesome and offensive water, and slovenly and costly management, have been the rule for years past throughout the city government.[40]

Such protests continued for decades. Well into the twentieth century, Philadelphia's water smelled and was rust-colored. Those who could afford it purchased bottled water; others travelled out to Fairmount Park, where they could be seen on Saturdays and Sundays waiting patiently in long queues to fill their jugs from the springs there.

Other matters of public health were presented to the College from time to time—the location of a slaughter house on the west bank of the Schuylkill, myopia and astigmatism among public school children, labelling and packaging of dangerous and poisonous drugs, the safety of illuminating gas. Some of these questions were pressed in cooperation with the County Medical Society; others, like dangerous drugs, were referred to the College of Pharmacy.

### *Profession and Public*

The more medical science improved after mid-century, the more was expected of it and its practitioners. By 1870 the increasing number of malpractice suits began to alarm some physicians. John James Reese, professor of medical jurisprudence and toxicology in the University of Pennyslvania, blamed "unscrupulous patients" and those who encouraged, even instigated them —unprincipled lawyers "& perhaps even . . . some unworthy members of the medical profession." He proposed that the College and other medical societies in the state petition the legislature for a law to protect physicians from frivolous suits. In case the charge was not sustained and the defendant was exonerated of all blame, the plaintiff should be assessed a portion of the damages he sought to compensate the doctor "for his expenses incurred, his loss of time, & the anxiety of mind & trouble to which he has been subjected in consequence of the suit." The plaintiff should also be required, before going to trial, to post a bond to pay such compensation, should it be awarded. The College approved Reese's proposal and prepared a memorial which was sent to the several county medical societies for their concurrence.[42]

A few years later the College addressed another professional concern. The Obstetrical Society in 1877 called on the College to join in memorializing the legislature to extend legal protection to communications between physician and patient. New York had had such a law for fifty years. Responding favorably, the College obtained the support of the County Medical Society, and together they rallied support from county societies throughout the state. The petition was presented to the Assembly in 1880, but no bill emerged.[43] But the issue was not settled; like unjustifiable suits for malpractice, it came up repeatedly in the following decades.

Two other subjects, both professional, both also scientific—the use of living animals in experiments and the need for human bodies for teaching and research—also came before the College frequently after the Civil War. The practice of animal experimentation became increasing visible, and the issues it raised became increasingly urgent, as medical knowledge and practice benefited from the results of laboratory research. In the records of the College of Physicians, the first evidence of the laboratories' need for animals was an appeal to the Philadelphia City Councils in 1871 to require that, on certificate from the president or vice-president of the College, condemned dogs be made available for physiological inquiry.[44] Five years later a bill was introduced into the state legislature to prohibit the use of animals for class demonstration or illustration. The College would probably have supported such a limitation, but the bill was so loosely drawn that some Fellows feared it would prohibit any use of animals for scientific purposes. Horatio C Wood, one of the College committee lobbying in Harrisburg, predicted "another tooth & nail fight." When the sponsors refused to alter the wording, Mitchell and Wood announced the College's opposition; and with the support of a physician member of the State Senate, the bill was easily killed.[45]

In these early measures in defense of vivisection, Mitchell, Wood, and Keen played leading parts. Individually and as a committee, they were impressive and persuasive. But their views did not have unanimous support even in the College. George Hamilton, for example, an elderly Fellow, who was known to love and keep bird and animal pets, addressed the College on vivisection in 1881. Reviewing the arguments for and against the use of animals in scientific experiments, he criticized the extremists of both sides; but nonetheless advocated a state law to regulate the practice.[46] Other Fellows who shared Hamilton's views were the surgeons Thomas G. Morton, Frank Woodbury, and John H. Packard.

Meanwhile, the American Anti-Vivisection Society had been formed. (It soon changed its name to the American Society for the Restriction of Vivisection.) The College, apprehensive of the Society's purposes, appointed a strong committee, headed by Mitchell, to investigate the group "and to take such steps as may seem to it best to guard the interests of the public and the profession." One of the Society's first acts was to get an anti-vivisection bill introduced into the state legislature. The College voted at once to oppose it.[47] On further thought, however, reckoning that more might be gained by cooperation, the College, through Wood, approached Thomas G. Morton, who was now president of the Anti-Vivisection Society; and the parties agreed on a substitute bill. This would have required that institutions and researchers obtain a license from the College, that records be kept of all experiments with animals, and that these records, deposited in the College, should be open to public inspection. Unlicensed persons were forbidden to perform scientific experiments on animals. In the hearing before the Judiciary Committee in Harrisburg, representatives of the College and the Society disagreed whether all changes in the substitute draft had been approved by both parties. Mitchell then asked whether the Society would regard the enactment of the bill as a final settlement of the whole question. To this Woodbury responded that if the law were faithfully observed and enforced, the Society would be satisfied; but that, of course, he could not bind the Society for an indefinite future. For their part, Mitchell and Wood spoke only as individuals and could not commit the College to the requirement of trusteeship. Presented with this impasse, which was exacerbated by an emotional speech by Horatio Wood in favor of experimentation, the Judiciary Committee adjourned the hearing, rejected the substitute bill, and recommended the original bill negatively.

The College and Society now each publicly blamed the other for failure to obtain a law.[48] On its part, the College passed a series of resolutions asserting that it had no knowledge of abuse of animals anywhere in the commonwealth, affirming its judgment that the existing laws provided adequate protection and that no more were needed, and directing that a committee be appointed to oppose the enactment of any laws on the subject. Accordingly, the president of the College appointed a Committee for the Protection of Scientific Research, with himself as chairman.[49]

Before 1867 there was no legal way in Pennsylvania to obtain cadavers for scientific purposes. Yet the large and steadily rising enrollments of medical schools, which regarded anatomy as the foundation of their science, made an adequate supply essential. William S. Forbes, who had founded a private school of anatomy in 1857 and was a demonstrator in anatomy at Jefferson Medical College, petitioned the legislature in 1867 to allow the schools to obtain bodies legally. The legislature, he pointed out, had chartered medical schools, yet denied them the material they required for instruction. The result was that doctors might be, and in fact were, sued for malpractice in surgical cases about which they had in effect been prevented from acquiring the knowledge their patients needed. In this situation, Forbes continued, medical schools had to resort to those "degraded and debased creatures" who plied the grisly and unlawful trade of resurrectionists and traffickers in human bodies.[50]

The bill was, predictably, denounced as a "ghastly act" and rejected by the Senate committee when one member objected that it was unworthy of the enlightened age in which Pennsylvania lived. At this point Forbes turned to the College of Physicians, which responded at once by naming him, Agnew, and Samuel D. Gross (the latter's place was taken by Henry Hartshorne) to lobby the legislature. They pressed all the arguments Forbes had already advanced and then one more:

> . . . it was gravely observed that, as it was impossible in the nature of things to prevent the examination of the dead body of man, and as there was no law of the Commonwealth regulating the matter, it was manifest the bodies of distinguished legislators themselves, after a life full of good works, were no longer safe, in their graves, but were liable to be rudely disturbed.[51]

The committee's arguments were persuasive, and the bill passed.

The Anatomy Act of 1867, however, proved to have serious limitations. It applied only to the city of Philadelphia and Allegheny County, which meant that officials in other parts of the state had neither obligation nor authority to provide medical schools with such unclaimed bodies within their jurisdictions as would otherwise be buried at public expense. Nor did the law require, but only permitted, the Philadelphia and Pittsburgh officials—superintendents of morgues, almshouses, prisons, and hospitals—to turn over such bodies; and some of them found excuses to frustrate the purpose of the law. At least one Philadelphia coroner, who was also a teacher of anatomy, was understandably disinclined to provide his competitors with an adequate supply of anatomical material. In 1881–82, Forbes pointed out, an estimated 796 bodies were required for the 1,493 students in Philadelphia schools; they had to make do with only 405.

After some years' experience with the law, Forbes in 1883 asked the College of Physicians to approach the legislature once more. This the College did, offering a draft prepared by the Association of Teachers of Anatomy and Surgery in Philadelphia. Opponents of an amended law, or of any law at all, abetted by a sensation-seeking journalist, succeeded in having Forbes arrested and tried on the charge of conspiring to rob graves in a Germantown cemetery. Forbes was acquitted, to general approbation; but the episode underlined again the importance of putting the supplying of cadavers on a legal basis. A new, stronger, and better law was enacted in June 1883. It extended over the whole state, created a board to which bodies were to be reported or consigned and by which they would be allocated to institutions requiring them, and directed the appropriate public official to notify the board of such bodies as became available in their respective institutions. A curious omission in both laws, in view of some often-voiced opposition arguments, was any requirement that the remains be buried or otherwise decently disposed of. Despite the new law and a further revision in 1911, the Anatomical Board complained in 1914 that the Philadelphia coroner was evading the law by certifying unclaimed bodies to be those of "travelers" and therefore exempted from its provisions.[52]

### *Women in the College I*

Getting a supply of cadavers for the anatomy laboratories of medical schools had been relatively easy. Getting even one live woman physician into a medical society was more difficult. The question first arose officially in the College in 1868, but some Fel-

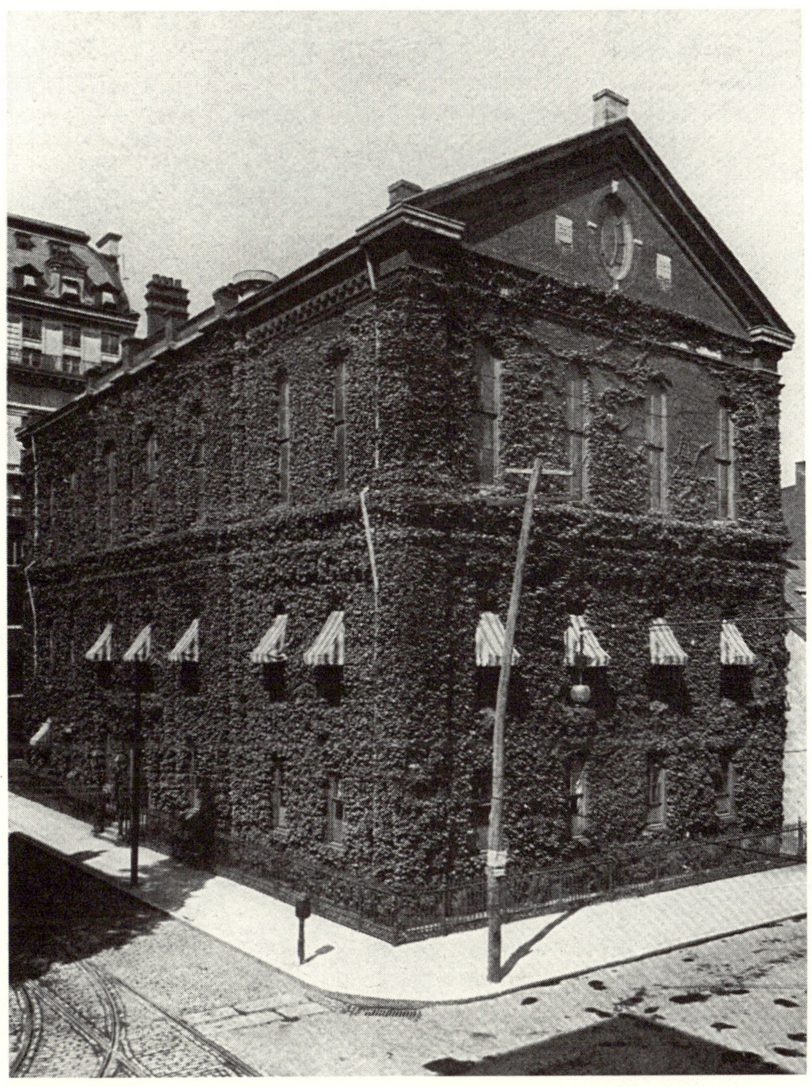

Hall of the College of Physicians, Thirteenth and Locust Streets, Philadelphia.

The College occupied the building from 1863–1909. The third floor was added in 1885.

lows, as members of the Philadelphia County Medical Society, had borne the principal burden of the fight over female doctors for ten years.

The Female Medical College of Pennsylvania (after 1876 the Woman's Medical College of Pennsylvania) opened in 1850 and graduated its first class of seven in 1851. Each year thereafter, the College turned out more graduates, more women entered practice in Philadelphia and Pennsylvania, acquiring success, reputation, and patients. Needless to say, this developoment was "not agreeable" to many established physicians.[53] They offered various reasons and rationalizations for their opposition, but, probably, most men regarded women in medicine simply as strange, disturbing, and improper, and therefore to them offensive, perhaps threatening. No concerted action against women physicians was taken until 1858, when the censors of the County Society (the censors' secretary was D. F. Condie) recommended that members of the regular profession not countenance or support the faculty and graduates of any female medical college, or consult or hold professional intercourse with the professors or alumnae of such schools. The State Medical Society approved this resolution in 1859 and urged the county societies to observe it.

The Montgomery County Society, however, dissented, and the Lancaster County Society also condemned the State Society's action as "premature, ill-advised, and injurious." When Hiram Corson (whose niece had recently graduated from medical school) began to read the Montgomery County resolutions at the 1860 meeting of the State Society, he was met with a storm of protest and rebuke. Discussion was foreclosed by a motion to table, and the Lancaster County Society's resolution was ruled out of order. In the ensuing years, opponents of recognition of women physicians offered a variety of arguments and employed an arsenal of parliamentary measures and tactics. They pointed out that the faculty of the Female Medical College included some irregular practitioners (which was true) and that therefore the institution could not be represented in the state or national associations. Alfred Stillé, who was not opposed in principle to admitting women into the profession, nonetheless pointed out that women were all graduates of schools that were by definition inferior at a time when leaders of the profession were endeavoring to raise the level of medical education. This and other arguments were employed by Squier Littell in resolutions presented to the College of

Physicians in support of the County Society in 1868.[49] After citing the efforts of the profession, particularly by the American Medical Association, to achieve "the highest possible standard of professional attainment" as being "essential to the welfare of the community," the resolution continued:

> whereas, from her mental, moral & physical constitution, it is as a general rule impossible for woman to receive the thorough instruction & training which such elevated standard requires, or even if, in exceptional instances, received, to discharge satisfactorily, in all conditions of weather & at all hours of the night as well as of the day, the varied & arduous duties which it involves . . . and whereas, for the reasons stated, her admission into the profession would give sanction & authority to an order of practitioners of inferior capacity & qualification, thus defeating an object so much desired & so steadily pursued; it is therefore
>
> *Resolved,* That the College of Physicians, following the example of the State & County Medical Societies, & disavowing every consideration other than a due regard for the public good, will neither recognize private female practitioners of medicine, Hospitals in which the sick are treated by female physicians, nor institutions in which medical instructionn,—necessarily partial & defective,—is given to females; & that its Fellows are hereby instructed & enjoined to govern themselves in accordance with this declaration, holding no connection with such institutions, & no professional intercourse with such practitioners.

The College voted thirty-two to eight to take no action on the resolution.[54]

The main area of battle was the State Society. Almost every year there was a long, heated, and noisy debate. Corson usually opened it, ably supported by Washington L. Atlee, who was to become in a few years president of the County and State Medical Societies, a man who, in Corson's words, "loved justice, courted battle with wrong, and was a stranger to fear."

Leaders of the opposition included Jacob Solis-Cohen, William H. Pancoast, and Nathan L. Hatfield. But year by year, support for the women increased, and the opposition weakened as it lost votes to experience, reason, and death. In 1869 the County Society once more voted that its members should not accept professorships in women's medical colleges or hospitals or engage in professional consultations with female doctors. The resolution was generally understood to be directed against Stillé, Atlee, and young Albert H. Smith.

None of these was intimidated. It was, in fact, too late to turn the tide. Reynell Coates, although no longer an active Fellow of the College, had accepted the chair of surgery at the Female Medical College in 1865, and in 1869, the year of the County Society's resolution, Charles H. Thomas and Henry Hartshorne, both Fellows, were appointed professors of materia medica and of hygiene and diseases of women respectively. Consultants included Smith, Hartshorne, Stillé, John Forsyth Meigs, Thomas G. Morton, and S. Weir Mitchell, all Fellows of the College.[55] Bowing to the inevitable, the State Society by a vote of fifty-five to forty-five in 1871 rescinded the offending resolution of 1859; and three years later the County Society removed from its by-laws all references to the admission of women.

Some, of course, continued to resist. D. Hayes Agnew, the distinguished surgeon of the University of Pennsylvania and of the Pennsylvania Hospital, who was hostile to any sort of higher education for women, strongly opposed the decision of the Hospital Managers in 1869 to admit women to the clinics. When the Managers reaffirmed that decision in 1871, he resigned. Littell in the College of Physicians brought in a resolution condemning the Managers for their usurpation of the physicians' authority and "peremptory dictation to the medical staff," and approving the action of Agnew, who, "rather than submit to such dictation, has vindicated his own dignity & independence." The College voted it down fourteen to five.[56]

Agnew returned to the hospital staff in 1877. The County Society was slower to accept women. After rejecting several nominees, they finally elected "a lady doctor" in 1888, the same year in which the Medical Society of the District of Columbia elected its first woman member.[57] The College of Physicians did not receive its first woman Fellow until nearly half a century later.

## *International Medical Congress, 1876*

The College might have been expected to take a lead in the International Medical Congress held in Philadelphia in connection with the Centennial Exhibition in 1876. Thanks in part to the deliberations required by the existence of the Council, however, it did not. The first suggestion that local medical societies and schools should participate in the celebration was made in the County Society in 1872.[58] The initial response was cool, but in 1874, as the city's plans for the anniversary began to take form, the Society renewed the suggestion and concluded that an international congress should be held. The College was one of the many institutions invited to appoint representatives to the Centennial Medical Commission. The invitation was referred to the Council; the Council asked its clerk to get more information; and by the time the clerk reported back to the Council, the Commission had been formed, as William B. Atkinson of the County Society explained:

> As the Commission is now fully organized, it is too late for any delegates from your body.
>
> As I saw Dr. Edw. Hartshorne & had a long talk with him on the whole subject, I am surprised that he did not mention it in some way.
>
> I find that we have invited & secured the acceptance of three of your Councillors and as we have your secretary & several of your prominent members, the College is perhaps as well represented as it could desire.[59]

This reply might have been thought unfriendly, if not actually offensive; but the College was, as Atkinson said, *de facto* represented: its Fellows filled most of the offices on the commission. Samuel D. Gross was president; Alfred Stillé and W.S.W. Ruschenberger, vice-presidents; Caspar Wister, treasurer; and Richard J. Dunglison, foreign secretary. Hartshorne explained that as he considered his conversation with Atkinson to have been informal and unofficial, he had not felt at liberty to make use of it in the College. The council voted that in the circumstances further action was precluded.

The International Congress, which met for six days in September 1876, brought together some 450 physicians and surgeons from most of the states of the Union and from nineteen foreign countries. From Philadelphia, in addition to Gross and I. Minis Hays, who were elected president and secretary-general respectively, were Alfred Stillé, president of the Section on Medicine, Isaac Hays, D. Hayes Agnew, Jacob M. DaCosta, J. Solis-Cohen, Thomas

S. Kirkbride, Isaac Ray, and W. W. Keen; from New York, Austin Flint; from Washington, Joseph M. Toner, who read a paper on American medical biography, and John Shaw Billings, who exhibited sample pages of the forthcoming *Index-Catalogue.* Henry I. Bowditch came from Boston; R. Palmer Howard from Montreal; and Nathan Smith Davis, president of the American Medical Association, from Chicago. Tokyo, St. Petersburg, and the Medical Society of Victoria, Australia, were also represented. By far the most distinguished delegate, representing the University of Edinburgh, was Joseph Lister, who presided over the Section on Surgery.[60] He was elected a Foreign Fellow of the College the next year.

### *Antisepsis*

Lister had an immediate and lasting influence on at least one Philadelphia surgeon. Until he spoke at the International Congress, William W. Keen recollected half a century later, "we knew almost nothing of germs," although Lister had published his first paper on the subject nine years before. Surgeons who did not understand the principle of antisepsis derided it as "only surgical cleanliness." Keen once—'but once only"—saw Samuel D. Gross test the sharpness of a knife on his finger, then, lifting his foot, strop it on the sole of his shoe, and finally "clean" the blade between thumb and forefinger. Convinced of the merit of antisepsis, Keen became Lister's "first disciple in Philadelphia" and introduced the new method on October 1, 1876, at St. Mary's Hospital, where he was one of the surgeons.[61] In fact, he was not quite the first.

On October 4, 1876, J. Ewing Mears, gynecologist at Jefferson Hospital and surgeon at St. Mary's, reported to the College on his successful use in July—before Lister's address in Philadelphia—of Lister's method in the case of a lacerated wound of the elbow joint.[62] The report would be the more acceptable, Mears thought, because, to judge from the few published reports, "it may be safely asserted that the antiseptic method of treating wounds, either simple or complicated, has not been largely employed in this country." Mears' statement is a reminder that, for many reasons, it took—as it still takes—some time for any improvement to be received, understood, and adopted.

Another decade was to pass before antisepsis was uniformly

practiced in Philadelphia. William J. Taylor, later president of the College, recalled that when he was a resident at the Pennsylvania Hospital in 1884, D. Hayes Agnew let him "use Listerism"—carbolic acid steam spray, catgut ligatures, and carbolic gauze dressings. They tried it on different patients in adjoining beds, and the results were so striking that Taylor was "converted."[63] Yet as late as 1887—twenty years after Lister's first announcement—a surgeon, newly appointed to the Pennsylvania Hospital staff, was so notoriously unsympathetic to Listerian principles that he was sharply questioned by newspaper reporters on the point.[64]

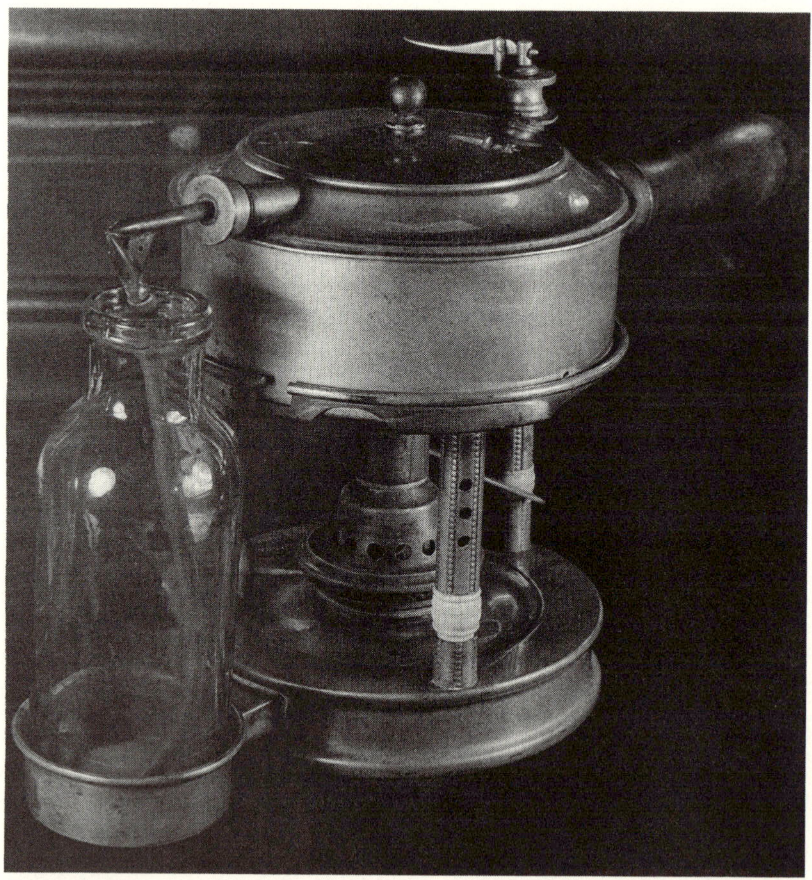

Lister's Carbolic Acid Spray Apparatus *(Abbe Collection, College of Physicians).*

CHAPTER VII

# *Interlude and Transition, 1863–1885*

FOR half a century after the construction of the hall at Thirteenth and Locust Streets in 1863, presidents of the College in their annual reports almost without exception described the work of the College in terms of three principal divisions—the library, the museum, and, after 1882, the Directory for Nurses. Other activities—publication of the *Transactions* and scientific sessions, for example—usually received less attention; but these three, prospering year after year, serving both the medical and lay communities, were recognized for their usefulness and their role in expanding the reputation of the College.

The small collection of anatomical specimens and surgical instruments, assembled in response to Isaac Parrish's proposal for a museum in 1849, expanded in 1863 when Thomas Dent Mütter's collection was installed in the new hall, with an endowment that enabled it to grow. After 1863 the library, too, grew rapidly and steadily from gifts and bequests of Fellows and their widows. In the 1870s, until overtaken by the Surgeon-General's Library in Washington, it was the largest medical library in the country. As for the Nurses' Directory, this brought the College into close association each year with hundreds of private families in Philadelphia; it also proved successful both financially and professionally. Each of these enterprises had its own committee in the College and its own history, but as the years passed their several activities converged on a common need—more room. Only twenty years after it was opened, the new hall had to be enlarged.

### *Mütter Museum*

Mütter's collection, which had been stored in Jefferson Medical College while his trustees awaited the construction of a fireproof building to receive it, was moved into the College at the end of 1863. It contained 1,139 specimens, including 518 bones and 289 calculi, as well as 363 water colors, forty-eight oil paintings, and about two hundred casts. Thomas G. Morton, curator from 1862 to 1866, who received an annual stipend of $300 under the trust, prepared a catalogue (on the principles of that of Guy's Hospital, London). The articles were hardly in their new cases before additions began to come in. Washington L. Atlee, for example, in 1867 gave the museum his collection of 250 specimens, mostly of ovarian conditions. Other donations were made in response to a general appeal. The curator arranged an exchange of duplicates with the Army Medical Museum, requesting particularly examples of gunshot wounds; but a similar request to the Smithsonian Institution for human crania was declined, with the explanation that any duplicates that might be available "must be reserved for institutions in less favored localities" than Philadelphia. Because it was expected that the materials would be closely studied by anatomists, surgeons, and others, the museum was opened regularly, with a supply of pens, paper, and ink for those wishing to make drawings.

Thanks to the Mütter endowment, the museum was also able to purchase specimens, models, and even whole collections. William W. Keen, going to Europe in 1866, was authorized to buy appropriate anatomical preparations. In the next few years the museum purchased specimens and preparations from the French anatomists Professor Philibert Constant Sappey and Louis Thomas Jerome Auzoux of Paris, and some 250 pieces from the osteological collection of Henry H. Smith, who had recently retired from the chair of surgery in the University of Pennsylvania. From Adam Politzer of Stuttgart the College bought the preparations of the ear that had been exhibited at the Centennial Exposition of 1876. The most important acquisition was the collection of Joseph Hyrtl of Vienna, which the College had been interested in since 1866. Thomas Hewson Bache, curator of the museum, finally secured it in 1874 for about $6,000, when Hyrtl was retiring from his professorship. The collection included specimens of the organs of hearing, microscopical and other preparations, seventy skulls of "all

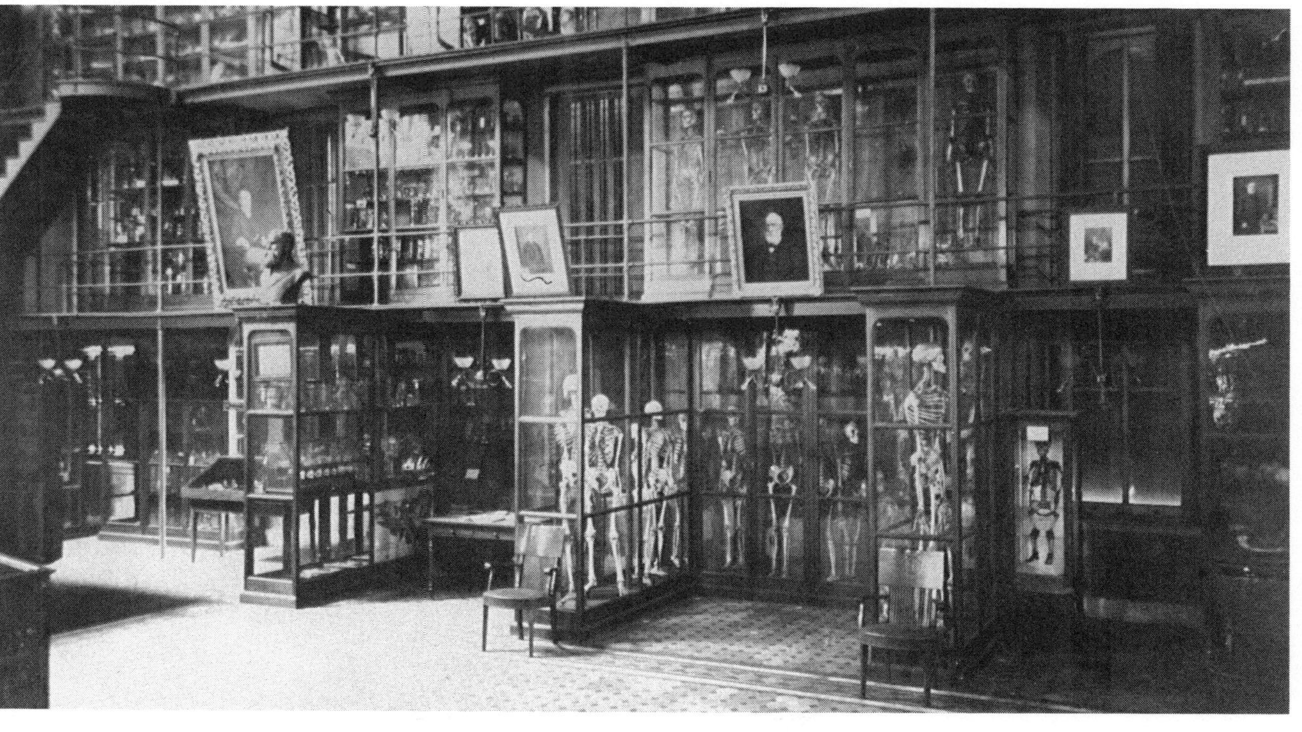

Mütter Museum, Interior, c. 1890. Photograph.

the tribes of Eastern Europe," and seventy other skulls. The "authentic" skull of Mozart, however, said to be in the collection, was missing.[1]

Bache was a tireless acquisitor for the museum. On his travels abroad he kept its needs in mind as he visited hospitals, museums, manufacturers, and dealers in anatomical materials. Old acquaintances from his student days in Paris helped him. Skeletons, they told him, were hard to find in London; he obtained one in Paris and sent it to England to be mounted by the man who did such work for the Royal College of Surgeons. Even small matters were never far from his attention. "I am worried about the mummy," he wrote the acting curator from Rome, " . . . lest it introduce moths into the Museum."[2]

Eager to make the museum a center for study and research, the Museum Committee improved its reference collection with anatomical atlases and other works on surgery and medicine. It also employed Robert Bridges, a Fellow of the College, who had recently catalogued collections at the Academy of Natural Sciences, to analyze the urinary calculi, with a view to publishing an illustrated catalogue. Despite these efforts, however, few persons visited the museum; none of the local professors used it in his teaching; and some Fellows dismissed it scornfully as something that survived and grew only because it had an endowed income that could not be diverted to more urgently useful projects. Such sentiments were voiced more frequently as the museum began to require more space. As early as 1874 the Museum Committee called for the construction of a third floor on the College building as "the only available method of accommodating the Museum and its probable increase."

In addition to the museum Mütter's endowment also supported a lectureship. The terms of the endowment required that the lecturer should be appointed for a term of three years, that he should deliver a course of lectures each year, and that for each course he should receive $200. The first lecturer was John H. Packard, a promising younger physician, who was surgeon to the Episcopal Hospital and had been secretary of the Pathological Society. His first series of lectures, in 1864–65, was on inflammation, his second on fractures of the upper extremities, and his third on fractures of the lower extremities. The first two series were published. Harrison Allen, professor of comparative anatomy in the University of Pennsylvania, was the second Mütter lecturer;

his subject was bones and their diseases. Allen resigned after one year. John H. Brinton delivered one course, on gun-shot wounds, and also resigned the appointment. It was clear that few men would commit themselves to a three-year obligation, especially for so modest an honorarium. Accordingly, with the consent of the executor and Mrs. Mütter, the lectureship was changed to a one-year appointment every third year, with the lecturer receiving the whole of the three-year stipend of $600. The first lecturer under this arrangement was Jacob Solis-Cohen, a recently-elected Fellow.[3]

Like the museum, the Mütter lectureship achieved less than either the donor or the College hoped. Although advertised to medical schools, hospitals, Fellows, other physicians, and even in the newspapers, the lectures had only a disappointing attendance and were seldom published.

### *The Library*

Although the decision to build a new fire-proof hall in 1863 was hastened by the College's desire to receive the Mütter collection on the testator's terms, the library's need for space was as urgent as the museum's and of longer standing. And the library, like the museum, soon outgrew its space, forcing the College eventually to enlarge the hall. Meanwhile, assurance of sufficient room for the book collection in the new building encouraged Fellows to make gifts. One of the first and most important was the donation in 1863 of nearly 2,500 volumes by Samuel Lewis.

A native of Barbados, Samuel Lewis was graduated in medicine from the University of Edinburgh in 1840, opened a practice in Philadelphia, and was elected a Fellow of the College in 1849.[4] His health was not up to the rigors of general practice and, in any case, he found the literature of medicine more congenial. As he had a sufficient private income, he closed his office and devoted himself to book-collecting. He was put on the Committee on Library in 1854, presented some books at that time, and after a few years decided to give his entire personal collection to the College. Thereafter, until his death in 1890, the library was Lewis' principal interest. He regularly ordered books from European dealers and personally scoured bookshops for titles to supplement the College holdings and fill gaps in its runs of periodicals. Weir Mitchell said that Lewis "disliked to see a man who needed a book unable to find it here." John Ashhurst, Jr., testified to the truth of this assertion. Once, writing to Lewis, who was then in Europe, Ashhurst mentioned that he had been unable to find a title by Paulus Barbette: in next parcel of books Lewis sent home there were three editions of Barbette's work.

Although he gave the College many volumes that were old, rare, or exciting to bibliophiles, Lewis was no mere collector, but had a scholar's appreciation of their contents and "real utility." "He could appreciate a beautiful book," Ashhurst wrote, apparently with someone or some example in mind,

> but he did not value it on that account alone. . . . He was a lover of books, a bibliophile in the truest sense of the word, but in no sense was he a bibliomaniac. He did not care for a book because it had an additional third of a line in height, nor did he value it more because it had rough, uncut edges, than if its edges were neatly trimmed and gilded.[5]

During nearly a quarter of a century Lewis gave the College about ten thousand volumes. They were formally designated "The Samuel Lewis Library."

Thomas Hewson Bache, librarian since 1855, resigned shortly after the library was moved into the spacious rooms in the Locust Street hall (only to return to the College in 1866 as curator of the museum). He was succeeded as librarian in 1864 by Charles Stewart Boker, a graduate of Princeton and of the University of Pennsylvania Medical School and a Fellow since 1859. Within a few months Boker had the books on their shelves. Arranged by size, according to the prevailing practice, their orderly appearance pleased him; but the College directed that the books be arranged by subject instead. Boker resigned, whether for this or another reason does not appear; and, despite some faint resistance to shelving by subject (as being wasteful of space and untidy as well), the new librarian, John Hamilton Slack, fell in with the College's requirement.

Slack was a bookish physician, who operated a private press in his house and had a taste and some talent for music and painting and the means to indulge them. He reorganized the general collection, made a card catalogue of the Lewis library, added bookcases and shelves. Satisfied with what he had done, the Library Committee recommended that the library should receive an annual appropriation of $100 from the general fund—raised in 1867 to $500. At the beginning of 1865 the collection contained 7,742 volumes, probably fewer than the Pennsylvania Hospital's but several times more than the 2,282 in the Surgeon-General's Library in Washington. "It may, with just pride," the committee asserted the next year, "be regarded as the largest, as well as the best collection of medical works belonging to any similar institution in the United States."[6]

The rapid growth of the library, and the demands that physicians made on it as the medical sciences advanced, brought calls for easier access. In this situation, in 1866 George Bacon Wood offered $500 a year to keep the library open several hours daily. Since this would add to the work of the librarian, making it unlikely that a Fellow could ever be found able to spend the additional hours at the College, it was decided that daily attendance at the reading room should be the responsibility of members of the Library Committee. Fortunately, the committee had someone in mind willing to take on the task. The committee was enlarged from three to five, and one of the new appointees was Robert Bridges. After Slack resigned as librarian in 1867 to cultivate fish at "Troutdale," his New Jersey farm, Bridges was elected the next year to succeed him.

Bridges was the last Fellow to conduct the library unassisted. A man of sixty-two when he succeeded Slack, he had been professor of general and pharmaceutical chemistry at the Philadelphia College of Pharmacy since 1842 and had previously and simultaneously taught the same subject in the Philadelphia Association for Medical Instruction and the Franklin Medical College. He had been a pupil of Thomas T. Hewson for four years and had had a long association with Franklin Bache at the College of Pharmacy and at Jefferson Medical College. He was on the committee to revise the United States Pharmacopoeia in 1840, and had been librarian and president of the Academy of Natural Sciences of Philadelphia. When he assumed his duties at the College on January 1, 1868, the library contained 13,043 volumes; when he retired in 1881 it contained 23,288. These two figures reveal much of the history of the library in Bridges' time.

The influx of gifts and bequests continued. Lewis gave another

1,124 volumes in 1865. "I do not know of any enterprise as popular in the Profession as the increase of the Library of this Institution," Joseph Carson wrote in 1869.[7] Alfred Stillé, chairman of the Library Committee, and Isaac Hays were constant benefactors. Charles D. Meigs left the College "all the books in my library that treat specially of the subject of midwifery"—ninety-nine volumes. Other books came from the estates of Francis West and Caspar Wistar Pennock, from the widows of Professor Samuel Jackson and William F. Jenks. From Carson's large library the librarian selected 278 volumes. The bequest of George Bacon Wood brought an additional 574 volumes as well as a legacy of ill feeling—a discrepancy was found between a list made after his death and the volumes actually delivered, and some Fellows charged Wood's nephew Horatio C Wood with having held them back.

Other volumes were received regularly in exchange for the College *Transactions,* notably from the Surgeon-General's Library, the Smithsonian Institution, medical societies, and publishers. There were also occasional informal exchanges. The College gave the Historical Society of Pennsylvania a copy of Thomas Cadwalader's *Essay on the West-India Dry-Gripes* (1745) in return for we know not what, and it gave the Library Company of Philadelphia a collection of non-medical pamphlets.[8] The favor was returned forty years later, when a copy of William Harvey's *Exertationes de Generatione Animalium* (London, 1657), which the Library Company had given Weir Mitchell "in Exchange," was given to the College by Mitchell's son John in 1914.

However valuable and welcome, the gifts were mostly older titles, with relatively few recent monographs or even late editions of standard works among them. Thus, library accessions reflected the achievements and practices of a passing generation rather than filled the needs of the present. With only a tiny budget for purchases, the Library Committee could do little to shift the balance. Of 870 volumes added in 1879, for example, only thirty-five were purchased by the Library Committee. In 1881 the figures were 1,259 and thirty-two respectively.

To the implications of these figures there was one exception. Impressed by the success of the private Philadelphia and Rush Medical Book Clubs, to which many of them belonged, Fellows formed the Journal Association in 1871 to purchase American and foreign periodicals. These were placed on the library tables upon receipt, then bound and given to the library. In its first year the Association had fifty-seven members, whose annual dues of $4 bought twenty-seven journals, American, British, German, French, and Indian. The next year there were seventy-two members, and, though the dues were reduced, the number of journal subscriptions increased. The Journal Association was of such obvious benefit that in 1880 Weir Mitchell gave $1,000 to establish a journal fund,which the Council named after him.

All this made clear that the library was in ever greater demand. In 1871, on motion of Mitchell, it was opened two evenings a week, but the innovation was dropped after a year because of "extremely limited attendance." After 1874 it was kept open during the summer, and in 1881 the daily hours were extended from 11 a.m. to 4 p.m. Inter-library loans with the Surgeon-General's Library were instituted in 1877. In 1885 Nathaniel Archer Randolph proposed that the College compile a catalogue of private libraries of Fellows willing to lend their books for brief periods for use in the College building under the rules of the College library.[9]

When Bridges fell ill in 1881, an assistant had to be found to keep the library open. Charles Perry Fisher, a graduate of a local academy, whom Samuel Lewis had engaged to catalogue his library, was a young man of great ability and promise, who quickly won the respect and confidence of the Library Committee. Self-taught in many subjects, he proved an intelligent and imaginative administrator and bookman, and eventually acquired a national reputation as a wise, pioneering medical librarian. When Bridges died early in 1882, Fisher was named assistant librarian. The obligations of the librarian, hitherto always a Fellow of the College, were now much altered and reduced. The post of honorary librarian was therefore created; the first to fill it was James H. Hutchinson. Thereafter the honorary librarian and the chairman of the Committee on Library were the principal links between the library and the Council and Fellows. Fisher, however, who was eventually named librarian and remained at the College more than fifty years, became increasingly influential in all library matters. For example, he prepared the annual reports which the chairmen of the committee presented, and saw to it, even when the College cut back on the size of the *Transactions,* that the reports were printed in full, usually with lists of recently acquired incunabula. In many respects the College library after 1885 may fairly be said to have been Fisher's creation.

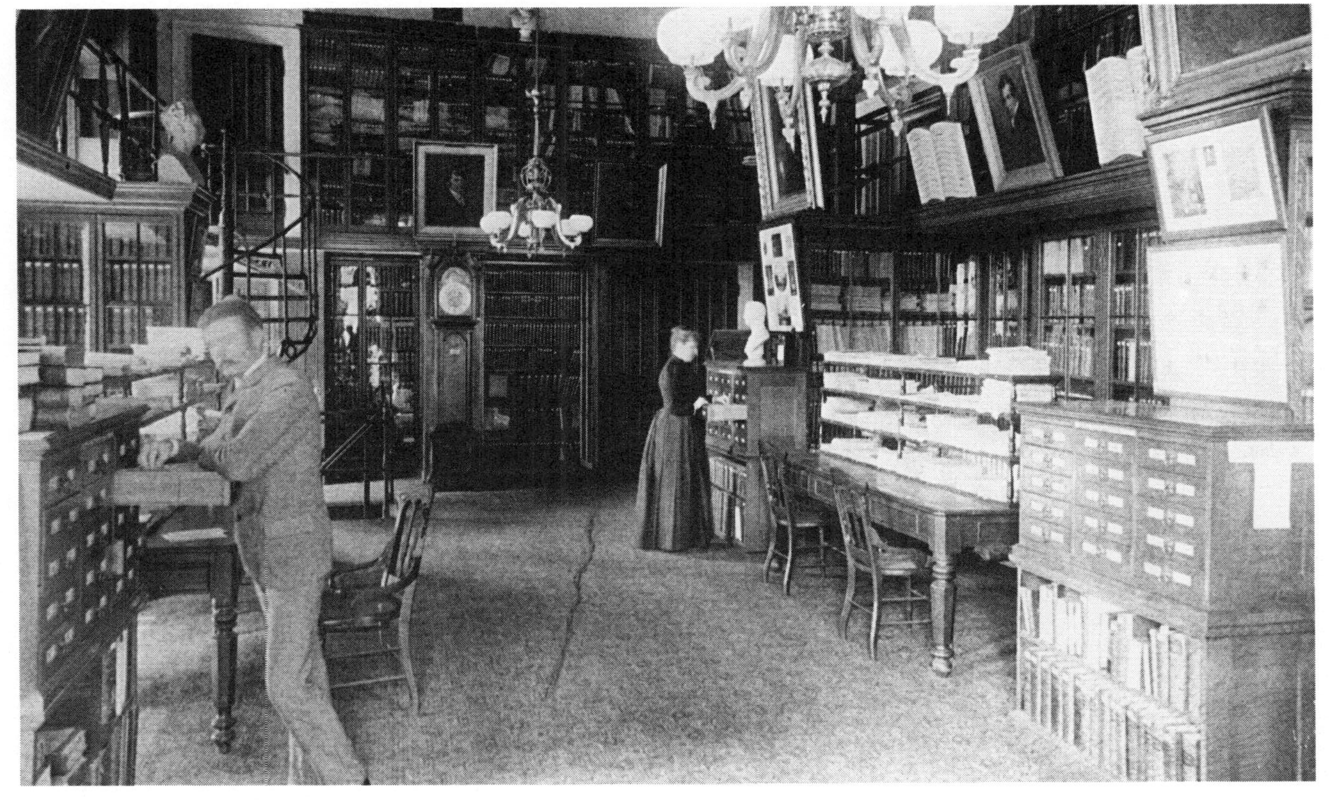

Library, Interior, c. 1890. Photograph. Charles Perry Fisher, librarian, is at the catalogue in the foreground.

### *Directory for Nurses*

Together the library and museum strained the limits of the College hall. Additional pressure was put on the available space by the Directory for Nurses, which required several small rooms.[10]

A nurses' directory had been operated by the Boston Medical Library Association since 1879. Impressed by its work, Weir Mitchell asked for details. "I can assure you," James R. Chadwick of the Library Association replied, "that our Directory for Nurses has proved the most useful institution that we have in Boston."[11] Mitchell enlisted the support of William W. Keen, who proposed a similar directory to the College on Mitchell's behalf on February 1, 1882. The need for a register of qualified nurses, Keen wrote many years later, was obvious:

> It is hard for those of you that have always had the Directory to call on, to realize the difficulties for doctor, patient and nurse before the existence of any such centre—the more so as those were the days before either telephones or taxicabs.
>
> Many was the time that I—and every other practising physician—would have to employ a horse hack, often in the night time, and drive for miles in search of a nurse. Quite often, our first choice would be out of town, or sick, or engaged. Usually the next on our list would live in quite another part of the city, and so we might have to spend precious hours merely in the search for a second, a third, or even a fourth choice.[12]

On March 1 the Directory was approved. It would have a secretary, who would also assist in the library. She would live in the hall, with a telephone and, if necessary, a telegraph, so as to be on call at any hour. The Directory would be supervised by a new committee of the College, and there would be an auxiliary committee of women. The ladies, led by Mrs. Mitchell, had already solicited their friends and raised $1,000 for initial expenses. The Directory opened on May 14, 1882, with Miss Emily Thomas, already employed in the library, as secretary.

From the start the Directory was a success. It covered all its expenses and produced income for the College as well. Nurses paid a small fee to be registered; and the Directory charged those who called for its services—$1 to $3 for information about available nurses, depending on the hour of the day or night when the inquiry was made; an additional dollar for finding and despatching the nurse; $5 for a wet nurse and $10 for a *certified* wet nurse.[13] In its first eight months the Directory sent out 342 nurses, and in 1883 it was able to turn over $200 to the library. In 1890 over seven hundred nurses were on the roll, 1,572 calls for nurses were answered, and $2,000 was contributed to the library after all expenses were paid. In eight years a total of $7,950 was given to the library. In their annual reports presidents of the College, without exception, expressed pride in the Directory and called on the Fellows to use it when their patients required nursing.[14]

The Nurses' Directory, however, was not merely an employment agency. It inquired into the character and capacity of prospective registrants, and its discipline was strict. Although it eventually included attendants and even physiotherapists, it accepted principally only trained nurses. The result was that for many years it did as much as, if not more than, any institution in Philadelphia to preserve and raise the standards of the nursing profession.

One of those impressed by this record was Abraham Jacobi of New York. He persuaded the New York Academy of Medicine to establish a Bureau of Nurses on the Philadelphia model in 1894; but after New York City required the bureau to be licensed, it was closed in 1906. In Baltimore the nurses' directory of the Medical and Chirurgical Faculty of Maryland was met with indifference, even hostility, and was discontinued after fifteen years in 1897.[15]

This is not to say that the Directory was universally applauded. It was criticised and attacked, as well as imitated. Nurses with little formal training, it was urged, might be as competent in the sickroom as the trained nurses the College admitted to its Directory. Furthermore, the College collected a fee from its registrants, profited from the operation, and made no public accounting. There were charges of favoritism in selecting and assigning nurses. In the 1890s some nurses withdrew from the College Directory and formed another. It failed after a few years; but a second attempt was made in 1900. This was by the School for Philadelphia Nurses, whose directory provided nurses who had received only a ten-week course of instruction.[16]

### *Building the Third Floor*

The Library Committee's annual report for 1873 first mentioned the approaching crisis of space. Echoing the warning next year, the Museum Committee looked to the construction of the third floor (provided for in the original plans) as the only way to meet the needs. Accordingly, the architect James Windrim was approached; a building committee was named, with George Fox as chairman; but nothing happened for seven or eight years.[17]

As so often, the obstacle was money. Canvassing the prospects, some Fellows looked longingly at the income of the Mütter endowment. With no space to exhibit or even store more specimens, the Museum Committee had stopped adding to the collection. As a result the unspent income amounted to $7,000 in 1883. Surely, it seemed to some Fellows, that money could be used to provide enlarged accommodations for the museum. However, a lawyer, consulted on the point, advised that it could not.

The College thus appeared to be held hostage by the Mütter trustees, who in effect required the College to enlarge its hall at its expense simply to provide for their growing, but little used, collection. Tension grew between friends of the library and advocates of the museum, between those who took a large view of the College and those who administered the Mütter trust as though they and it were independent of the College. From London in 1882 Bache wrote the acting curator an emotional defense of the museum's position:[18]

> The opinion of certain Fellows that the Museum is a white elephant should not influence the Museum Committee. A fine Library in the possession of a fool, who neither uses it nor allows others to use it is a white elephant. In the possession of a liberal and sensible man, a blessing. I well remember when some fellows thought *it was absurd to try and form a library.* Probably some of them thought me a fool for working a number of years to form a library when no one used a book which we possessed . . . . I begged books everywhere. Obtained all the journals received in exchange from all the editors of our Phila. journals . . . . The result was that in 1862, when we occupied our Hall, we had something of a library.
>
> The Museum Committee are not responsible for the

> bad accommodation of the Museum. It is *responsible for the* proper spending of the income of the trust . . . . The most melancholy thing is that those who now enjoy the College paid very little for what they enjoy and are not willing to be as liberal as those of the generation which has passed away. The College has nearly 200 Fellows. How many paid anything for the building? They outnumber the fellowship which built the Hall and there is not enterprize and liberality enough to add a 3rd story.

In these circumstances the College obtained another legal opinion, which proved to be contrary to the first. An amicable suit was entered into, and the court sensibly allowed the trustees of the Mütter fund to lend the College $5,000 toward the cost of enlarging the building and increasing accommodation for the museum, with no expectation that the loan would be repaid. The College then voted to add the third floor. A new Building Fund committee was named, with Mitchell as chairman. Jacob Da Costa, president of the College, gave the first $1,000.[19]

As Windrim was occupied with other commissions, the plans were drawn by another Philadelphia architect Theophilus D. Chandler, Jr. In addition to adding the third story for the museum and its adjoining laboratory, alterations were made in the original building, including provision for a smoking room, which it was expected would "add materially to the comfort and convenience of the Fellows."[20]

Fund-raising, which had languished under Fox, proved successful under Mitchell's energetic leadership. A few Fellows made generous contributions, but, unlike the campaign for the hall in 1863, most of the gifts came from the wealthy patients and friends of Mitchell, Samuel W. Gross, and other Fellows, from Philadelphia manufacturers, bankers, and businessmen like A. J. Drexel, William Disston, Edwin H. Fitler, and Charles L. Harrison. Through Mitchell, Mrs. Cyrus McCormick of Chicago donated $1,000.[21] When it appeared that the fund might fall short, Mitchell proposed taking out a mortgage, on which he offered to pay the interest for three years. As it turned out, this was not necessary: $26,976 was raised, which proved to be $400 more than the total cost.[22]

The final furnishings were installed in the next year or two. A magnificent rostrum was put in place. Marble tablets were mounted bearing the names of the founders of the College, of benefactors who were descendants of founders, of other benefactors, and of Fellows who died in times of pestilence. With a gift of $2,500 from the publisher George W. Childs, a monumental fireplace was constructed, with mantel and andirons. Mitchell gave a carpet and, with William Barton Hopkins, some desks and chairs; and "an improved closet" came from the sanitary engineer Colonel George Waring. The telephone was installed in 1887 and, after frustrating delays, electricity in 1896.[23]

Soon after the renovations and enlargement were completed, Mitchell spoke of the library and of all libraries with warmly imaginative understanding. He was especially proud of the constant supply of journals,

> of which we receive at least 325. This steady inflow of weekly and monthly publications represents for us the swiftly changing tides of knowledge, the floods and ebbs of opinion, the never-ending novelties, good or bad—all to be put on trial. By-and-bye the best of this matter, solvent in a hundred journals, crystallizes into more permanent shape in books. This vast accumulation and the multitudinous contributions it represents has, of course, its embarrassments, for not all new facts are valuable or correctly interpreted; but, be they true or not, we must at times have access to them all. Whilst in some very good ways our profession is unyieldingly conservative, as to matters of intellectual opinion and modes of practice it is, nowadays at least, alertly ready to accept the novel and as ready to give up the old.
>
> Books are the best tools of our business, and a great library like ours insensibly educates by tempting men with the noblest of opportunities. It is like an unfailing friend to whom we go for counsel and helpful advice, and a catalogue is its ready memory of all that our greatest knew and taught. Look around that great collection in all tongues. It is a vast presentation of the thoughts, the beliefs, the victories, the defeats of that profession which has been, as compared to any other, the purest, the most single-minded, the most simply devoted to its moral creed, the world has seen through all its changeful ages. It has its peerage, its lords of thought, its sturdy, practical com-

mons. Yet here is no set creed of dogmatic beliefs. We make and unmake our rulers, and time, which is more wise than Bacon, has a large vote in the matter; but while systems of medicine crumble, and doctrines have their little day, and men have been intellectually right or wrong, it is pleasant to remember that the lofty code of moral law our Greek Fathers taught has kept through all these productive centuries an invigorating control over the lives these gathered volumes represent. Thus, for him who loves his art, a great medical library is full of lessons in the conduct of life. There, side by side, the feeblest and the strongest meet. What a record of the follies and caprices of learning, of devotion, of martyrdom, of simple usefulness, of ambitious failures! Here are stately tomes unread for ages. Here is some little volume which has changed the great currents of thought, and brought hope and relief to a thousand bedsides. In yonder corner is a modest book-case, which groups the bric-a-brac of the bibliographer; the mad jesters, the cranks, the queer anecdotists, the priceless incunabula, the medical poems.[24]

### *Fellows*

Membership rose steadily after the Civil War, from 128 resident Fellows in 1863, to 195 in 1885, to 204 in the year of the College's centenary in 1887. Nineteen Fellows were chosen in 1864, fourteen in 1868, sixteen in 1870, 1883, and 1885, and twenty-three in 1884. The annual growth was about three.

The men elected in these years are those who gave the College its character and reputation for more than thirty years after 1885. They read papers, served on committees, donated books to the library, and endowed lectureships and prizes to encourage and reward research. Their attitudes and arguments often determined how the College responded to particular questions. From their number came the presidents of the last years of the nineteenth and the first decades of the twentieth century—John Ashhurst, Jr. (1867), 1898–1900; William W. Keen (1867), 1900–02; Horatio C Wood (1865), 1902–04; Arthur V. Meigs (1875), 1904–07; James Tyson (1866), 1907–10; George E. de Schweinitz (1887), 1910–

13; James Cornelius Wilson (1874), 1913–16; and Richard H. Harte (1885), 1916–19. Most of these men were influenced by Weir Mitchell, by his devotion to the institution, his knowledge of its history, his respect for its tradition, his taste for ceremony, and above all by his vision of the College's role and future.

Others elected in these decades who made distinguished contributions to medical practice, science, and education included Harrison Allen (1867), William Goodell (1868), William Pepper (1868), Isaac Ray (1868), William Thomson (1869), Jacob Solis-Cohen (1871), Edward O. Shakespeare (1887), John B. Roberts (1878), Theodore G. Wormley (1878), Charles K. Mills (1881), and William Osler (1885). Their reputations added to the reputation and usefulness of the College.

Professor of clinical medicine in the University of Pennsylvania, Osler was elected a Fellow only three months after coming to Philadelphia from Montreal. He proved to be an active, popular, and finally much-loved member of the College.[25] He was a frequent, almost regular, attendant at its meetings, participated in the discussions, and presented papers of his own.[26] As a member of the Committee on Library he gave sound advice and contributed generously to the collection; after leaving Philadelphia he continued to give the library rare and interesting volumes—works of Sir Thomas Browne in 1900,a first edition of Sydenham on gout in 1901, an Aldine edition of Galen in 1906, "an extremely fine copy" of *Astronomici veteres* of Marcus Manilius and others 1499 in 1909. His note to Weir Mitchell on finding at Quaritch's in London for £84 a superb copy of the first printed edition of Celsus' *De Medicina* has often been quoted: "Why not bleed the Fellows of the College? I will go $25." In May 1889, as he was leaving Pennsylvania for Johns Hopkins, the Fellows paid him the unusual testimony of a farewell dinner.

In November Osler was back in Philadelphia for a meeting of the College, and he continued to attend frequently during the years he lived in Baltimore. In 1893 he presented a lock of Jenner's hair and urged the Fellows to join an English committee in establishing a cottage hospital in Jenner's memory at Berkeley in Gloucestershire.[27] In 1901 he came to read a paper on his favorite author, Sir Thomas Browne; the next year he read a memoir of Alfred Stillé, whom he greatly admired; and but for his commitments and the First World War he would have delivered one of the Weir Mitchell lectures in 1913 or 1914. But the remembrances continued—books, a physician's pomander cane, and from Lady Osler in 1914 a splendid crayon portrait of Sir William by John Singer Sargent. In 1915 the College exempted him from further payment of dues "in consideration of his great distinction and attainments and of his high service to the College"—to which he replied in acknowledgment, "I would much rather remain among the ordinary Fellows."[28]

Osler died in Oxford in December 1919. Three months later, in March 1920, the College held a memorial service, at which Thomas McCrae, Hobart A. Hare, Charles W. Burr, Francis R. Packard, and George W. Norris spoke.[29] Osler remembered the College at the last, bequeathing it a 1348 manuscript copy of the *Lilium Medicinae* of Bernard of Gordon. It was received from the executors in 1929. Soon afterwards Lady Osler presented a silver dish which she and Sir William had been given by Dr. and Mrs. Mitchell.[30]

During this same period, 1863–87, thirty-seven Associate American and eighteen Associate Foreign Fellows were chosen. Of these, twenty-two were elected in 1876 in connection with the Centennial Celebration and the International Medical Congress of 1876, and nine were admitted on the occasion of the College's observance of its own centennial in 1887. The Associate Foreign Fellows, most of whom were British, included Joseph Lister (1877), whose address at the International Congress the year before had deeply impressed many Philadelphia surgeons in his audience.

In addition to resident and foreign Fellows, a class of Corresponding Member was created in 1880. Just how Corresponding Members differed from Associate Fellows is not clear; it can only be conjectured what the College expected from them. Associate Fellows were "distinguished foreign or American physicians residing beyond the limits of Philadelphia." Corresponding Members were foreign or American physicians residing beyond the limits of Philadelphia, who were selected "because of their devotion to medical science, and with a view to advance the interests for which the College was founded." A strict interpretation of the distinction might suggest that Corresponding Members need not be distinguished, and that Associate Fellows need not be devoted to medical sciences and likely to advance the interests of the College. Nothing firm can be inferred from the names of the Corresponding Members—only eight in all—elected between 1880 and 1899. In any event, the College soon lost interest in its

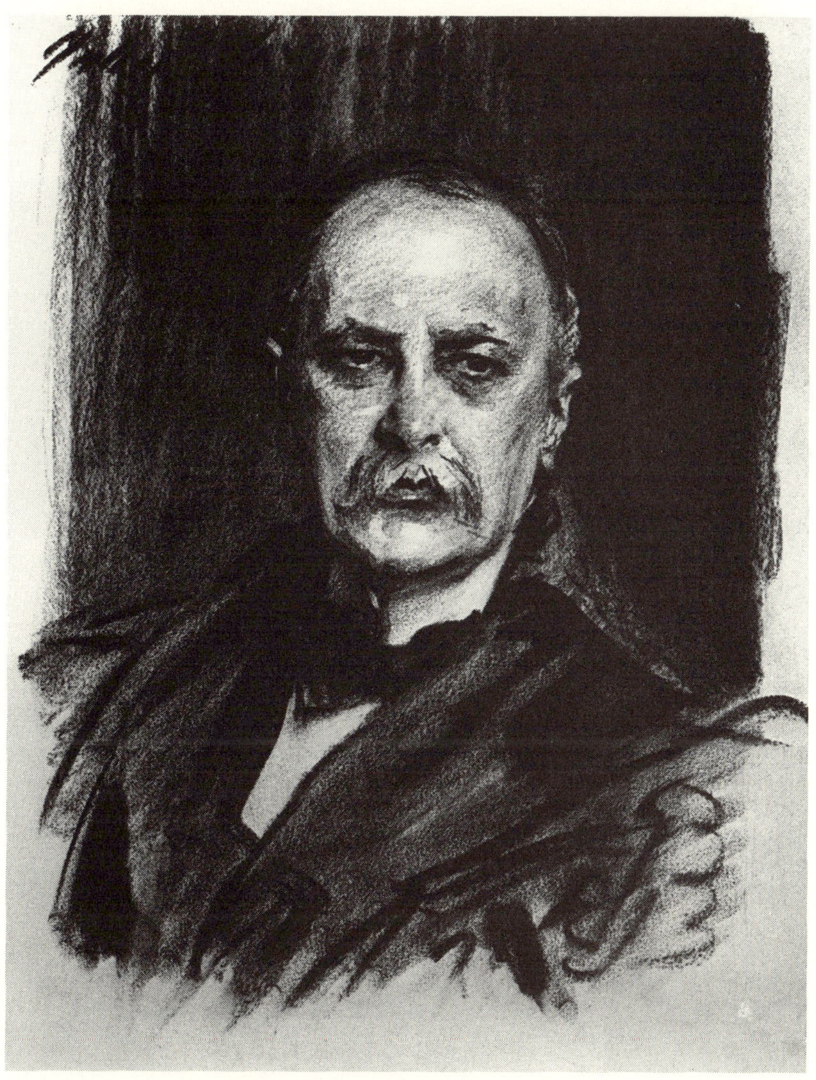

William Osler, (1849–1919). Charcoal drawing by John Singer Sargent. Presented to the College by Lady Osler, 1914.

Correspondents, failed to keep in touch with those it had chosen, elected five in 1915–17, mostly residents of upstate Pennsylvania, and dropped the class in 1925, transferring the survivors to Associate Fellowship.

### *Transition*

In 1879 George Bacon Wood had been president of the College for thirty-one years. During that period the College had moved forward strongly in many areas, and in many of the advances Wood had provided advice, encouragement, and timely financial support. In his latter years, however, he had given up his teaching and hospital posts, and after 1872 no longer attended meetings of the College. Nonetheless, he was reelected president annually until his death on March 30, 1879, at the age of eighty-two. The Fellows attended his funeral in a body, and on May 7 unanimously elected as his successor William W. S. Ruschenberger, who had been vice-president since 1875. Then, in an action which may be thought to have revealed their feelings about the twilight years of their late president, on July 2, 1879, they amended the by-laws to limit presidential terms thereafter to five years (reduced in 1882 to three).

A graduate of the University of Pennsylvania in 1830 in the same class with William Wood Gerhard, George W. Norris, and Joseph Carson, Ruschenberger was one of the young doctors with Paris training who had become Fellows of the College in the 1830s.[31] He had served fifty-three years in the naval service and now, at age seventy-two, held the commission of Medical Director with the rank of commodore. His taste was for natural history: he wrote several books about his long sea voyages in the Pacific, and during shore duty prepared a series of manuals on the natural sciences that did much to popularize those subjects in schools and academies. At the time of his election as president of the College, he was also president of the Academy of Natural Sciences of Philadelphia. He remained president of the College until January 1883, when he was succeeded by Stillé. He died in 1895 at the age of eighty-eight.

Stillé was a famous teacher and author, active in College affairs for many years, a forward-looking leader of the profession both in Philadelphia and the nation, who had been president of the

American Medical Association in 1867.[32] He took the opportunity of his presidency of the College to define the role of the institution. No other agency, Stillé asserted, challenging the Fellows with thoughts of the "great future" the College might enjoy, could do so much to instruct, enlighten and encourage both profession and laity:

> The day is passing when it is any longer necessary to hold a dark screen between physicians and educated laymen, and the better the world shall learn what are the aims and the achievements of a physician's life, the sooner will be dispelled the prejudices that antagonize the medical profession and the delusions under which the public become the victims of error and of fraud.

The same progressive spirit informed Stillé's address on leaving office a year later. Largely historical in content, it was a restatement of the purposes of the College. Citing past events, quoting the charter, Rush, and the founders, Stillé spoke once more of the institution's potential role:

> The history of this College justifies the belief that it will not readily fall from the high level it has occupied as a conservator of sound science and pure ethics. But there is nothing in this position inconsistent with its taking a more lively and effective part in the discussion of questions of contemporary interest; not, indeed, that it should play the part of a gladiator, and contend for the sake of the conflict merely, but the part rather of a mediator, or of a judicial tribunal in which the medical questions of the day can be debated with the sole object of arriving at the truth. Activity does not necessarily imply progress, nor does tranquillity necessarily denote stagnation; but the movement that proves strength is the movement that generates, fashions, and builds, because it is directed by a definite idea towards a fixed and definite end. The lines of action and the objects of the College are clearly defined in the words of its Charter . . . . They include all that the most catholic spirit could desire. But it can scarcely be claimed, even in a partisan spirit, that these lines have been completely filled. We need a deeper conviction of the value of

> this institution, for self-culture, for mutual improvement, and for the benefits it has conferred and confers increasingly upon the community.[33]

Samuel Lewis followed Stillé as president in 1884. His election was chiefly a recognition of his many valuable gifts to the College library in the preceding twenty years, for he was not a notable practitioner, held no professorship or hospital appointment, and had made no contribution to medical knowledge. Lewis resigned the office after only a few meetings, possibly because, as a stutterer, speaking in public gatherings was embarrassing to both himself and his audience. He was succeeded in mid-year by Jacob M. Da Costa, professor of theory and practice of medicine at Jefferson Medical College and a physician to the Pennsylvania Hospital.[34]

Born in 1833 in the West Indies of a Portuguese family long settled in London, Da Costa received his early education in Europe, came to Philadelphia at the age of sixteen, and then, after graduating from Jefferson in 1852, studied medicine in Paris, Prague, and Vienna, where he was a pupil of the great pathologist Rokitansky. A founder and president of the Philadelphia Pathological Society, often a delegate from the College of Physicians to the American Medical Association, and an original member and president of the Association of American Physicians, he was the author of a textbook on medical diagnosis that went through nine editions. Da Costa was an outstanding clinician who was sometimes called "a physician's physician." The first graduate of Jefferson to be elected president of the College, Da Costa served from May 1884 to January 1886 and again from 1895 to 1898.

Da Costa, like Stillé before him, used his presidential address in 1885 to review the current position and future prospects of the College. He cherished the same aspirations for it as his older colleague. He was as impatient with its conservatism as Stillé, who had gently rebuked it for so often "clinging to the old because it is old in spite of . . . its incongruity with the existing state of the world." But he spoke more sharply. The College, he pointed out, was now well known in professional circles:

> But does it occupy the position it should with the public? It is, I believe, neither rightly known nor sufficiently appreciated by them. It has not the influence to which it is

> justly entitled. This state of things is somewhat, I think, our own fault. We are chiefly a scientific institution, but we ought also to make ourselves heard on the questions of the day concerning which our profession is best qualified to judge. If we did so oftener, we would be appealed to as a final authority, and the community would learn to look to us for guidance in many things. This would give the College a hold on the public which would lead to general interest in its doings and its extension.[35]

Such complaints and appeals as Da Costa's were to be heard often in the ensuing half century—indeed, they are still heard—and almost as often the College made some response. Whether because of the criticisms of Stillé, Da Costa and others, or because—as is more likely—the College was already moving and being moved in the directions they pointed, the College was on the verge of a more prosperous and glorious period than it had yet enjoyed.

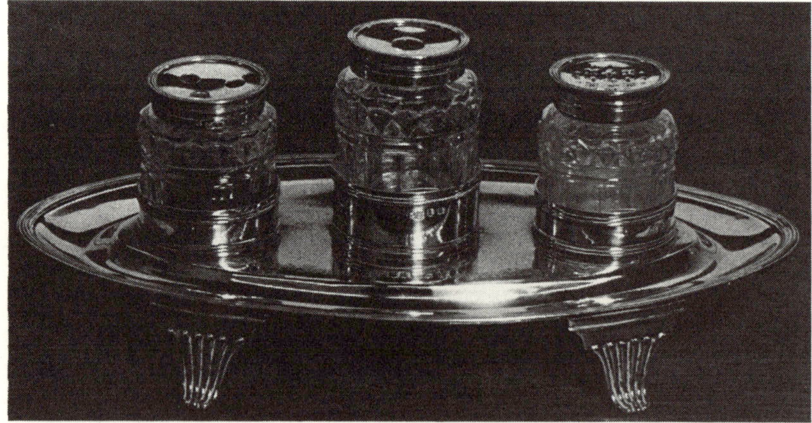

Edward Jenner's Inkstand. Used also by S. Weir Mitchell *(Abbe Collection, College of Physicians).*

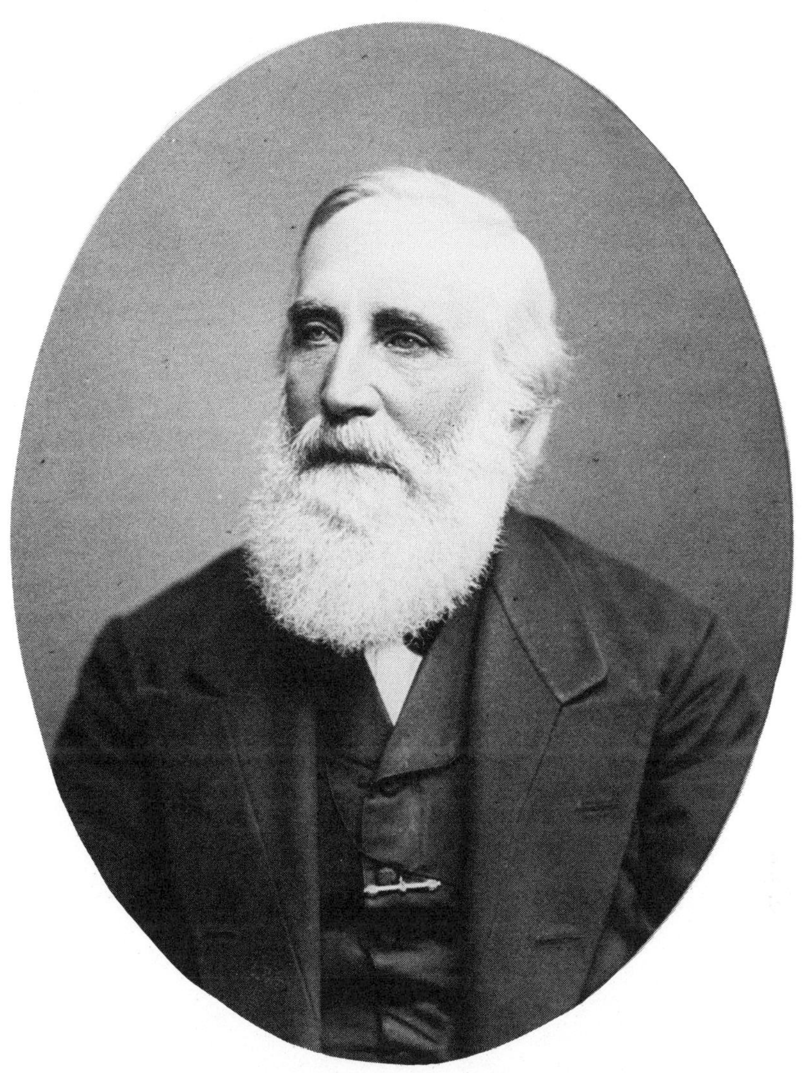

Alfred Stillé, (1813–1900). Photograph by Wenderoth & Co., Philadelphia.

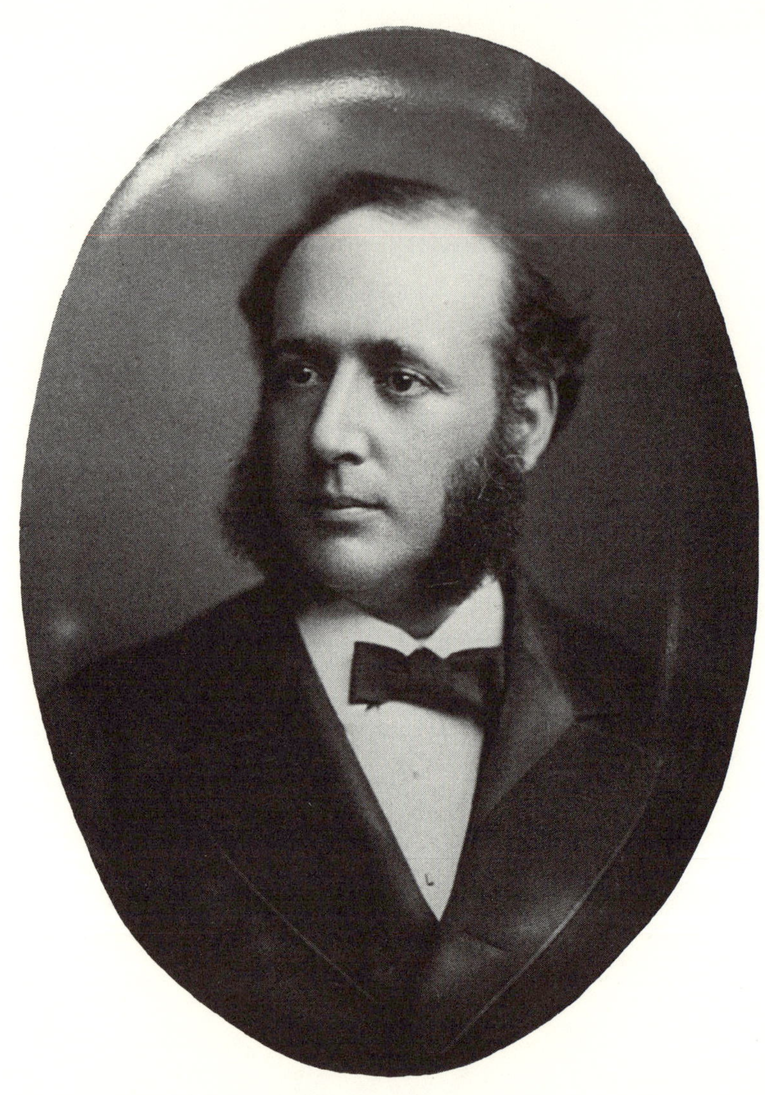

Jacob Mendez DaCosta, (1833–1900). Photograph by F. Gutekunst, Philadelphia.

CHAPTER VIII

# The Age of Weir Mitchell – I

NO man of his generation, perhaps no single individual in its long history, did so much for the College as Silas Weir Mitchell. A Fellow for fifty-eight years, he gave his first paper to the College, concerning protracted sleep, shortly after his election in 1856; his last, on marking the sites of Union and Confederate hospitals at Gettysburg, was read a few months before his death on January 4, 1914, in his eighty-fifth year. He served on a score of standing and special committees, represented the College frequently as a delegate to the American Medical Association, was elected a councillor in 1883, vice-president in 1884, and in 1886 president for the first of two non-consecutive terms. Mitchell proposed the Nurses' Directory, encouraged the creation of specialty sections within the College, and in his eighties was hoping that some Philadelphian would endow a laboratory of research, attached to the College, comparable to the Rockefeller Institute of New York. His concern for the library was unceasing. He contributed constantly to its collections, established its journal fund, and only a month before he died urged that a catalogue of its incunabula be published and that the College issue a monthly bulletin or newsletter that would include notes on books, portraits, and relics. In 1887 Mitchell presided with dignity and style over the observance of the centennial anniversary of the College; in 1909 he was the principal figure in exercises opening the new hall on Twenty-second Street, for which he was primarily responsible. The years between may fairly be called the age of Weir Mitchell.[1]

The son and grandson of physicians, a graduate of Jefferson Medical College, where his father was a professor, Mitchell early achieved distinction in experimental research. He was a founder of the Pathological Society in 1857 and read a paper at its first meeting. The next year, with Joseph Leidy, J. Aitken Meigs, Wiliam A. Hammond, and others, he organized the Biological Section of the Academy of Natural Sciences of Philadelphia, offering at its first meeting a paper on "Blood Crystals of the Sturgeon." Mitchell's early research on the venom of rattlesnakes—a subject that engaged him for years—was published in *Smithsonian Contributions to Knowledge* in 1860. His studies with William W. Keen and George R. Morehouse of *Gunshot Wounds and Other Injuries to Nerves,* published in 1864, won him a wide reputation and election to the National Academy of Sciences in 1865. In the twenty years after his first publication in 1852, Mitchell wrote over forty papers on physiology, toxicology, and pharmacology.

Despite demonstrated abilities and his own ambitions, Mitchell failed to get a residency at the Pennsylvania Hospital and was never on its staff. Nor did he receive an appointment from the University of Pennsylvania or from Jefferson, where he might be thought to have had some claim as a graduate. As a member of the staff of the Orthopedic Hospital and Infirmary for Nervous Diseases after 1872, however, he made that institution the principal center in the country for the study of nervous diseases and mental disorders.

Mitchell's little book *Wear and Tear: or Hints for the Overworked* popularized the concept of exhaustion from tension and over-work. Not a few physicians, however, were skeptical of the notion; some even complained that, as it was written in simple, straightforward prose that laymen could understand, the book was a sort of self-advertisement and therefore possibly "unprofessional." Many of the subjects Mitchell studied seemed mere commonplace occurrences—headache, eye-strain, disturbed sleep, knee-jerk, melancholia, fear of cats—and were sometimes dismissed as trivial. In fact, Mitchell's studies showed him to be a first-rate investigator and an acute clinical observer.[2]

Among the general public Mitchell was famous as a man of letters. His first short story—'The Case of George Dedlow," based on wartime hospital experience—appeared in 1866. Warned against the popular prejudice that no one who wrote novels and poetry could be serious about science, Mitchell published no more fiction for fifteen years. Then appeared *Hepzibah Guinness,* a tale of strong religious feeling; it was the first of several novels notable for their insights into the psychology of women, a subject unusual in contemporary fiction. Mitchell also wrote several volumes of poetry, innumerable verses for special occasions like the centennial of the College of Physicians, children's stories, historical works like *The Youth of Washington,* and such an astonishing *tour-de-force* as "A Madeira Party." His most successful and best-known book, for which his name is still most readily recognized outside the medical profession, was *Hugh Wynne: Free Quaker,* a tale of Philadelphia during the Revolution. Some critics and many readers compared it—too generously—to *Henry Esmond.*

A man of his own time, place, and class, who distrusted democracy, denied that all men are in fact equal, and had no sympathy for the growing women's rights movement, Mitchell was a patrician to his fingertips. His presidential addresses to the College had the lofty tone of majesty addressing the commons. But, judging persons as individuals, he recognized worth wherever he saw it, promoted the careers of able young men, made and kept friends as different as Sarah Butler Wister, Hideyo Noguchi, and John Shaw Billings. He lived by the code of gentlemanly honor: when an officer of the bank of which he was a director absconded, Mitchell called on his fellow directors to make good the depositors' losses, and paid his share from his own pocket. He was a man of commanding presence, his powerful personality tempered by grace and kindness. In his latter years his birthday was greeted with editorials in Philadelphia newspapers, as though he were an institution—which he was. "He was probably the most picturesque and many-sided physician of his time," Harvey Cushing wrote of him, "—and he knew it."[3]

Fond of the forms and ceremonies of social life, of good talk, good food and wine, he endowed a fund to enable the Fellows of the College to dine together from time to time; and his wife presented a loving cup, which passed from lip to lip on such occasions, until the implications of the germ theory prevailed over the ties of friendship. Saturday evenings found him "at home" at 1524 Walnut Street, where some of the best talk in Philadelphia might be heard. Cushing was taken there after a meeting at the College—"a memorable midnight session," he recalled, with William W. Keen and Mitchell's son John, where the men talked of Robert Burns, *Robinson Crusoe,* Samuel Johnson, and William Harvey until three o'clock in the morning, and drank Madeira that had been three times around the Horn.

## *Centennial, 1887*

Mitchell's professional distinction, his devotion to the College and knowledge of its history, his personal dignity and social graces all helped make observance of the one-hundredth anniversary of the College in 1887 a memorable event. It was another in the succession of centennials that had begun at Lexington and Concord in 1875, reached an early climax at Philadelphia in 1876, and would continue until 1889, when the inauguration of Washington and the new federal government was commemorated. Just as those anniversaries were a celebration of the success of American independence and union, so the College centennial came when physicians could point to indisputable advances in medicine. The carefully prepared program was an expression of pride in the College, its activities and achievements, its history and traditions; it also reflected increased confidence in medical science and the medical profession.[4]

I. Minis Hays, always aware of historical associations and sensitive to the importance of preserving ancient landmarks, in 1884 made the first suggestion that the College centennial be marked.[5] The committee appointed to make plans offered several recommendations: that the hall be enlarged by the addition of a third floor, that the ranks of Associates be filled, and that an exhibition be held of portraits of deceased Fellows. On these suggestions there was little discussion. But the proposal that the celebration be held in April rather than on January 2, 1887—the anniversary of the first recorded meeting, which had always been accepted as the founding date of the College—met with spirited and prolonged opposition. A position paper setting out the reasons for and against the two dates was ordered prepared and circulated; and with this in their hands the Fellows voted sixty to forty-one (the total was larger than the number who attended the centennial events) to celebrate on January 3–4 (January 2 being a Sunday).[6]

In one sense the centennial celebration opened at the stated meeting in October 1886, when W. S. W. Ruschenberger read a history of the College, based on minutes and publications, other printed sources, and careful research in the papers of Benjamin

Rush. Greatly expanded, with appendixes and biographical notes on all the Fellows, the history was printed in both the Centennial Volume and separately as a book.[7]

The Fellows felt a good deal of pleasurable excitement as the anniversary day approached. "Big time—Big time!!!" Samuel W. Gross exclaimed in a letter outlining the program to John Shaw Billings.[8] The leisurely two-day exercises opened with a carefully prepared, eloquent, often moving address by Weir Mitchell. Although primarily historical, with vignettes of the founders and recollections of his own early years in the College, it also noted the College's involvement in public affairs, spoke with pride of the library and museum, and concluded with a tribute to the 104 Fellows who had served in the Union forces during the Civil War. In another historical address the venerable Alfred Stillé described the College as it was forty years before, when he was elected a Fellow.

Nine distinguished physicians and surgeons were admitted as Associate Fellows; they included Hunter McGuire of Richmond, Virginia, Nicholas Senn of Milwaukee, Henry P. Bowditch and George C. Shattuck of Boston, and R. Palmer Howard of Montreal. A special feature of the centennial was an exhibition of 103 portraits from collections of the College, other Philadelphia institutions, and private individuals, mostly descendants of the subjects. Some of these paintings were donated to the College on this occasion or soon afterwards.[9] The anniversary celebration was capped with a formal dinner at the Union League, attended by 120 Fellows and guests. In the fashion of the day an appropriate quotation—each from Shakespeare—accompanied each course, from oysters on the shell ("Gape open wide and eat him quicke." *Richard III,* I, ii) to roquefort and brie ("Sullen presage of your own decay." *King John,* I, 1). There were seven toasts, verses by Henry Hartshorne, and a final salute by Mitchell:

A grander morning floods our skies
With higher aims, and larger light,
Give welcome to the century new,
And to the past a glad good-night—!

The total expense for the two days was $2,806.06.

The Centennial brought the College to the attention of Philadelphia. Though the College was a local organization, observed the *Medical News,* its members—Morgan, Shippen, Rush, Chapman, Wood, Gross, and many others—belonged not to the College or to Philadelphia alone, "but to the history of the profession in this country."[10] More gratifying, because it came from a rival city, was an editorial in the *Boston Medical and Surgical Journal:* the College of Physicians, it said, was just such an institution "as we . . . would like to see flourishing in our large cities, especially in such as are centres of medical thought and education."[11]

### *Fellowship*

The membership of the College grew more rapidly after the mid-1880s. Six Fellows were elected in 1880, and five in 1881; but in the next three years the numbers were nine, sixteen, and twenty-three. In the fifteen years from 1885, when sixteen were chosen, through 1899, when thirteen were elected, 217 resident members were added to the rolls, an average of 14.5 every year. The total resident membership of the College in 1885, the year before Weir Mitchell became president, was 195; at the end of 1900 it stood at 292. Membership was increasing at more than six a year—twice the rate in the two decades before 1885.

In the centennial year of the College sixteen Fellows were elected. They included Howard A. Kelly, soon to go to Johns Hopkins, the surgeon John B. Deaver, and three—George E. de Schweinitz, Thomas R. Neilson, and William J. Taylor—who became presidents of the College after 1910. Their elections were followed in the ensuing years by those of James M. Anders (1888), an early advocate of public health and industrial medicine; Lawrence F. Flick (1888), whose name is inseparably associated with the prevention and control of tuberculosis and the care of tubercular patients; Joseph Price and Charles S. Penrose (both 1889), famous obstetricians, who were the principal figures in a notorious case of professional misconduct; Charles W. Burr (1892) and William G. Spiller (1897), followers of Weir Mitchell in neurology; David L. Edsall (1899), whose plans for reform of the University of Pennsylvania Medical School were unappreciated and who went on to become dean of the Harvard Medical School; and Francis R. Packard (1897), a successful otolaryngologist, who achieved more

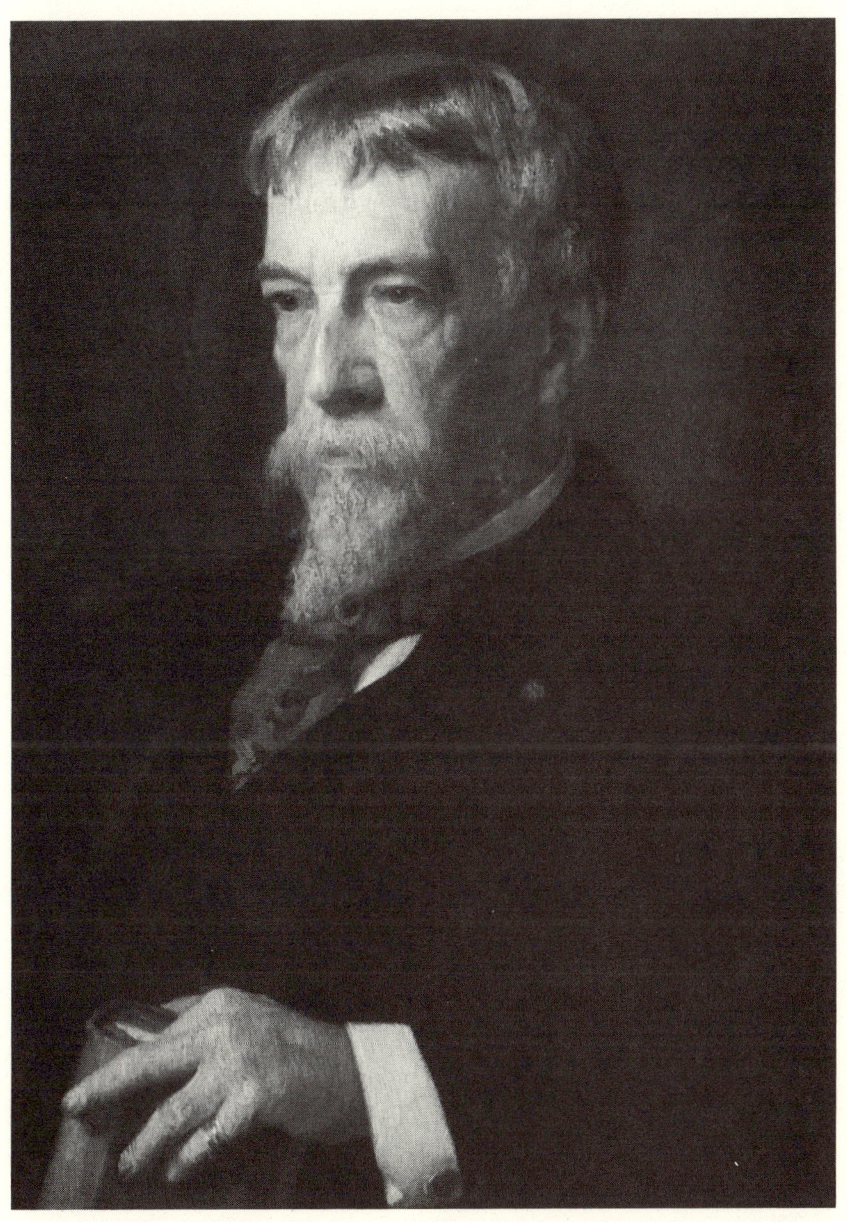

S. Weir Mitchell, (1829–1914). Portrait by Robert W. Vonnoh.

lasting reputation as the historian of American and Philadelphia medicine.

The last fifteen years of the century saw also an increase in the number of Associate Fellows, both American and foreign. The list contains the names of Abraham Jacobi of New York (1891), distinguished pediatrician and friend of the College and of Weir Mitchell; Oliver Wendell Holmes of Boston (1892), whose portrait was presented to the College, he and Mitchell exchanging graceful verses on the occasion; William H. Welch (1892) and William T. Councilman (1893) of the new Johns Hopkins Medical School; Reginald H. Fitz of Boston (1892) and Charles McBurney of New York (1895), whose names are linked in the history of appendicitis; and Robert Fletcher (1895), the scholarly assistant editor of the *Index-Catalogue* of the Surgeon-General's Library. From Europe Rudolph Virchow was chosen an Assocate Fellow in 1891, T. Lauder Brunton of London and Sir Thomas Grainger Stewart of Edinburgh in 1894 and 1896 respectively.

### *Public Health: Cholera*

Stillé and Da Costa in their presidential reports had claimed an important role for the College in matters of public health. Mitchell shared their view. "We are not merely physicians meeting to hear and to discuss facts and theories," he told the Fellows in 1888. Their most important duty was "that of incessant watchfulness of all public interests in which questions of health are concerned," and he mentioned matters that had engaged the College's attention in the preceding three years: quarantine, sanitation, water supplies, sewerage, sales of poisons, abattoirs. Some of these specific concerns arose from the threatened outbreak of cholera in 1884 and 1885, just before Mitchell was elected president of the College.

The appearance of the disease in Asia and Europe in 1883 and 1884 alarmed physicians and public health officials in the Atlantic port cities of the United States. Cholera appeared to be moving across Europe in much the same way as in previous epidemics; sooner or later it was expected to reach North America. Many physicians had had personal experience in earlier epidemics; others had read or heard accounts from their teachers and preceptors of the terrible mortality of 1832. All knew what they might expect.

Accordingly, the College of Physicians on February 4, 1885, called on the Philadelphia City Councils to prepare for the emergency before it was too late. In particular, the College asked that the Board of Health be strengthened, that it be empowered to appoint committees to make house-to-house visits in areas at risk, and to clean up the city, establish dispensaries, and prepare hospitals to receive the sick. There was a tone of urgency in the memorial: "The work should be done now and with great care . . . ."[12]

Although the recommendations about cleanliness, overcrowding, water supply, diet, and prompt treatment were like those made in former years, there was a difference—physicians were now acquainted with bacteriology and knew something about the cause of the disease, its prevention and methods of treatment. At the same meeting of the College when its memorial to the City Councils was approved, Edward O. Shakespeare, who was deeply interested in epidemiology, exhibited a specimen of the cholera bacillus together with microphotographs made by his young colleague George A. Piersol, demonstrator in histology at the University of Pennsylvania.[13]

A few months later, as a result of a personal approach by Weir Mitchell to Secretary of State Thomas F. Bayard, President Cleveland on October 1, 1885, commissioned Shakespeare to visit Spain to investigate the outbreak of cholera there. To prepare for his work Shakespeare visited Berlin, where he became acquainted with the comma bacillus of Koch, which he later described as "a diagnostic sign of the greatest practical value for the early recognition of the presence of the true Asiatic cholera." During a year abroad Shakespeare observed the disease in a score of Spanish and Italian cities, and in the spring of 1886 made a short trip to India. Immediately on his return home, he was invited to address the College. So that the Fellows could examine his slides for themselves, he brought along a number of microscopes. Eventually, Shakespeare produced a long, detailed account of his observations and findings.[14]

In the next year, the fall of 1887, the first cases of the long fearfully awaited cholera appeared among newly-arrived immigrants. Both the fears and the preparatory measures of the preceding three years now seemed justified. The College named a special committee composed of James C. Wilson as chairman, Richard A. Cleeman, and Shakespeare to investigate quarantine arrangements in Philadelphia, New York, and Baltimore. The committee reported promptly on October 28, 1887; and the report was printed in the *Medical News* the next day.[15] After endorsing a long series of recommendations about prevention and treatment, the committee described the organization and administration of quarantine laws in the several cities, judged them all deficient, and concluded that such matters should be placed in the hands of the federal government. The committee asked to be continued to prepare an appeal to the medical societies of the country.

This second report was submitted to the College on December 7, printed and distributed to the Fellows, and approved and ordered circulated on December 18. It was a masterly review of public health legislation and enforcement in the several port cities. These laws and regulations, the report pointed out, "have seldom or never been drafted with a full recognition of the need of adequate and constant protection of the health of the general public," but had been adopted piecemeal in response to particular emergencies. The committee explained why the laws were inadequate, recommended that a national system of maritime quarantine be adopted, and asked the several medical societies in the country to endorse the proposed reform. "Never since I have known the College," Weir Mitchell remarked with satisfaction as he reviewed the year's work, "has it been more usefully active."[16]

The late winter of 1893 witnessed another cholera scare. The disease appeared in Hamburg, and a few months later there were a few cases of "choleraic disorder" in Jersey City, New Jersey. The College responded swiftly. A committee headed by Shakespeare conferred with the mayor and heads of city departments, and received assurance of cooperation to prevent the disease and improve the health of the city. To these ends the committee enlisted the cooperation of the physicians of the city, who were asked to report to the College committee not only "filth, foul water, garbage, faulty pavement, obstructed gutters, faulty sewers, foul smells," but also all cases "of Suspicious Bowel Disturbance." As it turned out, cholera did not appear in Philadelphia. Although the committee received many complaints about the physical conditions of streets, alleys, and tenements, no case of bowel complaint was deemed sufficiently dangerous or suspicious to warrant its being reported to the College or the Board of Health. As far as cholera was concerned, the summer passed uneventfully.[17]

### *Public Health: Tuberculosis*

The programs of the stated meetings of the College in these years are virtually a record of advances in medical science. A part of that record of acceptance—and resistance to acceptance—of new developments and techniques is preserved in the printed *Transactions.* The reception of Robert Koch's discovery of the tubercle bacillus in 1882 is one example. Koch's paper was published in *Berliner klinische Wochenschrift* on April 10. In September James T. Whittaker, professor of medicine in the Medical College of Ohio in Cincinnati, addressed the College on the subject. After reviewing the work of Villemin, Cohnheim, von Tappeiner, and other investigators, Whittaker described Koch's research, with its evidence of the transmissibility of tuberculosis through sputum, concluding that this was the "clue" to control of the disease. "When the phthisical patient pulls out his sputum-saturated handkerchief," Whittaker warned in a mixed figure, "he opens the box of Pandora on the public highways."[18]

Some Fellows at once acclaimed Koch's discovery. Shakespeare went abroad the next year to work with both Koch and Pasteur,[19] George A. Piersol exhibited to the College photographs that he had made of the bacillus .[20] William H. Webb denounced the skeptics in spirited terms:

> The discovery of the tubercle-bacillus is a scientific fact. . . . To doubt its existence in tuberculosis is to doubt the utility of scientific medical research, and to abandon further progress to the unstable dreams of theorists. The sputa of the phthisical contain these germs; the air they exhale is loaded with them or their spores, and their introduction into the system of animals will always produce tuberculosis, *while nothing else will.* These are not speculations, but demonstrable facts![21]

The facts were not demonstrable to everyone, however. Arthur V. Meigs, son and grandson of Fellows and himself destined to become president of the College, never accepted them. Although he had studied in Paris and was generally considered to be a successful physician, he had little confidence in medical science. "It is my belief," Meigs wrote of tuberculosis in 1911, the year before his death, "that the proof is still wanting that this microorganism is the one and only cause of the disease."[22] The sentiment was only another expression of that "intense conservatism" which contemporaries noted in him. His son explained it in terms that might also have been applied to other Fellows who, while resisting medical innovations, were nonetheless able, successful, and respected:

> . . . throughout his life he stood opposed to most of his contemporaries on certain fundamental medical questions. He had little belief in the view, which came to be almost universally accepted toward the end of his life [1912], that microorganisms are the causes of many if not all of the infectious diseases. . . .
>
> To me my father's position on this subject seems not so very surprising; I can understand how it was brought about by his conservatism and by his independence of judgment. We had many discussions on this subject from my first year in the medical school onward, and the storm centre of these was always the subject of tuberculosis. In looking back I can see how his unwillingness to admit that the tubercle bacillus was the chief cause of tuberculosis was connected with many other things—with his dislike of new theories and of new ways of doing things, with his respect for what he had learned from his father and his grandfather, with the small ground which his actual clinical experience gave him for believing in the contagiousness of tuberculosis, and with his unwillingness to accept important views on hearsay evidence, without some kind of definite confirmatory experience of his own.
>
> His mind had a peculiar quality of exactness; he never deluded himself into thinking that he understood a matter until he had thoroughly grasped it. This quality was connected with a dislike of most kinds of theorizing, and his attitude toward many of the great scientific generalizations of the eighteenth and nineteenth centuries was one of scepticism. He was a great admirer of Darwin, and accepted the doctrine of the transmutation of species. But he always adopted a waiting attitude toward the conclusion which to most minds seems to follow directly from that doctrine—the conclusion, namely, that all animals on

> the earth, including man, are only the different members of one great family group. His attitude toward the atomic theory was more or less similar; though he had the greatest interest in the facts on which that theory is based, it always seemed to him to be going too far to imagine matter as made up of fifty or sixty kinds of little particles, all eternally different from each other. The recent great discoveries in physics and chemistry seem to more or less justify this attitude on his part.[23]

Although contagiousness of tuberculosis continued to be discussed, the debate now turned more frequently on problems of control and prevention. In a paper to the College on February 5, 1890, Lawrence F. Flick called for establishing special hospitals for the treatment of tuberculous patients. In a broad survey of the history, organization, and operation of such institutions, especially in England and Germany, Flick concluded that these hospitals had materially reduced the incidence of the disease: "What we want is large, commodious, well-equipped special charity, or semi-charity hospitals for the treatment of tuberculous diseases in convenient proximity to our large cities, and the sufficient in-patient capacity to accommodate all who may apply for admission." The discussion was long and thoughtful; those who took part, though differing with Flick on particular points, accepted the desirability of segregating tuberculosis patients.[24] This was one of the earliest steps in the crusade Flick initiated and led for forty years to reduce and eliminate tuberculosis in the United States.

Tireless, energetic, not always a tactful advocate, Flick was a superb organizer and a master of publicity. In the College, however, he never held office and in fact seems to have had little influence there .[25] His proposals for a municipal hospital for consumptives were repeatedly rejected. His suggestion that Herman Biggs of Bellevue Hospital Medical School, who had done so much for the prevention of the disease in New York, be invited to address the College was turned down. A motion that the College cooperate with the County Medical Society and the Philadelphia Veterinary Society to inquire into tuberculosis in animals and the food supply was judged by the Council "inadvisable." "No action was taken" on an invitation from the Women's Health Protective Association to a meeting at which the contagiousness of tuberculosis was to be discussed.

Yet the question could not be ignored or dismissed. In 1893 the

County Medical Society called on the Philadelphia Board of Health to place pulmonary consumption on the list of contagious diseases and to order all cases to be registered and the measures usually observed in such instances to be enforced. The proposition was strongly opposed in the College. Owen J. Wister, presenting a resolution to this end, denounced registration as "cruel, unnecessary and impracticable," and argued that as far as it was communicable at all, pulmonary consumption might be handled by "the careful observation of the ordinary rules of cleanliness and decency together with efficient sterilization of sputa." Mitchell added the weight of his influence to opposition to registration.[26]

Flick responded with a substitute for Wister's resolution:

> 1. That tuberculosis has been demonstrated to be a contagious disease.
>
> 2. That tuberculosis can be prevented by proper sanitary measures.
>
> 3. That the contagiousness of tuberculosis need inspire no fear and preventive measures need produce no hardship, because the contagion resides only in broken down tissue, a thorough sterilization of which makes the consumption harmless.
>
> 4. That, for the protection of the consumptive poor, tuberculosis ought to be placed upon the list of diseases returnable to the Board of Health.
>
> 5. That the City of Philadelphia ought to establish a special hospital for the treatment of persons suffering from tuberculosis who voluntarily seek admission into a hospital, and who are now being turned away from other hospitals.

Presented with two opposing recommendations, the Council approved instead a third, submitted by the vice-president Jacob M. Da Costa, and called a special meeting of the College to discuss it. Da Costa's resolution rejected registration as a practice that "could not lead to any measures of real value not otherwise attainable," expressed confidence that "strict attention" by the attending physician to disinfection, ventilation, and the separation of the sick from the well could do more than the Board of Health, and urged City Councils not to enact the proposed ordinance, except to require disinfection of rooms.

Wister opened the special meeting on January 12, 1894.[27] The proposed registration, he remarked sardonically, regarded tubercular patients "as criminals guilty of consumption," their miserable lives "haunted by the familiars of the Inquisition," which was how he described the inspectors of the Board of Health. Flick responded with more statistics and new resolutions, which, taking into account criticisms of registration, proposed that infected houses, not persons, be registered and disinfected. He repeated his call for a municipal hospital for consumptives:

> The College of Physicians should now take a firm stand and do something in aid of these people. It is not necessary to do everything at once. Let us make a beginning. Experiments have been made, let us now come to action. It is not fair to the public that the medical profession, with the knowledge it possesses, should do nothing. The laity cannot act because they have not the knowledge. If we who have the knowledge do nothing we are certainly responsible for the deaths of those who otherwise might be saved.

Many of those who discussed the issue believed that tuberculosis was not "markedly contagious," that it was hereditary, and that any scheme for its total extirpation "under present conditions of civilized society" was, in the words of Frank Woodbury, "entirely impracticable, and . . . chimerical." Solomon Solis-Cohen feared that registration would divert attention from the need to cleanse and widen streets and alleys, drain and ventilate houses, provide proper food and clothing to the poor. Control and elimination of tuberculosis, he declared, depended on personal and community hygiene. John Shaw Billings in a written statement raised some practical questions about enforcement, as did Horatio C Wood. Other physicians, such as James Tyson, simply had no confidence in the Board of Health and resented its involvement in matters they believed physicians were fully competent to deal with. "Let it [the Board of Health] leave the care of the individual where it belongs," Da Costa said, "—to the conscientious physician." Only Osler, who had come from Baltimore for the meeting, and John B. Roberts supported Flick and registration. "Not the physician," declared the latter, "but some central body should have the authority to ascertain the facts and enforce such measures as will limit the spread of the disease among the poor. If we limit it among the poor, we limit it among the rich."

The sentiment of the meeting was clearly against Flick's proposals. The discussion concluded with reference to the cautious conduct of which so many Fellows were so proud. "I feel sure," said Charles W. Dulles, who in addition to being a surgeon on the staffs of the Rush and Presbyterian Hospitals, was lecturer on the history of medicine at the University of Pennsylvania,

> that the College will act in keeping with its traditions of a hundred years, and give new illustration of the fact that it is a body in which prudent and conservative counsels prevail, and I have no fear that it will hastily commit itself, as a sister society has done, under the ingenious arguments of those strongly infected with the idea of the infectiousness of tuberculosis.

Dulles' confidence was well-founded: the College rejected Flick's motion and approved the Council's resolution opposing registration and the establishment of a hospital for consumptives.[28]

Less than twenty years later the College reached another conclusion and formally recorded its opinion "that Tuberculosis is a contagious disease transmissible from one person to another," and that the Director of Public Health should be empowered to remove "to suitable hospitals or sanitaria" sufferers from the disease who were "a menace" to family and neighbors.[29]

### *Public Health: Overseas*

Sometimes the stated meetings reflected America's expanding political and economic role in the world. An account of the educational work of John C. Berry, a recent graduate of Jefferson Medical College and a medical missionary at Kobe, Japan, was presented by William W. Keen in 1878. The next year Robert P. Harris described foot-binding in China, with illustrative specimens obtained from Flemming Carrow of a missionary hospital at Canton. (Carrow was elected a corresponding member of the College in 1880.) In 1887 H. W. Boone, surgeon of St. Luke's Hospital in Shanghai, reported on the introduction of Western medicine into China and appealed for books, apparatus, anatomical preparations, and other teaching materials. An illustrated lecture on the leper colony on Molokai by Benjamin Sharp of the Academy of Natural Sciences of Philadelphia, elicited a lively discussion led by Louis A. Duhring. Simon Flexner of Johns Hopkins and Louis F. Atlee, late surgeon of the U.S.S. *Olympia,* reported on conditions found by the Philippine Medical Commission in 1899.[30]

At the same meeting at which Boone spoke, Weir Mitchell commented briefly on the researches and publications of Carlos Finlay on yellow fever.[31] Finlay was a graduate of Jefferson Medical College, where Mitchell's father had been one of his professors. In 1886 he published in the *American Journal of the Medical Sciences* an account of some experiments on the transmission of yellow fever by mosquitos. In 1887 he sent Mitchell cultures he had prepared; Mitchell turned them over to William H. Welch in Baltimore and Osler at the University of Pennsylvania. In Philadelphia they were examined also by George Dock and Edward O. Shakespeare, who, like other reviewers of Finlay's work, pronounced his procedure defective and his evidence unconvincing. "We are far from having any unassailable proof that the organism presented here has anything to do with the etiology of yellow fever," they reported.[31] Fifteen years later the proof was in; and on January 7, 1903, Finlay and William C. Gorgas, the Army medical officer who controlled yellow fever in Cuba, were elected Associate Fellows of the College.

Walter Reed, whose Army Yellow Fever Commission proved that it is the Stegomyia (now *Aedes aegypti*) that transmits the disease, would also have been elected on January 7, but he died on November 23, 1902, before his election could be completed. The College informed Reed's family of its intention, and "heartily" supported a bill in Congress to give Mrs. Reed a pension "as a most desirable and commendable recognition of Major Reed's splendid work for his country and for science." At the same time, citing the sanitation achievement in Cuba, the College urged that the Panama Canal Commission include a medical officer, and that "the amplest powers should be given to the medical officers in charge of the Sanitation of the Canal."[32] This reasonable suggestion was ignored and opposed by the political and military appointees on the Commission. Disease seriously impeded construction work, until finally President Roosevelt, after a personal visit to Panama, named Gorgas to the Commission.

### *Practice: Appendicitis*

While the treatment of tuberculosis and the cause of yellow fever were being debated, another advance was made in the surgical medical world. Addressing the Association of American Physicians in 1886, Reginald H. Fitz of Boston described in careful detail symptoms of the inflamed vermiform appendix and concluded that the condition should be treated by surgical removal. On April 27, 1887, in an operation in the Pennsylvania Hospital done in response to diagnosis of a diseased appendix, Thomas G. Morton removed the organ. That same evening Morton's colleague Frank Woodbury reported the case to the Philadelphia County Medical Society. A few weeks later at a stated meeting of the College on June 1, he and Morton described this and two other operations.[33]

Thereafter, removal of diseased appendixes became increasingly common, especially in Philadelphia, where John B. Deaver at the German (now Lankenau) Hospital made the operation his specialty, performing several operations almost daily. In 1899 he reported to the College on 460 operations done in the preceding two years: of 264 acute cases, he lost forty-six or 17.4%; but of 196 chronic cases not one failed to recover.[34] Arthur V. Meigs, however, was unconvinced, deprecating such surgical intervention in what he regarded as essentially a medical condition. It is ironical that he should have died a victim of his principle in this matter. His friend and colleague Robert G. LeConte, attending Meigs in what proved to be his last illness, diagnosed a ruptured abdominal abscess and urged immediate surgery. The patient refused on the ground that he had never approved such operations.[35]

### *Practice: X-Rays*

No medical discovery in the last quarter of the century was so quickly reported or so universally adopted as Röntgen's discovery of x-rays. He presented his paper—"Eine Neue Art von Strahlen"—in mid-December 1895; preprints were available by January 1; and the proceedings of the medical society of Würzburg including the article appeared a few days later. An English translation was printed in the British journal *Nature* on January 23. In the next two or three weeks, other articles, scientific, descriptive, and popular, appeared in journals and newspapers in the United States as well as in Europe and Britain. The succession of dates alone indicates the intense excitement the Philadelphia scientists felt at the reports. The *Nature* translation was reprinted in the March issue of the *Journal of the Franklin Institute.*[36] On February 19 in a session of the College devoted to intracranial tumors, William W. Keen cited inability to diagnose the location, size, nature, and number of such tumors as "unquestionably" the chief obstacle to their treatment by surgery. Then he added, "Possibly the recent discovery of Röntgen may assist us."[37]

Even as Keen spoke, the assistance was forthcoming. At the University of Pennsylvania Arthur W. Goodspeed, assistant professor of physics, who had been doing research with Crookes tubes, repeated Röntgen's experiments successfully on February 5; he reported on his work in *Science* on February 14.[38] At the Franklin Institute, on the same evening on which Keen addressed the College, Edwin J. Houston and A. E. Kennelly, partners in their own firm of consulting electrical engineers, presented a long paper on "The Röntgen Rays." Two nights later, on February 21, the American Philosophical Society suspended its regular order of business so that Goodspeed might present "the entire subject in detail." Attendance was two or three times greater than usual; and there was a lively discussion by Houston, William Pepper, and others.[39]

The College now organized a program on the clinical application of Röntgen rays; it was held on March 4, 1896, only two months after the discovery was published. William F. Magie, professor of physics in Princeton University, described and demonstrated the instrument; Keen spoke on the value of x-rays in surgical diagnosis; and Edward P. Davis read a paper on the use of x-rays to study the infant's body and the pregnant woman's womb. The session attracted seventy-nine Fellows and uncounted guests and strangers. During a scheduled intermission they inspected the equipment, watched a demonstration, and examined the "skiagraphs," as x-rays were then called.[40] On June 3 Robert G. LeConte reported to the College on his removal that morning of a bullet imbedded in a man's neck; he illustrated the report with an x-ray taken by Professor Goodspeed. Jefferson's professor of surgery John H. Brinton, who had attended the operation, testified that he had never seen such an operation performed more boldly and confidently. "I realized what an immense boon had been given to us in this process, which throws light in dark places."[41]

Within six months x-rays were in general use in the principal hospitals. Medical journals were flooded with notes, cases, and reviews of the subject. Several appeared in the *Transactions* of the College in the first few years after the 1896 symposium. Deaver, who x-rayed about five hundred patients in 1897 alone, nonetheless warned of the danger in "absolute dependence upon the x-ray" to the neglect of diagnosis by touch.[42] Charles L. Leonard, who had worked with Goodspeed and White in 1896 and was now "Skiagrapher" to the Hospital of the University of Pennsylvania, used x-rays to diagnose calculi in the urinary tract. "The diagnosis it affords," he assured the Fellows, "is absolute, both positively and negatively, and has the advantages of mathematical accuracy."[43] Like other pioneers in the development of x-rays, Leonard fell a victim to them, losing first his fingers, then a hand, finally an arm; and died prematurely at fifty-two.

### *Sections for Specialties*

By 1892, when Weir Mitchell was elected president of the College for his second three-year term, physicians had for some time been separating themselves into specialties, no longer identifying themselves simply as physicians, surgeons, or obstetricians, but more precisely as pediatricians, laryngologists, urologists, ophthalmologists, dermatologists, neurologists, and the like. The creation of sections within the College was thus a recognition, albeit tardy and reluctant, of one of the striking developments in medicine in the last third of the century. In winning acceptance for the specialties, Mitchell's support was here, as so often elsewhere, significant, even decisive.[44]

In fact, division into specialties had already taken place in Philadelphia, not to mention Boston, New York, and the nation generally.[45] In 1890 there were or had been Philadelphia societies devoted to pathology, obstetrics, ophthalmology, laryngology, neurology, surgery, and medical jurisprudence. There was a children's hospital, a lying-in hospital, a hospital for diseases of the eye, and an orthopedic hospital and infirmary for nervous diseases. The existence of these societies and institutions, many felt, afforded sufficient scholarly and clinical opportunities of a specialized nature; in their view the College should remain a general medical society where practitioners and researchers in every specialty might address scientific and professional concerns of common interest.

The first request for a section came from the ophthalmologists. In 1890 Edward Jackson, a surgeon at Wills Hospital, asked that a room be reserved, one evening each month, for such Fellows as desired to meet there.[46] Permission was given and the meetings were organized, with William F. Norris as chairman; they proved successful and well-attended. The next year Jackson proposed that the College consider a general plan of sections "for the better cultivating of special branches of medical & surgical science." Weir Mitchell warmly supported the idea, not only because it had scientific merit but for the practical reason that the sections would relieve stated meetings of the College from the pressure of too many papers—a condition that relegated College business to the late hours, when only a handful of Fellows remained to discuss and vote. The Council, however, rejected Jackson's suggestions, saying that the fellowship was too small—it numbered 234 residents in 1891—to divide.[47] Doubtless a more basic reason was the widespread prejudice, especially among older Fellows, against specialization. They belonged to a tradition in which physicians took all medicine for their province, and regarded specialists, especially "eye-doctors," as only a step removed from quacks and charlatans.[48]

A year later, at the end of 1892, Jackson renewed his appeal. This time he presented the College with concrete rules and regulations for sections and the names of sixty-three Fellows who wished to join one or more—fourteen ophthalmologists, twenty-seven gynecologists, twenty-two orthopedists. Several discussions by the Fellows and the Council ensued, until finally the Council acceded to the wishes of the former, making it clear, however, that the change did not have its approval.[49]

The terms authorizing sections accommodated the opposing views. The specialists might establish sections, but only by permission of the president of the College, who was now Weir Mitchell, and only for three years. The College kept the sections under tight rein. The president of the College was the president of every section and appointed its executive committee. The clerk of the section had to send the secretary of the College a monthly report of the section's proceedings. The work of the section was to be "wholly and only scientific." Any Fellow might become a member of any section simply by signifying his wish to the clerk. Non-Fellows might attend meetings only if properly introduced by a Fellow; they might not speak unless invited to do so; and they must leave before the section opened its business session. The sections could meet only in the hall of the College, which would provide light, heat, and janitorial service. The College might abolish any section by a two-thirds vote.

Before the end of 1893, sections on ophthalmology, orthopedics, and otolaryngology were instituted. A section on gynecology was formed in 1895, and one on general medicine in 1897. Medical history was added in 1905. All the sections began with great enthusiasm. "There has been so much material brought forth," Jacob M. Da Costa reported in his presidential address in 1897,

> that it would have been impossible for the College, as a whole, to manage it, and the sections have proved themselves indispensable as fields for the working spirit of the College and in preventing the stated meetings from being overcrowded.[50]

In seventeen meetings over two years, thirty-three papers were read in the section on ophthalmology, fifty cases were presented, and nineteen specimens and eighteen instruments shown.[51] At some section meetings the number of Fellows in attendance exceeded the average attendance at the stated meetings of the College. Unfortunately, as Da Costa several times remarked, there was no room in the *Transactions* for the papers read in the sections, and no money to inaugurate a supplementary publication to print them. Authorization of the sections was extended in 1896, and they became a permanent feature of the College thereafter.

Within a few years, as was to have been expected, there was some falling off in interest. This was likely owing to the existence of larger, more representative specialist societies in the city. Orthopedics lasted only two years; in 1895 it was pronounced "dead beyond any hope of resuscitation."[52] General surgery expired in 1899, and gynecology in 1907. Those that survived seem to have done so by acquiring a life of their own. They invited speakers from outside the fellowship and from out of town. They came to regard non-Fellows who attended their meetings regularly as fellow-members of the section. They often planned their programs without reference to the College. Francis R. Packard, when president of the College in the 1930s, complained about this lack of deference and cooperation: the sections, he charged, were too independent and too casual about observing the terms of their creation.[53]

## *Two Failures of Collegiality*

As guardians and enforcers of canons of professional conduct, the College censors were called on from time to time to act in cases of alleged violations. Understandably, they were cautious, even reluctant, in such matters. An Associate Fellow was dismissed from the naval service for uttering falsehoods and other offences; the Censors judged such conduct unbecoming, but concluded they could take no action as they could not obtain his attendance at a hearing. For advertising a "New Elixir of Life," William A. Hammond was pronounced a "charlatanoid," but perhaps out of consideration for his real abilities and reputation and for his considerable services as Surgeon-General of the Army, no action was taken against him. But two other cases involving Fellows and the spirit of collegiality were too flagrant to ignore.

The first was a bitter personal attack of one Fellow on another. Joseph Price, of whom Howard A. Kelly wrote admiringly that he "found gynecology and abdominal surgery twin babes in swaddling clothes and left them, after a life of extraordinary activity, full grown specialties," was physician-in-charge of the lying-in hospital Preston Retreat. Although generously devoted to the poor, who then made up most of his practice, Price, as the event showed, possessed a wide streak of envy and jealousy and could be unrelenting in his enmities. Despite indisputable talents as a surgeon, he was never a professor.[54] With Charles B. Penrose, a recent graduate of the University of Pennsylvania Medical School, he was one of the first attending physicians of the Gynecean Hospital in 1888. Two years later the two men, until then close friends, were candidates for an appointment at the German Hospital. Price actively opposed Penrose's candidacy. In a bitter, intemperate letter to the president of the Hospital board, he alleged that his rival was "a blasphemer, an infidel and a libertine; that he had no respect for women and [that] he [Price] would not invite him to his house." Price made similar statements to others in institutions with which Penrose was connected. He charged there was "something rotten in the obstetrical teaching in the University," where Penrose was a professor, and derided the physicians and surgeons of the Pennsylvania Hospital as "damn stupid chumps."[55]

Despite this campaign against him, Penrose received the German Hospital appointment. In 1891 he formally charged Price with unprofessional behavior.

Charles B. Penrose was one of the most striking personalities who was ever a Fellow of the College.[56] The son of a Fellow, he was the brother of Richard, Boies, and Spencer, whose achievements were as outstanding as his own. He was graduated from the University of Pennsylvania Medical School at the age of twenty-two in 1884 and in the same year received a doctorate in physics from Harvard, where he had been an undergraduate. As a young man he once swam from Philadelphia to Chester, a distance of thirteen miles. Despite this display of athleticism, his health was not always strong, he developed pulmonary tuberculosis, and made several trips to the West to restore it. In Wyoming he was once mistaken for a rustler and escaped lynching only by the timely arrival of the United States marshal; and he was also attacked and mauled by a grizzly bear—his account of the experience is vivid and memorable. Six feet tall, powerfully built and strikingly handsome, unemotional and undemonstrative, he was an aristocrat who used his considerable power and influence in constructive ways for medicine and the public good.

After hearing Penrose's statement, the Censors recommended that Price be censured. Their report opened a discussion and debate so prolonged that at last it seemed as though the Censors, not Price, were on trial. Price demanded a hearing; when it was granted, he refused to speak. There was loose talk of legal rights, counsel, jury, and court-martial: "The whole thing is contrary to common law and everything else." Hoping to postpone a decision, the College directed the Censors to reconsider the case. This they did, extending their inquiry and returning a stronger recommendation that Price be "publicly censured . . . for his malevolent and unprofessional conduct," and asked to resign. Advised by its ever-cautious lawyer, the College took no action, but tabled the resolutions; whereupon the Censors resigned. The Fellows refused the resignations, but the Censors held firm in their decision. Summer vacations intervened to cool feelings and provide opportunity for an adjustment. It was offered by Weir Mitchell. "Public" censure, he suggested, need mean only an action within the College and made known to the Fellows; and he deplored the effect a repudiation of the Censors might have. Gratefully accepting this solution, the College approved the Censors' recommendations, and, relieved to put the sorry business behind them, voted to censure Price and request his resignation, which he offered. Now vindicated, the Censors withdrew their resignations; and the College amended its by-laws to define the Censors' authority in such cases in the future.[57]

The other case of censure a few years later was perhaps more serious than the Price-Penrose incident, for it involved the entire Fellowship and brought out a potential source of tension and disagreement that had long lurked below the surface of College business. It was rooted in the long-standing rivalry of the University of Pennsylvania and Jefferson Medical College.

From the moment Jefferson Medical College was established in 1824, members of the two institutions regarded one another with reserve, if not active ill will. Every faculty member in each school viewed his opposite in the other as a competitor for student fees and professional reputation and preferment. Jefferson resented Pennsylvania's assumption of superiority and its faculty's claim to the most prestigious professional appointments. Pennsylvania men regarded Jefferson as an upstart, and sometimes treated its faculty with ill-concealed contempt. William P. Dewees, adjunct professor of obstetrics at Pennsylvania, for example, refused to acknowledge the gift of a book by Samuel D. Gross of Jefferson, explaining to a mutual friend that "the Faculty of the University could take no notice of anything that emanated from the Jefferson School." George Bacon Wood of Pennsylvania, though a large-minded man, was surprised that Robley Dunglison of Jefferson, with whom he was thrown for several days in Washington, "proved himself to be . . . a very pleasant fellow;" and he thought it "somewhat singular" that two of his closest friends, Franklin Bache and Charles D. Meigs, should both be members of the rival school. "My feelings are in no respect altered towards them," he wrote; then added that he was not sure what his feelings would be if Jefferson should "triumph" over the University.[58]

In this situation it was inevitable that the fellowship and offices of the College should be not merely evidence of professional achievement and acceptance, but prizes for which the two parties contended. None of the first faculty of Jefferson, for example, were or ever became Fellows of the College, except George B. McClellan—but that was years after he had been dropped from Jefferson. Graduates of Pennsylvania were often elected Fellows within four or five years of receiving their degrees; but not until twenty years after Jefferson's first class was graduated was an alumnus of that school elected a member of the College. Weir Mitchell believed that his election was delayed a year or two because of this anti-Jefferson sentiment.[59] On the other hand, Jacob M. Da Costa of the Jefferson faculty was elected president of the College in 1884—which, given the long tenure of Wood and the inevitable succession of Ruschenberger,the vice-president, was about as early as a Jefferson graduate could have hoped to be considered for the post.

By the mid-1880's the mutual prejudices of the institutions, their faculties, and their graduates had considerably abated. One of the speakers at the Centennial dinner in 1887 contrasted the harmony currently prevailing in medical circles with the contentiousness, antagonisms, and violence of earlier periods; and he quoted a guest, "a physician from a neighboring town," as saying of Weir Mitchell's address, "I do wish that Dr. Mitchell had abused somebody."

That, of course, was not Mitchell's style. A great believer in the emollient effects of a good dinner, wine, and cigars, he proposed as early as 1877 that the president of the College give a reception annually in the Hall. Lacking funds, the Council laid the proposal aside as "inexpedient." In 1883, judging the time ripe to strengthen nascent sentiments of respect and good will, Mitchell gave the College $5,000 (subsequently increased to $7,000) for an Entertainment Fund to provide agreeable social occasions when members of the several schools and societies might meet. The first such occasion was a reception for the medical members of the American and British Associations for the Advancement of Science, meeting together in Philadelphia in 1884.[60] The dinners and receptions proved eminently successful, not only because Mitchell carried them off so well, but because, as a graduate of Jefferson and a trustee of Pennsylvania, he belonged to neither faction or to both. "One of the noblest functions of this College," he said years later as he reflected on what had been achieved, "has been to put an end to the quarrels between the two great institutions of learning, which kept them so actively hostile for years."[61]

Yet old loyalties and prejudices died hard. Until well into the twentieth century the Fellows of the College were aware whether it was a Penn or a Jefferson graduate who held the presidency. The election of January 2, 1895, was a revealing illustration of this.

Da Costa was finishing a term as vice-president and, according to the current practice, would be nominated unopposed for the presidency (his second non-consecutive term). As was also the custom, there would be a contest for the vice-presidency. William W. Keen of Jefferson and Horatio C Wood of Pennsylvania were the likely nominees, the winner of this election succeeding to the presidency in three years. Because Pennsylvania graduates outnumbered Jefferson alumni in the College, it was expected by many that Wood would be chosen, thus preserving the Penn/Jefferson balance. But Wood was not acceptable to all the Penn Fellows: old Robert P. Harris, for example, raked up the charge that Wood had kept back books intended for the College under his uncle's will. Accordingly, John Ashhurst, Jr., the professor of surgery allowed his name to be put forward. Thus, there was a possibility that the Pennsylvanians' votes would be divided, Keen would be elected, and both the president and vice-president would be Jefferson men. Furthermore, Keen would succeed to the presidency as the third Jefferson president in succession.

This alarming prospect moved one of the Fellows to action. Henry Beates, Jr., a graduate of Pennsylvania, soon to become president of the State Board of Medical Examiners, in a remarkable letter alerted his fellow-alumni to the danger and urged them out of loyalty to alma mater to concentrate their support on Wood, lest "the Jefferson candidate outflank us" and be elected. "This would give the total appointing power . . . to the Jefferson College."

A copy of Beates' letter came into the possession of a local newspaper, which promptly revealed the affair to the public—'Doctors Pull Election Wires" read the headline. The result of all this was that 156 Fellows attended the election, the largest turnout ever for such an event. At the meeting Owen J. Wister presented Beates' letter to the College, denounced its author's conduct as "unbecoming a member," and turned the matter over to the Censors. Beates defended himself on the ground that electioneering was a common practice and that, in any case, he had not begun it. The Censors were unpersuaded. Beates was censured by a vote of thirty-two to twenty-four, Harris by forty-four to one.[62]

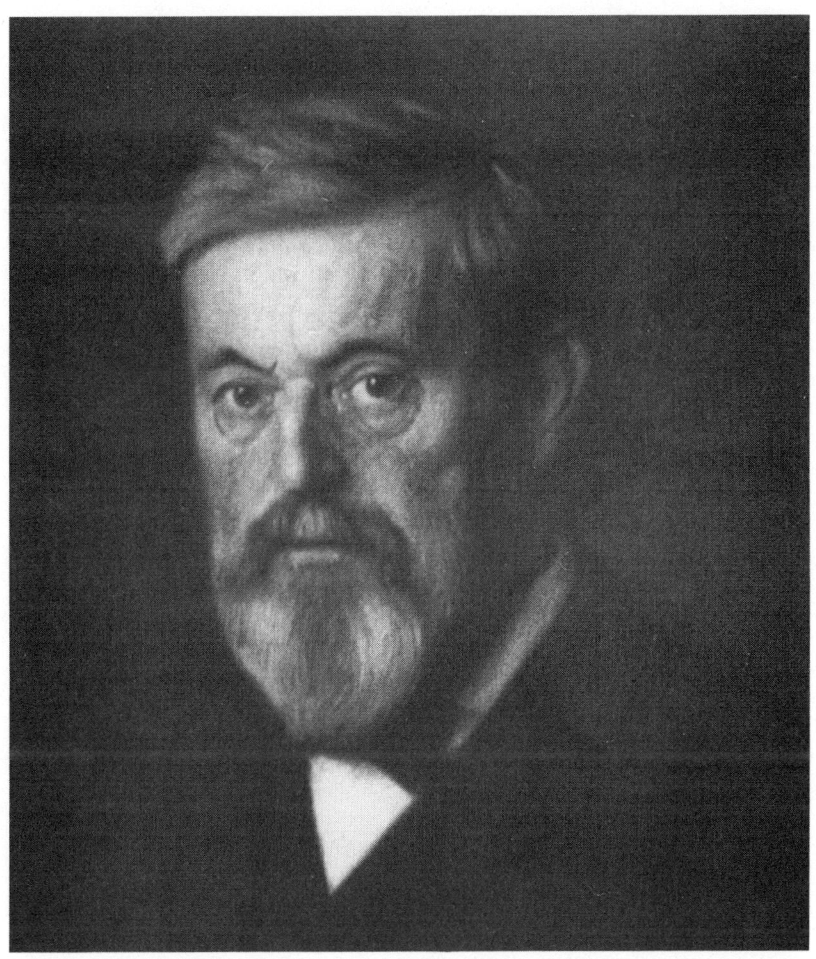

Horatio C Wood, (1841–1920). Painting done in 1905 by Dr. Wood's artist son, James Longacre Wood.

As for the election, despite, or because of, Beates' efforts, his candidate lost; Ashhurst was chosen vice-president; and the Jefferson/Pennsylvania balance was preserved. In time, however, all the candidates achieved the presidency. Ashhurst succeeded Da Costa in 1898; Keen followed Ashhurst in 1900; and Wood followed Keen in 1902.

·1787· ·1887·
The
Centennial
of
The College of Physicians
of
Philadelphia
Dinner
· Tuesday · January · 4th · 1887 ·
"Feasts so solemn and so rare,
Since, seldom coming, in the long years set,
Like stones of worth they thinly placed are,
Or captain jewels in carcanet."
—Shakespeare, Sonnet 52.

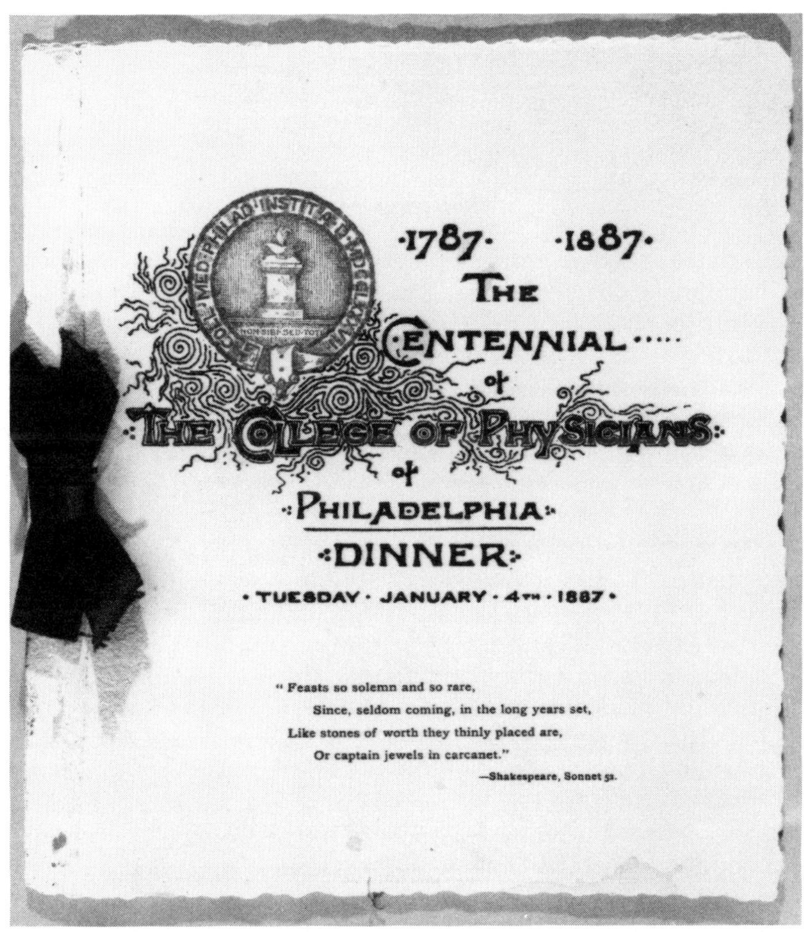

College of Physicians of Philadelphia, Centennial Dinner Menu, 1887.

CHAPTER IX

# *The Age of Weir Mitchell – II*

As the College moved into its second century, it was increasingly clear that its administration needed reform. The old, informal way of handling College business—by officers and committee chairmen out of their private offices—was no longer adequate to an institution with several hundred members, an annual budget of several thousand dollars, and endowments and trust funds. The College needed bankers and brokers, occasionally a lawyer. Its treasurer, always a Fellow, needed clerical assistance, and in 1889 he was finally authorized to spend up to $50 a year for that purpose.

To strengthen the administrative role and influence of the president, as Weir Mitchell wished, the by-laws were amended to allow him to appoint the committees on finance and entertainment and to attend meetings of standing committees. Proposals by Mitchell, or made in his behalf, that the presidential term be lengthened from three to five years were, however, always rejected. The Council's control of College business was extended in 1896 when all business of standing committees was required to be first laid before it; and a few years later all expenditures in excess of $500 were required to be approved by the Council or proposed at one meeting of the College before being voted on at another. Changes were also made in the office of treasurer, although not without injured feelings: when the College required that that officer be bonded, Horace Y. Evans, who had agreed to be treasurer, refused to serve, regarding the requirement as personally insulting. In 1909 the College authorized the employment of an accountant to audit the treasurer's books annually. Meanwhile, in 1899 a trust company was engaged to invest, collect, and keep safe the College's securities, moneys, and income.[1]

Nonetheless, in 1902 Fellows were complaining of "unbusinesslike" administration and "the mystifying methods" the College practiced.[2] The Committee on Finance in that year proposed that all accounts thereafter should be consolidated in the treasurer's office, that the records be kept in the College hall, and that a bookkeeper be hired.[3] These measures, however, would have cost money and reduced the independence and prestige of the committee chairmen, and they were promptly rejected. President Meigs, however, favored reform, and secured appointment of a Committee on Financial Methods with the able, progressive-minded John B. Roberts as chairman. Roberts' committee in 1905 made essentially the same recommendations to modify and modernize the accounts as had been made three years before—and with the same result.[4] But in 1908, with a new building to supervise, ampler funds to invest and disburse, and President Tyson charging that the accounting was "difficult to grasp or comprehend by the average mind," the College cautiously approved the centralization of accounts in the treasurer's office and the appointment of a bookkeeper and a building superintendent.[5] The first superintendent was the librarian, Charles Perry Fisher, who received an additional $300 in compensation. But the College refused to print the annual reports of the secretary and the treasurer in the *Transactions* on the ground that this was "private business," which should not be revealed to public eyes.[6]

New rules or procedures were also adopted or proposed for the stated meetings. Weir Mitchell in 1898 proposed that, "in order to save time," the secretary be authorized to cast a single ballot for nominees at the annual elections; but the suggestion was not adopted.[7] It was in any case impractical as long as nominations could be made from the floor by any Fellow. In 1899, for example, six men were nominated for two vacancies on the Council; it required two ballots to elect one and four more to choose the second. To speed business, it was agreed in 1907 that the reports of the Honorary Librarian and the Curator of the Mütter Museum should no longer be read. (They consisted principally of lists of acquisitions, which were included in the regular meeting notices anyhow.)[8] Similarly, proposals for fellowships were no longer read in the stated meetings, but posted, "as is customary at present in most of the social clubs." But every effort to limit papers to twenty minutes was rejected or ignored.

Physicians who were not Fellows were now attending the regular meetings in increasing numbers. They were supposed to do so, however, only on invitation of a Fellow, who would introduce his guest formally to the president. This requirement was only laxly observed and never enforced, to the stern disapproval of members who felt that attendance by strangers was a privilege that should be acknowledged.[9] Accordingly, the printed meeting notices for some years bore the reminder that "strangers can be present at the meetings of the College only by invitation of a Fellow." A motion to make this rule less off-putting—'Visitors are welcomed at meetings when introduced by or presenting the card of a Fellow"—was voted down.[10] The meeting notices carried the sterner warning until 1910.

Both Mitchell and William W. Keen, who became president in 1900, were interested in promoting change and efficiency in other respects. Keen proposed in 1901 that membership on the standing committees should rotate, that the senior member should go off each year and be ineligible for reappointment for one year.[11] Such a practice would have brought the energy and ideas of more Fellows into the governance of the College. But the Council, as might have been expected, rejected the idea since many of its members would have been affected. It also rejected a proposal to make ex-presidents members of Council.[12]

Such reactions to suggestions for even slight changes, when added to the cautious views of many Fellow on matters like contagion and antisepsis, confirmed the College's reputation for conservatism. J. William White, able, impulsive, outspoken, but never active in College affairs, characterized the institution in 1893 as "perhaps the most conservative in America." Mitchell in a private letter damned "this Quaker conservative spirit. It has been fatal to our civic life." To outsiders the spirit was especially noticeable. A visiting lecturer once described the College as an institution complacently contemplating its incunabula.[13]

### *Anti-Vivisection*

Use of animals in scientific experimental work was an issue repeatedly presented to the College as medical science and education continued to expand in the latter nineteenth century. The College had helped defeat a bill in 1886 that would have restricted animal experimentation in Pennsylvania. It quickly learned, however, that no decision on this increasingly emotional topic was ever final. Rebuffed or defeated one year, the advocates of regulation or prohibition returned the next, with new arguments or the familiar ones uttered with greater fervor. The physicians responded to each effort, and eventually mounted a permanent guard against the humane societies.

At the beginning of their campaign, officers of the American Society for the Prevention of Cruelty to Animals and similar groups did not deny that some animal experiments were necessary and justifiable. They wanted, they said, only to stop "useless repetition of cruel experiments," and they appealed to like-minded physicians to join them.[14] No such alliance was ever formed. Both the humane and the medical societies contained members of absolutist opinions; their relations quickly became antagonistic, with mutual abuse the normal tone of communication. The two groups simply did not trust one another.[15]

In 1893 another effort was made in the Pennsylvania legislature to regulate experimentation on living animals. Flatly denying there was any abuse and asserting that existing laws provided sufficent safeguards, the College was instrumental in defeating the bill. A more serious threat was put forward in 1899, when Senator Jacob Gallinger of New Hampshire, who had once practiced medicine for a few years and was therefore assumed to know about such matters, introduced a bill in Congress that would have severely limited animal experiments in the District of Columbia. Should it become law, this bill would set a standard the states might follow. Its passage, declared the College in a strong protest submitted by Weir Mitchell, would hamper and arrest scientific progress, "and hence it will perpetuate and increase suffering and death in man and the lower animals. Hence it is inhumane to the highest degree."[16]

A vigorous campaign was waged against the Gallinger bill nationwide, and in the end it failed of enactment. President Eliot of Harvard advised the opponents on strategy; their principal spokesman was William W. Keen. He had first assumed that role in 1897, when, addressing the American Medical Association on the progress of medicine and surgery in the preceding half century, he ascribed the advances to a number of causes: improvement in teaching, establishment of libraries and journals, the application of anesthesia and antisepsis, the use of precision instruments—and animal experimentation.[17] Keen was president of the Association in 1900, when the Gallinger bill was under discussion, and he helped defeat it by testifying before Congress, writing articles in popular journals, corresponding with other organizations, committees, and individuals. With the stupid and uninformed, Keen could be short and sharp; to those who acted from personal and religious conviction he spoke in the terms and tones of the devout Christian he was. To one who claimed it was immoral to save a man's life "by the torture of animals," Keen replied, "If you are consistent, you should never eat meat; you should never ride on street cars drawn by horses, or otherwise use them . . . for your advantage."[18]

In the next dozen years, the College took a stand against other anti-vivisection bills introduced into the Pennsylvania legislature. Of one such bill in 1909, the College expressed its "emphatic disapproval" and sent a committee to Harrisburg. The bill died. Four years later another bill was quietly introduced into the Assembly that would have prohibited any experiment by drugs, harmful substances of any kind, instruments, inoculations or injections on any human patient without his permission or that of parents or guardians. President Wilson of the College denounced the bill as "atrocious" and predicted that enactment would be a "calamity." The College and the County Medical Society sent a joint committee to Harrisburg to lobby; and though the bill passed the House, it failed in the Senate.[19]

Research physicians in Philadelphia now concluded that they must organize a continuing explanation and defense of their position. Accordingly, William Pepper, a Fellow and dean of the University of Pennsylvania Medical School, and some of his colleagues formed the Society for the Protection of Scientific Research in 1914. Charles H. Frazier, professor of clinical surgery in the University, and Richard M. Pearce, professor of research medicine there, both Fellows of the College, were president and secretary respectively; Keen was honorary president. The honorary vice-presidents included the presidents of Lehigh University, Haverford, Bryn Mawr, and Pennsylvania State Colleges, the provost of the University of Pennsylvania, the chancellor of the University of Pittsburgh, the president and vice-president of the State Federation of Women, and the superintendent of the Philadelphia Roman Catholic parochial schools.

The new society asked the College for $500 towards the expenses of a secretary, legal advice, and printing. The Council judged that the appropriation would establish an unwise and dangerous precedent. Regardless of that, the College did not have the sum, and so the Council called on the Fellows to contribute as individuals. Within a month six did so.[20] To present the subject to a wider audience, the College then invited Victor C. Vaughan of Ann Arbor, Michigan, president of the American Medical Association, to speak at a special meeting. In a somewhat anecdotal account of the Spanish-American War, Vaughan ascribed particular recent advances in medicine to animal experiments.[21]

The subject arose repeatedly. When the American Red Cross in 1918 decided to withhold funds from armed services laboratories that used animals for research in pneumonia, gas gangrene, trench fever, and other diseases, the College voiced its strong condemnation.[22] In 1922, on the motion of Keen, it "emphatically protested" the Johnson bill in Congress, which would forbid gas experiments on animals "because its passage would assure horrible cruelty to our troops and, it might well be, serious military disaster to the Nation."[23] In 1921 the College took the unusual step of contributing $100 and co-sponsoring with the County Medical Society a public lecture by one E. H. Baynes, whose defense of animal experiments in the *Woman's Home Companion* had been fiercely attacked and had elicited an appeal by anti-vivisectionists to boycott the magazine.[24]

### *Library*

Charles Perry Fisher, named assistant librarian in 1882, had begun at once to organize the College's large, growing, and sprawling collections of books and pamphlets. He had two assistants, one of whom, Emily Thomas, though engaged as a cataloguer, gave part of her time to the Nurses' Directory. They had valuable help and guidance from I. Minis Hays, chairman of the Library Committee, and from Fellows like William Osler who appreciated libraries or had bibliophilic interests. During the ensuing ten years, while the library's holdings doubled, the collection was catalogued according to a modified version of the Surgeon-General's Library's plan. The hours of opening were extended to a full day (9 to 6 daily, including Saturdays); duplicates were identified and sold; such modern library aids and procedures as call slips and charge cards were introduced; and borrowing regulations were drafted and published. After 1900 the entire catalogue was revised and copied on typed cards. Many Fellows, like Osler, formed the habit of stopping at the College on their way home at the end of the day to look at the latest journals and books. In fact, what Osler missed most in Baltimore was the library and fellowship of the College. He worked to fill the gap by helping to rejuvenate the Medical and Chirurgical Faculty of that city.[25]

The flow of books from Fellows and their estates, which had begun so noticeably in the 1860's, swelled in the last decades of the century. Samuel Lewis continued to make gifts until his death in 1890: one of his last was a complete set of Nicolas de Blegny's *Zodiacus medico-gallicus* (1680–82), a Latin translation of the first medical journal. In all, Lewis gave about ten thousand volumes. Like his father before him, I. Minis Hays sent along books and journals received for review or other notice by the *American Journal of the Medical Sciences.* The son of H. Lenox Hodge in 1895 finally made a gift of his father's library, which had been on deposit for several years—1,740 volumes, 1,011 pamphlets (including reprints), and 1,516 numbers of periodicals. Richard J. Dunglison presented some hundreds of books that belonged to his father. Other donations came from the estates of Addinell Hewson, N. Archer Randolph, Albert H. Smith, and John F. Weightman. Jacob M. Da Costa, Alfred Stillé, Horatio C Wood, and Weir Mitchell were constant donors; and Da Costa's library of 2,466 books came after his death. William Osler, appointed to the Library Committee within a year of his election as a Fellow, was a benefactor of the library throughout his life. He is reported on May 28, 1887, as having given ten volumes, eight pamphlets, and ninety-eight numbers of journals. A few months later he brought in four volumes, forty-two pamphlets, and 568 numbers of journals. By the terms of the will of John Ashhurst, Jr., the College was allowed to select fifteen hundred volumes from his library. Fisher, who was acquiring a considerable knowledge of incunabula and other rare books, chose some important rarities: the 1491 edition of *Hortus*

*Sanitatis, De Balneis* (1553), sixteenth-century editions of Dioscorides, Jerome Cardan, and Rhazes, early editions of the works of Kenelm Digby, Celsus, Thomas Bartholinus, and Steno, and Culpeper's *Pharmacopoeia Londinensis.*

In addition to gifts and bequests, there were permanent deposits from sister institutions, which now regarded the College as a safe and appropriate depository. The Academy of Surgery placed its Gross Library in the College in 1885. The library of the Obstetrical Society—359 volumes as well as pamphlets and journals—came in 1886. In 1899 the County Medical Society deposited its archives at Thirteenth and Locust Streets, and in 1905 the Episcopal Hospital gave the College its library of 1,982 volumes. From time to time some Fellow would asked whether the Pennsylvania Hospital should not add its old library to the College's growing collection.

Only occasionally, however, was the Library able to purchase a collection of books or even a single volume. It spent $200 at the sale of George Hamilton's library. It made its largest purchase in 1901—the library of J. Stockton Hough, 2,402 titles. Hough had valued his books at $8,000; the executor hoped to get $5,000 for Mrs. Hough; but Fisher and William W. Keen negotiated the purchase for $3,000, to which the executor added $1,000 of his own. Had the College not acted with unwonted speed, the books might have been purchased by the New York Academy of Medicine or been sent to auction in London. Much interested in the library, as was Mitchell, Keen in 1900 secured nearly seven thousand theses and inaugural dissertations from French and German universities, and,during a long visit to Europe in 1907–08, set up an exchange that brought in hundreds more.

Even small purchases usually required special action by the Library Committee. In 1893 it authorized a bid of $5 for a copy of Benjamin Rush's *Enquiry into the Natural History of Medicine among the Indians in North-America* (1774), and three guineas (about $15) in 1898 to buy in London a copy of William Harvey's *Exercitationes Anatomicae* (London, 1653).

Doubtless it was Weir Mitchell who brought the Harvey item to the committee's attention. Throughout his long association with the College he was a constant and generous supporter of everything connected with the library. He gave $300 in 1887 to catalogue the pamphlets and $100 in 1890 to complete journal files; and in 1892 he gave $100 to purchase incunabula, and promptly donated forty-two ancient volumes from his own library—works of Albertus Magnus, Arnold of Villanova, Bartholomaeus Anglicus, Celsus, and three editions of the *Regimen Sanitatis* of Salerno. He had already established the Journal Fund with a gift of $1,000; additional large gifts for the library brought the Weir Mitchell Library Fund up to $5,000. He reminded the College repeatedly of the need to preserve its own archives and manuscripts, and got the Secretary to transfer these records to the library.[26] He presented the W. Kent Gilbert collection of autograph letters of physicians, and had them properly arranged and bound. He and J. M. DaCosta acquired in 1895 John Morgan's Edinburgh diploma, and in 1898 they bought a collection of seventeen autograph letters of Edward Jenner. In 1905 Mitchell presented some manuscript notes of Morgan's visit to Rome in 1764. Generous himself, he did not hesitate to ask others for gifts. He begged a file of the *Proceedings* of the American Association of Public Health from his friend John Shaw Billings—"Or how else can we get it."[27] He even provided furniture for the reading room—tables, book cases, a tall case clock.

Valuable as the old books were, current journals were more useful to the physicians. According to Fisher's statistics, they were consulted four times as often. In 1889 the library received 392 periodicals (196 American, forty-three British and Canadian, sixty French, thirty-three German, and thirteen Austrian). In 1890 the total had risen to 491; and in 1896 more than six hundred journals were received regularly. By that time the book collection had long since outgrown the available space. In the concluding pages of his *Account of the College of Physicians* (1887), Ruschenberger had suggested that a building fund be started to meet the need, "possibly afar off," but likely to break over the College in ten or fifteen years. In 1890 the Library Committee took note of the approaching crisis. Each year thereafter the familiar warning became more insistent. In 1897 books were reported stacked on the floor. "Something radical" had to be done, the committee cried out in 1901. In 1906 books were "piled and crowded, and scattered in fifteen rooms and galleries." In 1907, thanks to filling one of the meeting rooms with thirty thousand volumes, the committee was able to spare the Fellows the "usual jeremiads about the distressing want of shelf-room." By then, however, there was the prospect of a new building.

As the library grew in size and usefulness, Fellows and their officers increasingly mentioned it with pride. Indeed, by 1900 many regarded the library as the principal function and obligation of the College. Those who could not give books, gave money. Book funds were created—by Mrs. Lewis Rodman and Mrs. Elizabeth B. Judson in memory of their husbands, by Clement A. Griscom in memory of his father, by George Fales Baker in memory of Henrietta Rush Fales Baker. "Yet," Weir Mitchell warned the Fellows in 1892, "you must in reason expect your library to make even larger demands for money. It is an expensive necessity."[28] At the suggestion of the honorary librarian Frederick P. Henry in 1896, a committee was appointed to solicit endowment gifts from the public; but it did nothing and soon asked to be discharged. Another suggestion, that the College ask the legislature for an annual appropriation for books, was promptly rejected by the Fellows.[29]

### *Museum Needs*

The history and problems of the museum in these years were similar to the library's—a steady increase of holdings, unyielding limitations of space. Anatomical specimens and models, books, and photographs flowed in from the surgeons John B. Roberts, John M. Baldy, and Joseph Price, and from other Fellows. John B. Deaver and A. O. J. Kelly offered 1,008 appendixes removed at the German Hospital; it was, they said, "an initial installment" to which they expected to add. Others presented single artifacts with historical associations—Thomas D. Mütter's gold-headed cane came from Weir Mitchell, the death mask of John Hunter from William W. Keen, Edward Jenner Coxe's cupping apparatus and scarificator from Miss Mary Clapier Coxe. Jacob M. DaCosta, donating a number of surgical instruments, recommended that the museum collect such articles.[30] His suggestion was promptly taken up: a year later Mrs. William H. Pancoast presented over one thousand instruments that had belonged to her late husband and her father-in-law. Like the library, the museum received but a small appropriation and could only rarely buy anything. Taking what was given it, but encouraging gifts to illustrate particular systems and conditions, in 1898 it contained more than five thousand specimens as well as 160 illustrated texts and atlases, not to mention the great many instruments. To display these articles, additional cases and shelving were erected until all the wall space was filled. A catalogue was begun in 1899.

A constant purpose of the Committee on the museum was to encourage the use of the collections for study and teaching. To this end a dark room for photographic work was built in 1893. Although foreign visitors praised the general appearance of the museum, conditions worsened and became more cramped as the collection grew. Storage facilities were wholly unsatisfactory. Kept near the roof, wax models were damaged and destroyed in the sweltering summer heat. "One hundred degrees might be tolerated," the Curator complained earnestly, not for the first time, in 1893, "but 110° and 120° are inexcusable."[31] Installation of a barrier ceiling two years later afforded some protection, but was a temporary expedient. Like the library, the museum required more space and better care.

### *Removal or Non-Removal*

Speaking as a private member, Weir Mitchell presented the matter bluntly at the regular meeting on December 5, 1900. "It must be clear," he asserted, "that we are to be soon hopelessly cramped for room . . . . Within a year something must be done to give more library room."[32] There were, he went on, three alternatives. The first two—to buy the property adjoining the College's hall and erect an annex for books upon it, or to use the meeting room on the first floor for books—seemed neither practicable nor attractive to Mitchell. The College had no money to buy the adjoining building, much less the additional $40,000 the construction of an annex would cost; while the use of the small meeting room for book storage would deprive the College of $330 a year in rent from the County Medical and other societies and leave the College with but one meeting room for all occasions.

Mitchell's third alternative was a startling one—to give up the Mütter Museum and use the space for books. The income from the Mütter bequest, once $1,800 a year, was now only half that and, after obligations under the will and necessary charges for maintenance and insurance were met, nothing remained for acquisitions. "In plain words," Mitchell concluded, "the Museum is stranded as its founder never dreamed it would be." Unable to fulfill the donor's intentions unless it appropriated $1,000 from its own funds, the College would do better to place the collection in another institution able to achieve Mütter's purpose.

The committees on the Museum and Hall, the Council, and the College at large responded promptly. Everyone recognized the "imperative need" of the library, but almost no one except Mitchell, it appeared, wanted to give up the museum to meet it. Accordingly, it was proposed that a small room attached to the museum should be given to the library; and when engineers reported that the floors and walls would not support the weight of books, other space, taken from the Nurses' Directory, was assigned. This, however, was only an expedient. "Soon or late," Mitchell insisted "we must double our library space." A special committee "to consider the whole question of the needs of the Building in its present condition, and the future needs of the College," contented itself with proposing some minor adjustments of space.[33]

Here the matter rested for a year or so. But Mitchell, determined to provide adequately for the library, was not idle. He knew that funds must be raised, that the Fellows alone could not contribute all that was required, and that any campaign must have an objective of general appeal—such as a new building in another location. In 1902 he approached his friend Andrew Carnegie, and on January 3, 1903, was able to report that Carnegie promised $50,000 "to provide increased accommodations for the Library" on condition that the College raise an equal amount. This forced the Fellows seriously to consider the library's problems and their solution.

Horatio C Wood discussed the matter fully in his first presidential address two weeks later, and surprised most of the Fellows by presenting an architect's sketches showing how the existing hall might be enlarged. Two committees were appointed: one, with Mitchell as chairman, to collect subscriptions to meet Carnegie's offer; the other, headed by Wood himself, to consider the sketches he had just displayed. Mitchell lost no time in canvassing his rich friends and the wealthier Fellows; within six weeks he had raised $53,000 to match Carnegie's gift.[34]

Wood, too, moved swiftly, and at a special meeting on February 24, 1903, made a detailed report for his committee:[35]

> The solution of the problem before the Fellows of the College is surrounded with difficulties, but it is clear that

action must be taken. . . . At present the income of the College is no more than sufficient for its needs, and it would seem, therefore, that building upon a new site would require the College to sacrifice the growth of its Library or to face a yearly deficit of from 21 to 35 per cent. of its income (according to the site selected). It is not at present apparent how this deficiency of income could be made up, except by increasing the annual dues from $20 to $30. The President of the College, believing that the dues are as high as they ought to be, at present deems it unwise to put up a new building, but on this point your Committee was divided. At the final meeting of the Committee—six members in all being present—it was unanimously decided that the College ought to take action within a reasonable time, and should not demolish the present building and rebuild on its site; but the motion that the alteration of the present building is inexpedient received three votes in the affirmative and three, including the Chairman, in the negative.

In laying before the College the information contained in the report just given, the President desires to state that he most earnestly hopes that the College will not *load itself with a mortgage or other serious debt.*

Whatever the final decision of the College may be as to the character of the improvements to be made in its housing, it is very evident that more money than has been obtained is necessary to make the present movement thoroughly successful. There have been some surprise and much congratulation at the success of the money-getting, but the work has so far been done by a few persons. Twenty-one thousand dollars have been obtained from persons not members of the medical profession by the solicitations of ten Fellows. Over $30,000 have been contributed, in sums ranging from ten dollars to five thousand dollars, by *less than one-half* of the membership of the College. Certainly the time has come when every Fellow of the College should give according to his means, and when every Fellow should try to obtain assistance from the laity,—i.e., those who constantly receive by transmission benefits from the College Library.

If the Fellows "could be widely aroused to earnest effort," Wood believed,

> it would be easy to buy the site on Twenty-second Street, below Market, and erect thereon, free from all incumbrances, a handsome edifice, with space around it for future enlargement, sufficient for any probable needs of the College for centuries. On the other hand, if the burden of improvement is to be carried by a portion of the Fellows, and no more funds are forthcoming, it would be better to remodel the present building.

Thus was opened a discussion that continued almost without interrruption for six years, until at last in 1909 a new College hall was erected and opened. The debate was often confused and contradictory, with the College rescinding at one meeting what it had approved at an earlier one. Motions were made, tabled, rejected, approved, and repealed. Attendance rose to unprecedented heights as advocates and opponents of particular proposals rallied in force. There was scant time for scientific papers. "Whole evenings," one participant remembered, "were consumed in endless debate, usually punctuated with bitter remarks and recriminations."[36] Passions ran so high that some Fellows feared permanent harm to the College. This was avoided in part because President Arthur V. Meigs, although strongly opposed to moving the College, presided over the most heated exchanges with strict impartiality and courtesy.[37]

There was general acceptance that the library needed and should have more room. The disputes were over how and where this space should be provided—whether in the old hall remodeled and enlarged or in another building bought or erected at another site. On the one hand were men like Mitchell, who believed that a large, spacious, modern building would meet the needs of the library, benefit the other activities of the College, and increase the institution's prestige. On the other, were men strongly attached to the old Hall and its associations, who were dismayed at the probable cost of a new hall and the problem of raising funds, who believed that some sites proposed were too remote from their homes and offices and from the center of the city generally. Some frivolous reasons also had their supporters—that such a mass of books as the library's collection could not be moved; that Carnegie's gift was tainted money from a wicked rich capitalist and should not be accepted.[38]

With reports from the Mitchell and Wood committees before the College, action now accelerated. A committee on alterations in the building was named. Wood obtained an option on properties adjoining the hall on Thirteenth Street; but as the owners required an answer within five days, the College could not take it up.[39] It did, however, authorize the expenditure of $100,000—the building fund—to purchase a suitable building or a piece of land on which to build. Wood, who at this time favored extension at Thirteenth and Locust Streets, tried to obtain two properties to the east of the hall on Locust Street, but the owners refused to sell. In May 1903 the College appointed a committee on removal or non-removal, with power to secure an option; it was instructed to report by November 1, 1903.[40] With Mitchell urging it on, the committee did not delay; and before the end of the month obtained an option to purchase the property at Twenty-second and Ludlow Streets. At a special meeting the Fellows voted seventy-two to thirty-eight to buy the lot for $80,000.[41] On leaving office on January 6, 1904, Wood, now an advocate of the move to Twenty-second Street, reviewed the probable financing of the building. The sale of the Locust Street building, he pointed out, would bring in a large sum. "For complete success," he concluded in an exhortation to the Fellows, "but one thing is necessary: enthusiasm—an enthusiasm so virulent that it will infect the whole mass. Who will furnish the microbe?"[42]

Someone proposed that the fund-raisers might solicit the general public, even city and state authorities. This suggestion was received coolly when it was pointed out that the receipt of gifts from such sources might require the College to open its library to all. Nonetheless, in connection with the fund-raising effort, Frederick P. Henry wrote a long article for a Philadelphia newspaper under the accurate but uninspiring title, "Second Greatest Medical Library in the World."[43]

As Arthur Meigs assumed the presidency of the College in January 1904, the College was owner of a piece of land at Twenty-second and Ludlow Streets, but had neither means nor plans to build, while a strong minority was unreconciled to the purchase and all it implied. Mitchell and the supporters of a new hall, nevertheless, pressed forward. On March 30, 1904, after a full meeting attended by 157 Fellows and a long and often confusing discussion, in which not fewer than twenty-nine Fellows, including Mitchell, spoke, the College voted to move to Twenty-second Street. "200 M.D.'s decided by 96–62 to move to 22st.," Mitchell wrote in his diary that night. "The Pa. Hosp men were as usual stay still folk. There is a local infection there of unenterprise . . . great election work."[44] The next month the general description of a building that might be erected was presented and approved, and a building committee was named.

The battle was not over. The minority had other stratagems to deploy. Arguing strongly that the College should consider alternative locations, they obtained appointment of a special committee to identify them. For six months matters remained *in statu quo;* then in November 1904 the committee of the minority presented three alternatives to building at Twenty-second Street: erect a new building at Thirteenth and Locust Streets (for which they presented plans drafted by the New York firm of McKim, Mead, and White); build on Eighteenth Street between Rittenhouse and Manning Streets; or acquire a public school building at Seventeenth and Pine Streets.[45] An option on the Eighteenth Street property was actually taken, but was given up when the committee learned what the building restrictions were. On December 13, at a special meeting attended by 105 Fellows, the College rejected the alternative of remaining at Thirteenth and Locust Streets and voted to sell the Twenty-second Street property. On January 4, 1905, it recommended the purchase of the Grant School at Seventeenth and Pine Streets for $50,000, provided the Board of Education could give possession within three years. Someone on the Board offered "absolute assurances" and the City Council approved the agreement of sale, but the School Board ultimately proved unable to meet the condition.[46]

Meanwhile, no purchaser for the Twenty-second Street lot had appeared; and with the collapse of the Grant School purchase agreement, the College appeared to have no other option than to build at Twenty-second Street. The Fellows reaffirmed that intention on February 6, 1907, by a vote of sixty-three to forty-five. The Philadelphia architects Cope and Stewardson were engaged; Mitchell got another $50,000 from Carnegie; plans were drawn and presented; and on March 6, 1907, with 178 Fellows present, they were unanimously approved.[47]

One final effort had been made to delay or defeat the majority.

Robert G. LeConte, who had been chairman of the minority committee, moved on February 6, 1907, that the officers of the College consult with "three eminent financiers" on the advisability of investing a large sum of money in a building on Twenty-second Street. The "eminent financiers" approved the location both as "a Financial proposition" and in the light of all other circumstances.[48]

On April 29, 1908, the cornerstone of the new College building was laid by Weir Mitchell.

## *New Hall Built*

The new hall cost, as new buildings do, more than was expected. The Fellows had set a limit of $250,000.[49] On January 1, 1908, before construction began, the architects estimated costs at $227,101, with additional charges for paving and new curbing, electric fixtures, book stacks, and their own fees bringing the total to $267,401. The College approved this figure, increased its authorization to $270,000, and then authorized another $25,000 for furnishings. "The College is rising and will be very fine," Mitchell assured Osler in January 1909. "At present I want for it to finish—about 40,000$."[50]

A calculation made the next month showed estimated expenses of $292,095 (actual expenses proved to be $289,266) and funds in hand or collectible at $215,292, leaving a deficiency of $77,803. As the College did not want to mortgage either its old or new building, there were but two ways to get the money: obtain more large gifts or sell the Locust Street property. Meanwhile, the College might have to borrow from its own unrestricted funds.[51]

The new Hall was formally dedicated on November 10, 1909, with an academic procession, greetings from other medical society libraries, conferring of honorary fellowships, and an address by the president James Tyson. For the occasion a commemorative medal designed by R. Tait McKenzie was struck. That evening a great dinner was held in the Bellevue-Stratford Hotel, attended by 452 persons, including 311 Fellows and Associate Fellows. Among the guests were not only many of the principal medical figures in the nation—John Shaw Billings, Harvey Cushing, Simon Flexner, George W. Crile, Abraham Jacobi, William H. Welch, and Reginald H. Fitz—but also a score of civic and business leaders of the city and commonwealth—Governors Beaver, Pennypacker, and Stuart, Mayor Reyburn, George F. Baer, J. B. Lippincott, Joseph G. Rosengarten, Charles Custis Harrison, Daniel Baugh, Charlemagne Tower, Cyrus H. K. Curtis, Eckley B. Coxe.[52]

Weir Mitchell responded to the toast "The Old College and the New," and Andrew Carnegie to that of "Libraries." Carnegie's remarks were in a light and happy mood—'I have done rather a wholesale business in libraries"—and were interrupted repeatedly by "(Applause)" and "(Laughter)." He paid particular tribute to Mitchell, for whom, as he fully appreciated, the completion of the hall was the culmination of more than half a century of devotion to the College. "I believe this to be the apotheosis of his career .... nothing, no triumph, no ceremony, no honor can be bestowed upon him that can quite equal this night, at the very apex of his life . . . ."[53]

Next day the building was open for inspection, and there was a reception for Fellows and guests. The principal rooms had been furnished by families and friends of distinguished Fellows, for whom they were named—John Ashhurst, Jr.,[54] William F. Norris, Thomas Cadwalader (the gift of Mrs. Mitchell, a descendant), and William Thomson. Subsequently other memorial rooms were named, one by the Hutchinson family for James Hutchinson, a founding Fellow, and his grandson James H. Hutchinson; another for Frederick A. Packard by his brothers; a third by the Wood family in memory of George Bacon Wood. The great meeting room, called the Hall of Portraits, was now renamed Mitchell Hall. Mitchell spoke a brief welcome, thanking the contributors to the building fund, "who understood that the history of medicine in this city is national property," and concluding with a wry confession that the Fellows entered their new home with "a certain amount of debt," which he was confident some public-spirited Philadelphians would come forward to discharge.[55]

Mitchell soon brought one forward. In January 1910, only a few weeks after the new College was opened, the financier E. T. Stotesbury donated $75,000 "to relieve it from debt & leave it free to pursue its career of honorable usefulness." The pledge, expressed in Mitchell's words, was written in Mitchell's hand, on Mitchell's office stationery. "Now you are out of debt," Stotesbury is said to have admonished as he signed, "keep out."

"Thus ends my 7 year struggle," Mitchell wrote in his diary on January 28, 1910. "Thank God."[56]

## *Sale of the Old Hall*

Thanks to Stotesbury's gift, the College had no debt on its new hall, but neither had its income risen to meet the increased costs of maintenance. Opponents of the move from Locust Street had warned of this, but the warnings were lost amid debates on the greater issue of removal or non-removal, and in confidence that the sale of the old hall would provide a substantial addition to the endowment. As it turned out, however, that did not happen. For forty years the property remained unsold. Not only did it generate no income, it was a drain upon College resources year after year. The failure to sell was sometimes due to general conditions of economic depression and war; but it was always and primarily a consequence of bad advice and short-sighted decisions by men who, though understandably motivated by a desire to realize the most for the College, held unreasonable expectations and simply lacked knowledge and decisiveness when they did have the chance to sell.

As early as 1903, while the College was still debating whether to move from Thirteenth and Locust Streets, an offer of $150,000 was received. Had the Fellows been closer to consensus about moving, this offer might have been accepted; but they were not, and the offer was declined. A second offer in the same amount in 1907 was also declined in the belief that the property was worth $160,000, if not more.[57] Fortunately for the College, the Free Library of Philadelphia was willing to rent the building in 1910, paying $7,000 a year in addition to all taxes, utilities, insurance, and maintenance. The Free Library remained a tenant for fifteen years, its rent rising to $10,500, until it moved to its new home on the Parkway. During this period the College received several offers to purchase—of $300,000 (it wanted $350,000) and $350,000 (it wanted $400,000).[58]

For four years after the Free Library vacated the premises the building remained empty, a liability for taxes, insurance, and basic maintenance. In 1929 the building was razed and the ground rented as a parking lot for $4,500 a year. The parking operation apparently proved profitable, for the garage management in 1930 wanted to buy the lot for $275,000. The deal was not consummated, however, and in 1932 the College leased the lot for $8,000 a year.[59] In 1937 the income to the College after taxes was only $1,940. In that year and the next offers of $150,000 were declined.

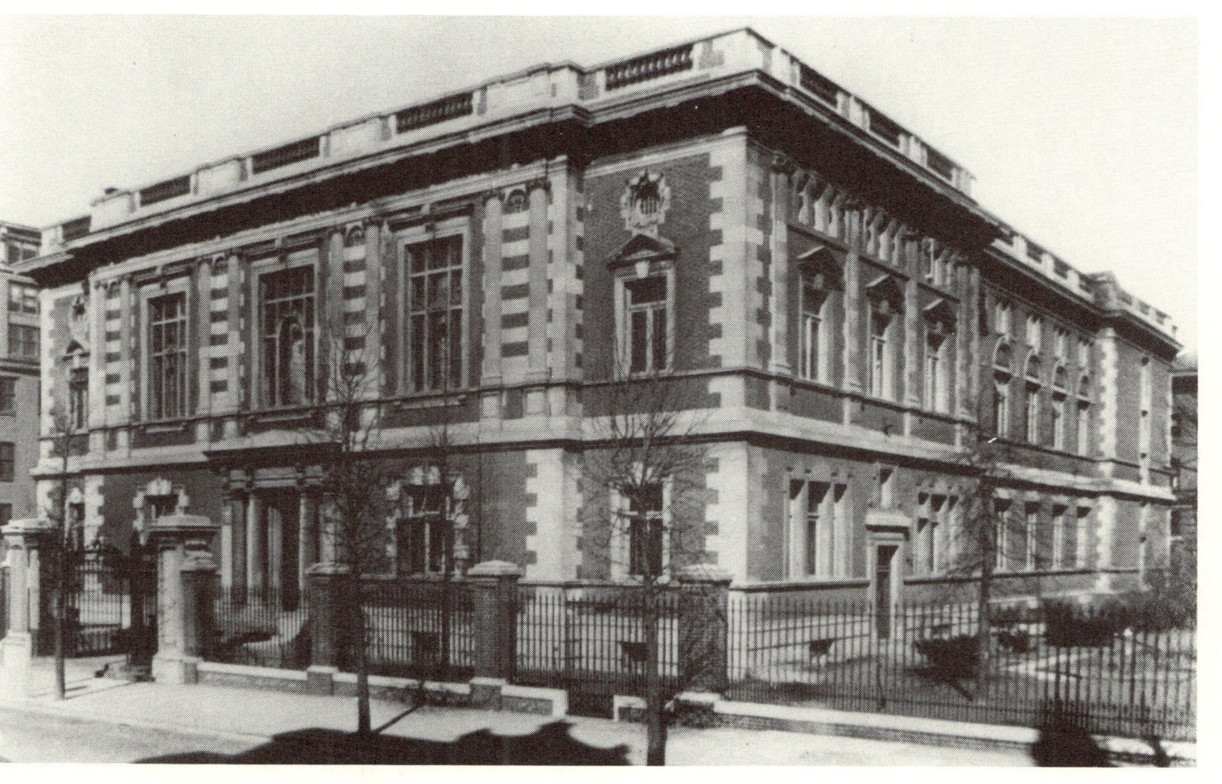

College of Physicians, 19 South Twenty-Second Street. Erected 1909.

"This land," the Finance Committee reported, "continues to be a source of trouble to the College."[60] Throughout the Depression and the Second World War, the parking lot remained in College ownership, with only a rare inquiry from a not-too-serious prospect. An offer of $70,000 in 1946, when the rent was $6,000, was declined. Two years later, however, when hardly any Fellow was left in the College who remembered the old Hall, the College determined to sell, was offered $100,000, and took it.[61]

But all this lay in the future. In the general celebration in 1909, as the Fellows and their guests inspected and admired their new home, not a hint was uttered that the new hall might be the source of unrelenting financial problems for the College for half a century to come.

### *Furnishing the Hall*

The great fireplace that George W. Child had provided twenty-five years before was brought from Locust Street and installed in the Norris periodicals room, a reminder of past associations. The old portraits, busts, and tablets were put up. Additional tablets were mounted in the vestibule, carrying the names of the College's recent benefactors and "eminent benefactors." Gifts to embellish the building soon followed. Richard H. Harte, treasurer of the College, who had already furnished the Ashhurst Room, gave a statue of Aesculapius to fill the niche at the head of the grand staircase, and a year later he presented a bust of Galen.[52] Hampton L. Carson, the College's legal counsel, presented silhouettes by Joseph Sansom of three founding Fellows. A portrait of Nathaniel Chapman came from Mrs. Henry C. Chapman, a painting of Adam Kuhn from C. Hartman Kuhn, and busts of George Bacon and Horatio C Wood from their families and friends.[53] It was much as he had predicted, Mitchell wrote Osler, "that our move would so excite attention as to even trouble us with gifts and now my son John [chairman of the Hall Committee] is bothered by people who want to present busts and pictures of doctors for whom nobody cares a penny."[64]

The formal elegance of the new hall invited additional embellishments. With a view to entertaining guests, President James Wilson and George E. de Schweinitz presented several handsome pieces of silver for a dining table. De Schweinitz, the new president, gave a flagpole and an American flag; and a College flag was designed. It was decreed that College officers henceforth should wear gowns at all stated and special meetings,[65] and that the Censors and Council were similarly to attire themselves at special functions. Democratic principles and prejudices, however, made the officers reluctant for some years to don robes; and gowns were never provided for the Council and the Censors, doubtless for reasons of cost. Another kind of tradition was inaugurated by Robert Abbe, a New York surgeon and Associate Fellow. In 1910 he presented a gold watch that had belonged to Benjamin Rush, directing that it should be put in the custody of a succession of distinguished physicians, each naming his successor. Abbe's inspiration may have been "the gold-headed cane" of the Royal College of Physicians of London. From time to time mementos of other great physicians and scientists—Jenner, Pasteur, Lister, Mme. Curie—were added to the cabinet, and in 1921 Abbe provided an endowment of $5,000 "to perpetuate and enhance the collection." He named Mitchell the first custodian of the Abbe cabinet; Mitchell named Simon Flexner as his successor; and other early custodians were William H. Welch, William W. Keen, and William J. Mayo. In later years the custodianship sometimes lapsed, and since 1943 income from the endowment has been used for general College purposes, as the deed of gift permits.[66]

### *Uses for the Hall: Lectures*

The completion of the Hall afforded means to realize another object Mitchell had long cherished for the College. That was to present public lectures and other programs of general interest to acquaint the laity with the College, its work and members, and with medicine and the history of medicine. Tyson recommended the idea in his presidential address in 1910. The first series of such lectures was delivered in the winter of 1910–11 on "Great Doctors and Achievements in Medical Research." The first lecture was by Mitchell on one of his favorite subjects, William Harvey; and this address was followed by Simon Flexner of the Rockefeller Institute on Pasteur, William H. Welch of Johns Hopkins on Jenner, and James G. Mumford of the Harvard Medical School on Paré. In subsequent years Mitchell's son John lectured on Jerome Cardan, the journalist Talcott Williams on "The Doctor from the Standpoint of the Layman," and Owen Wister, son of a fellow, on "Superstition and the Doctor." Although attendance was said to have been gratifyingly large, the task of arranging for three or four lectures each winter proved burdensome; the number of lectures fell to two, then one; none was given in 1914 and 1915; and after 1916 they were abandoned, only to be re-established from time to time in the following half century.

Another lecture series that was to have made use of the enlarged facilities of the Hall suffered a similar fate. To honor Mitchell a lectureship was established in 1910 which the Fellows hoped might enjoy the prestige of the Harvey Lectures of the New York Academy of Medicine.[67] President de Schweinitz asked Richard M. Pearce, a Fellow of the College, who was about to return, after several years in Albany and New York, to the University of Pennsylvania as professor of research medicine, to learn how that series was organized and supported. Pearce's reply revealed the deep cleavage that now existed between older members of the profession, most of them successful clinicians who also taught and wrote, and younger men dedicated to experimental research. "Please do not let the clinicians control it," Pearce advised de Schweinitz about the lectureship.

> Let the laboratory men control it and get laboratory men to lecture. If clinicians control it and I am afraid they will if the committee on scientific business of the college has charge of it, it is dead from the start, both as to lecturers and audience. It must be educational and can only be made so by research workers. The clinicians need educating and can but be educated by *laboratory men* giving *clinical lectures.* Paradox, but true.[68]

If the Mitchell lectures should number six or eight a course, Pearce went on in another letter, and if one or two "active investigators" were on the program committee, he saw no reason why the results he looked for might not be achieved through the College. "Otherwise," he warned, "it might be advisable to take some other action," such as establishing another society with its own course of lectures by laboratory men.[69] De Schweintiz rejected Pearce's notion: no lectureship under the College could be put in the hands of "any one set of men, were they laboratory men or clinicians."[70]

The first Mitchell lecture was delivered on January 17, 1911, by the pharmacologist Arthur R. Cushny of the University of London. He spoke on "Heart Irregularity from Auricular Fibrillation." De Schweinitz wrote Osler about the paper: "His science was good, and I think the clinicians, especially those who concern themselves with diseases of the heart, were very much interested."[71] Cushny was followed by Edmund B. Wilson of Columbia University, Svante Arrhenius of the Nobel Institute of Stockholm, and William T. Porter, professor of physiology in the Harvard Medical School. The lectures were well attended, medical and graduate students and their professors in neighboring universities and colleges being invited. But, like the public lectures, organizing the Mitchell lectures soon proved to be a burden, especially on the president. Both William C. Gorgas and Theobald Smith were invited to speak, but declined; Osler accepted, then withdrew. After the first year only two lectures were offered annually, and they were unrelated—far short of what Pearce had recommended. After 1914 the lectures were given up for many years.

### *Completing the College Lot*

The new Hall was undeniably handsome,[72] but some of its neighboring buildings were unattractive and offensive. Adjoining the property on the south, between the College and the Swedenborgian and Unitarian Churches, on lots running from Twenty-second Street east to Van Pelt, were three unsightly houses and a stable. All the Fellows were sensitively aware of them; all were dismayed when they learned that the properties had passed into the hands of a real estate developer and might be converted into a garage. But this space had more than aesthetic value. The College needed it, President Tyson explained, not only to enlarge and beautify its own property, "but also to give us an opportunity to extend our Hall by adding a laboratory where research work and clinical and bacteriological examinations may be carried out under the auspices of the College . . . ."[73]

Through the influence of a Fellow, James Thorington, the new owners offered the houses and stable to the College for $46,000. The College, however, had no money for the purpose, even if the Swedenborgian Church adjoining should put up half the sum.[74] In this situation Wharton Sinkler, vice-president and prospective president of the College, persuaded his nephew Eckley B. Coxe, Jr., to purchase the buildings to protect the College from "undesirable encroachments." Coxe promptly did so, with the understanding that the College, while under no obligation, might purchase them at any time. He offered them for approximately $6,000 and an annual ground rent of $1,600 (four per cent on $40,000). The College accepted the offer, razed the "unsanitary dwellings," tore down the stable, and proceeded to landscape the lots.[75]

Meanwhile Sinkler had died, and the College was considering the construction of some kind of memorial on its newly acquired property, when Mr. Coxe offered the College the ground rent free on condition that any building erected in the space should be a memorial to his uncle. No serious thought was given to erecting a laboratory building. Mitchell proposed making a flower garden and putting a memorial fountain in the middle of it. "A monument would not do," he continued; "the thing would look too much like a cemetery. But we could show Philadelphia, as we have in our building, how such a thing ought to be done."[76] The garden was planted in 1914, a sundial (not a fountain) was placed at its center, benches were placed along the walks and paths; and the Sinkler Garden became, as it has remained, "the source of great pleasure to the Fellows and the general public."

What Mitchell wrote de Schweinitz about the acquisition of the stable property applied equally to the entire achievement of a new home for the College: "Between luck and pluck we have done for the profession a most valuable thing."[77]

### *Transactions*

The third series of *Transactions,* which had begun auspiciously in 1875 with reports on the Siamese Twins, was not firmly established until 1885. Filling the volume was often a problem; in 1882 no volume appeared. To prevent another such failure, the chairman of the Committee on Publications obtained pledges from thirty Fellows that each would present and publish a paper within three years.[78] Further to encourage authors, it was arranged that each paper would be printed immediately after presentation and that "pre-prints" would be sent to professional journals.[79] Within three years another crisis developed: printing costs were greater than expected, unpaid bills amounted to

$822.33 (which President Da Costa paid), and another volume was missed.[80] Publication was resumed with the eighth volume in 1886. Thereafter the *Transactions* were published uninterruptedly, in an established format, the content and character of the volumes, with occasional aberrations, basically unchanging.

A welcome innovation was the inclusion of full discussions of papers, recorded by a stenographer. Occasionally an entire meeting was given over to discussion of a single topic, with no formal paper. Such a discussion was held on February 3, 1897, on "The Relation of Nervous Disorders in Women to Pelvic Disease." Barton Cooke Hirst, Edward E. Montgomery, Charles P. Noble, Weir Mitchell, James Tyson, Charles K. Mills, Wharton Sinkler, and others participated. Solomon Solis-Cohen and Lewis W. Steinbach reported on a case in their practice; but the College directed the Comittee on Publications not to include this presentation in the published volume.[81]

## *Fellows and Their Presidents*

There were 195 resident Fellows in the College in 1885; by 1909 the membership had more than doubled to 486. The growth was a reflection of the growing number of physicians in Philadelphia and of the decision made in 1886 to extend eligibility to those living up to thirty miles from the city. Although the increase made the College more representative of the profession and had obvious financial benefits, it did not please all the Fellows. There were frequent calls to safeguard elections by creating an election committee or empowering the Censors to pass on all candidates. In the end the Council was given the duty.[82] But even the Council was charged with admitting persons for other than demonstrated achievement in their profession. "Are the requirements for Fellowship as high as they should be?" D. Hayes Agnew asked as he stepped down from the presidency:

> Are its doors of admission thrown too widely open? Is there not some danger that the matter of emolument may come to outweigh other and weightier considerations? These are questions which I think may be asked with propriety. The College was designed to be, and should be, a thoroughly representative body, and its seats should be

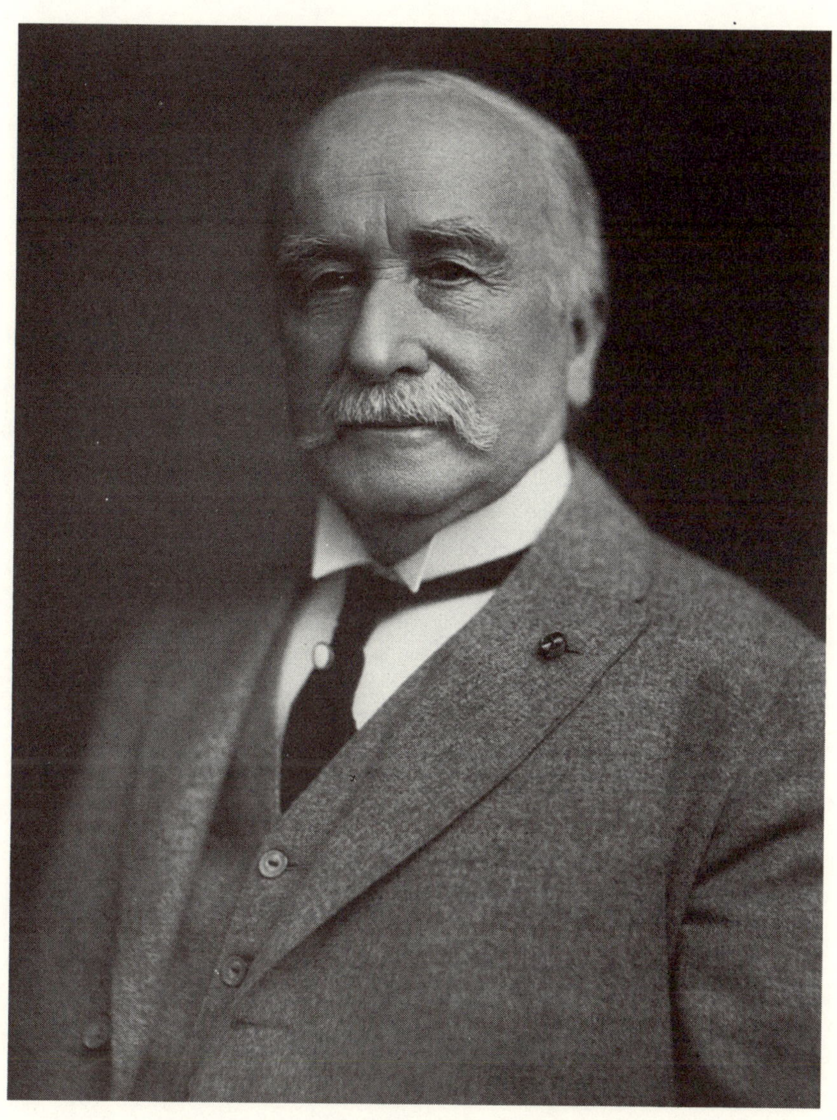

William W. Keen, (1837–1932). Photograph.

> occupied by those who, after years (perhaps nine or ten) of professional toil, or by literary labors or original research, have achieved distinction in one or several of the departments of medicine.

If this would make the College an "aristocracy," so be it: the Fellowship *should* be an aristocracy, not of wealth, family or social consideration, but of merit, an aristocracy "as accessible to the humblest as to the most favored member of our noble profession."[83]

Weir Mitchell shared these views: he would restrict membership to those over age thirty and require evidence of professional achievement.[84] To allow such persons to obtain admission, he urged that five votes, not three, be required for rejection; but although strong voices in the College supported it, the proposal was rejected by Fellows who regarded the College much as they might a social club. Candidates for admission whose sponsors did not appear to speak on their behalf at elections were likely to be dropped.

Debate over admission requirements was in part a reflection of the College's uncertainty about itself, its character and purpose, even the meaning of the Fellowship. Mitchell, always seeking new ways to extend the usefulness and influence of the College, in 1901 raised the question whether a graduate in medicine whose practice was principally in dentistry might not be considered for election.[85] The matter was referred to the Council and was not heard of again. Equally radical suggestions by President James Tyson in 1910 also came to nothing. Excellent candidates for membership, he thought, might be found among "well-educated practitioners past middle life" in the city and suburbs, "who may not have been authors or original investigators, but who are eminently respectable and honored by their patients and fellow citizens." The College, he went on, was not a social club; it might be desirable to require Fellows to offer evidence of continuing qualification, by attendance or otherwise, to justify retention of their membership.[86]

For more than a quarter of a century after George Bacon Wood died in 1879, the College had a succession of presidents of strong personality and memorable achievement. Stillé, Da Costa, Mitchell, Agnew, Ashhurst, Keen, and Horatio C Wood made basic advances in their sciences and fashioned reforms in medical education and standards. All were men of personal force and presence, who had national, even international, reputations. Agnew was called in to look after President Garfield when the president was shot in 1881. Keen, who performed the first successful operation for removal of a brain tumor, was one of the surgeons who removed President Cleveland's cancerous jawbone in an operation kept secret until some years after Cleveland's death. Mitchell was world-famous as a physiologist and neurologist. Wood took a leading part in the reorganization of the University of Pennsylvania Medical School. All seven who served as president between 1883 and 1904 are in the *Dictionary of American Biography.* They established a character and standard for the College at the turn of the century that Fellows took pride in and long remembered.

Their successors in the next quarter century served a well-established institution and a profession reformed or reforming. Arthur V. Meigs, James Tyson, George E. de Schweinitz, James C. Wilson, Richard H. Harte, William J. Taylor, Thomas R. Neilson, and Hobart A. Hare, learned, skillful, and successful practitioners all, were on the whole neither pioneers in medical science nor representatives and spokesmen of their profession nationally. Their influence was more limited than their predecessors'. Only three of the eight are in the *Dictionary of American Biography.* Content with a local reputation, they performed many useful services that made and kept Philadelphia an agreeable city, giving time and thought generously to the church vestry, the board of the Library Company, or the affairs of the American Philosophical Society. Richard H. Harte, active in local politics, was elected councilman from the city's Eighth Ward in 1907, and, as director of the Department of Health and Charities, developed plans for the reconstruction of Blockley Hospital. Others were pleased with the distinctions they won from substituting at the organ of St. Stephen's Church, rowing on the Schuylkill, playing cricket, or taking a seat regularly at the Orchestra. In the College they were heirs of a tradition which they cherished and protected but did not extend.

CHAPTER X

# *Holding Its Own*

AT the close of his three-year term of office on January 1, 1913, President de Schweinitz reported with satisfaction that the College had no debt and that its budget was balanced.[1] The old hall at Thirteenth and Locust Streets, now rented to the Free Library, and the new hall with its adjoining properties, had been valued in 1911 at $521,091, and the College's invested funds amounted to $180,304, not including the Mütter bequest, which was controlled by external trustees. The income from all sources in 1911 was $42,-104, and projected expenses were $39,721.[2]

George E. de Schweinitz was the leading ophthalmologist in Philadelphia, possibly in the United States. Born in Philadelphia but reared in Bethlehem, Pennsylvania, he attended Moravian College, of which his father was president, and read medicine with a country doctor until he could afford to go to medical school. He was graduated from the University of Pennsylvania in 1881. De Schweinitz was a successful teacher and practitioner and the author of a textbook on diseases of the eye that went through ten editions. He was professor of ophthalmology in Jefferson Medical College from 1896 to 1902, then moved to the University of Pennsylvania.

The College, to which he had been elected in 1887, was one of de Schweinitz's continuing loyalties. He had been chairman of its Section on Ophthalmology and for many years was also chairman of the Committee on Entertainments. Sharing Mitchell's belief about the uses of social occasions, he supported a plan to furnish a small dining room in the new hall where speakers and other guests of the College might be entertained, and contributed a silver punch bowl and six cups to dress its table. As president, he involved himself in every aspect of College business, even helping to plan programs of the stated scientific meetings. John B. Roberts, who was not free with compliments, told de Schweinitz after his first year in office, that he had "made the business of the institution so business-like, and the science of the body so scientific that now it is indeed a living thing to stimulate the medical men of Philadelphia to higher and better professional work. What a privilege Fellowship has become," he exclaimed.[3]

Three years after de Schweinitz presented his confident report in 1913, however, the College faced a deficit of nearly $1,400.[4] Thus began that condition of financial stringency which, occasionally relieved but never cured, remained an urgent concern of the officers and Council for many years.

Embarrassed by the situation—perhaps because it might be thought to reflect on their financial acumen and trusteeship—the Finance Committee and Council in 1917 directed that the treasurer's reports should not be printed and distributed, although, of course, Fellows might examine them in the secretary's office if they wished. Another reason for not publishing was given by President Harte: that most Fellows and the public, if they were to know the total worth of the College—more than one million dollars—might conclude erroneously that it had no need of financial help.[5] The result of this secretiveness was that most Fellows, not to mention the public, remained unaware for years of the true state of affairs.

### *Stated Meetings*

Meanwhile, the work of the College continued essentially unchanged. Three or four papers were read at each meeting. The Fellows' attendance averaged between sixty and seventy, with two or three times that number of non-Fellows. The Council frequently tried to increase these numbers, with varying success.

Throwing open the meetings to the public, however, was not without risk. Sensing the possibility of a good story, newspaper reporters also attended. They were not usually identified and could not be asked to leave. The stories they wrote were often inaccurate, sensationalized, and embarrassing. Reports on radium treatment by Howard A. Kelly of Johns Hopkins University and Robert Abbe of New York were headlined in the *Public Ledger:*

"Radium Hailed as Cancer Cure/Eminent Doctors Proclaim Conquest at College of Physicians/Acts as though by Magic."[6] To guard against such notoriety, the College sometimes resorted to ingenious but innocent deception. Certain that Judson Daland's paper on "Dr. Ehrlich's Remedy for Syphilis" would bring out the reporters, the College persuaded the author to retitle his paper "Dihydroxydiamino-arsenobenzene as a Therapeutic Remedy for Lues."[7] The journalists were baffled and successfully misled.

Concerns of a general sort were also sometimes presented. R. Tait McKenzie, a medical graduate of McGill University, professor of physical education in the University of Pennsylvania, and a sculptor, discussed the physical development of young men. Another Fellow, concerned about the moral, as well as the physical, improvement of "the race," believed that Mendel's laws of heredity provided a scientific basis for the great sociological challenge of the age—to encourage the marriage of persons with desirable qualities and to eliminate undesirable traits from society by forbidding those possessing them to marry.[8] This appears to have been the only paper on eugenics ever read to the College.

## *World War I*

Problems of the College budgets, even the regular meetings of the College, were overwhelmed by the First World War. Nearly half the Fellows served in the army or navy; and College meetings and several volumes of the *Transactions* from 1915 through 1919 became avenues through which military medical experience was communicated to the profession at large. In the spring of 1915, George Morris Piersol left his practice to attend the first Plattsburg Summer Training Camp and a special meeting was called to hear about camp and military hygiene and sanitation "in relation to war mortality." From time to time there were other lectures and papers on national health and preparedness.[9] As the war continued, representatives of international boards and commissions came to the College to describe medical conditions among the civilian populations of France, Italy, and Russia. James P. Hutchinson and President Richard H. Harte went to France as volunteers in the American Ambulance, about which the Fellows and their friends were informed in an illustrated public lecture in 1916.

By mid-winter of 1916–1917 popular sentiment in support of

the Allies had pretty well crystallized. In February the College urged young physicians to volunteer; and, in a departure from its long tradition of neutrality in political matters, it publicly endorsed President Wilson's tougher policy towards Germany.[10]

Within a few weeks of the United States' entry into the war in April 1917, Fellows began to leave their practices and posts, as hospital units were called into active service. In May the Pennsylvania Hospital unit—Base Hospital No. 10—took away the president, vice-president, and secretary of the College, as well as a score more. Of eighteen captains and lieutenants on the professional staff of Hospital No. 10, sixteen were Fellows. De Schweinitz was elected acting president of the College, but within a few months he, too, was called to duty. Of 463 active Fellows, 216 served in the armed forces before the war ended.[11]

Stated meetings were now devoted principally to war medicine. American, British, and French military surgeons related their experiences in the camps and hospitals in France. Single papers and entire symposia dealt with the nature and treatment of wounds or with particular topics and diseases, such as nutrition, psychiatry, sanitation, neurosurgery, syphilis, tuberculosis, and pneumonia. One speaker from overseas was Sir Berkeley (later Lord) Moynihan, chairman of the British Army Advisory Medical Board. His warm reception by the College and other Philadelphia medical institutions in the fall of 1917 was described as a "Patriotic Rally."[12]

Most of the papers printed in the *Transactions* in 1918 and 1919 came out of the war. There were articles on research on aviation medicine, the re-education of blinded soldiers, and reconstructive surgery at Queen's Hospital at Sidcup in England. The volumes contained the results of nutritional surveys, an account of psychological testing by Major Robert M. Yerkes of the Sanitary Corps, and A. Newton Richards' report on physiological experiments with poison gases. John H. Gibbon's paper on "Advancement in the Treatment of Wounds and Infections resulting from the War," read to the College on April 5, 1919, was printed in the *Transactions.* Wartime experience, as George W. Norris told the Fellows in a paper of his own in 1919, had "profoundly influenced and broadened" the doctors.[13]

In contrast to the emphasis on military medicine, hardly any notice was paid to the influenza that swept through the population in the fall of 1918. David Riesman, discussing a paper on pneumonia, spoke briefly of conditions in "this epidemic time," and Lawrence Flick urged that the clinical records of the emergency flu hospitals be collected and preserved for future study; but that was about all. The flu disappeared as quickly as it came, and, overshadowed by the momentous events in Europe, ceased to be a subject of concern or inquiry after the winter of 1918–19. The College declined to study the disease, and no paper on it was presented at any College meeting.[14]

The war left other legacies. William W. Keen moved in 1919 to expel three German and Austrian Associate Fellows. "At no time," said President Harte, supporting the motion, had they "protested or raised their voices against the many abuses, and, I may say, crimes against humanity, practiced by their respective governments . . . ."[15] Another piece of war-related business was to erect a memorial to those Fellows who had been in military service, particulary two who had died on active duty. The Germans were duly expelled, although not without objection by some Fellows; but the memorial plaque was never installed, because the College had no money to pay for it.[16] By then thoughts had turned to the future: Alonzo E. Taylor, professor of physiological chemistry in the University of Pennsylvania, delivered a Newbold lecture in 1920 on "Post-war Conditions of Civic Organizations in Europe."

With the return of peace, meetings were devoted once more to civilian cases, diseases, and medical and surgical conditions. Strong efforts were made to restore a sense of collegiality with College dinners and other social events. But the world after 1919 was changing, and the College changed with it. Fewer Fellows now than before the war were willing to present papers—only eight in each of the years 1922 and 1923, only four in 1926. Of fifty-four Fellows approached for a paper in 1925, none acceded to the request. One reason for this lack of response was that Fellows preferred to present papers to the sections, where discussion was livelier and more pertinent, or send them directly to the specialized journals. Attendance also fell—sometimes to an embarrassing level—as physicians moved to the suburbs and found it inconvenient to attend evening meetings in town.

To offset these conditions, the endowed lectures were scheduled to fill the stated meeting programs, and special invitations were sent to physicians generally and to the faculties and students of the local medical colleges. In addition, a lecture series, addressed primarily to medical students was organized; it was continued for several years.[17]

Thanks to the endowed lectureships, the College was able to bring distinguished foreign physicians and surgeons to Philadelphia. These included Frederick G. Banting and J. J. R. Macleod, who spoke on insulin (in 1923), Charles H. Best, who spoke on liver function (in 1938), Sir Wilfred Grenfell, famous as "the Labrador doctor," Sir Thomas Lewis of University College Hospital, London, C. M. Ariens Kappers of the Institute for Brain Research in Amsterdam, and Professor F. J. Lang of the University of Innsbrúck. The great public reputations of some of these men filled Mitchell Hall to overflowing. Sir Humphry Rolleston of London, Sir Andrew MacPhail of McGill University, Arturo Castiglioni of Padua, Charles Singer of London, and Karl Sudhoff of Leipzig lectured on topics in medical history, but to smaller audiences than the famous clinicians commanded.

Sometimes a foreign visitor tried his hosts' patience. The distinguished physical chemist and Nobel laureate Svante A. Ahrrenius, after accepting an invitation, changed both the subject of his lecture and the date on which he would appear, and then demanded that the "economical conditions" be settled before he spoke. De Schweinitz regarded this last as insulting, flew "into a blind fury," and almost replied sharply in kind. In the end he paid Ahrrenius' fee from his own pocket and resolved to have nothing to do with foreign scholars again. Alfred Stengel sympathized with him: "May we be protected from such high scientists for all time to come."[18]

Although Richard Pearce had been rebuffed in 1910 in his call for a series of lectures by laboratory men, the number of papers by researchers did increase in the post-war years. David Riesman, Rufus Cole of the Rockefeller Institute Hospital, and M. Howard Fussell discussed pneumonia, which had replaced tuberculosis as the cause of the greatest number of deaths from infectious diseases in Philadelphia. Peyton Rous, Alfred E. Cohn, Thomas M. Rivers, and Simon Flexner, all of the Rockefeller Institute, appeared on College programs; so did Hans Zinsser, Walter B. Cannon, and William B. Castle of Harvard Medical School. One of the most significant papers was A. Newton Richards' Mary Scott Newbold lecture in 1925 on "the nature and mode of regulation of glomerular function." Nor were the social relations of the medical profession and medical science neglected: Charles-Edward A. Winslow of the Yale University Medical School addressed the College several times on the subject, which was to force itself increasingly on the Fellows' attention.

In contrast to the stated meetings, the sections flourished, with numerous up-to-date clinical reports, stimulating discussions, and respectable attendance. The sections welcomed non-Fellows, were less constrained by traditional College attitudes and practices, and enjoyed some effective independence, including control of their own bank accounts. The Section on Ophthalmology even wanted to establish its own museum. Section proceedings were fully reported, often filling more than half of each volume of the *Transactions* in the 1920s. In 1922, for example, the papers and abstracts of papers on ophthalmology filled sixty-two pages, those on general medicine ninety-one pages, and those on the relatively new Section on Industrial Medicine and Public Health nineteen pages. The figures the next year were much the same, with the Section on Medical History claiming an additional forty-nine pages for its papers. In 1927 the *Transactions* contained fourteen general papers, of which three were endowed lectures and two were Lister anniversary addresses; but the Section on Ophthalmology had forty-three papers and abstracts, and the Section on Otology and Laryngology had twenty-two.

The Council viewed the success of the sections with mixed feelings and took some steps to curb them. In 1921 the number of pages they were allowed in the *Transactions* was limited to 250; and a few years later an unsuccessful effort was made to limit section reports to titles and abstracts only. Some thought was also given to eliminating the Section on General Medicine, which had 123 members in 1923, on the ground that papers read there might equally properly be presented to the whole College. President Hare admitted that section programs were often better than those of the College.[19]

### Public Health

In the three decades after 1909 the College was notably active in public health. To consider and speak out on such questions was consistent with the conviction, strongly held by Mitchell, Agnew, and other presidents at the turn of the century, that the College had an opportunity and a duty to advise, and be consulted by, public authorities. Through its standing Committee on Public Health and Preventive Medicine, established in 1912, and through the complementary section, created a few years later, the Fellows individually and the College as a whole expressed their views not only on matters for which there was general public support, like vaccination,[20] but also on such controversial issues of growing concern as child labor and health insurance.

In 1909 the College formally condemned long working hours for women and children and urged the Fellows to write their representatives in favor of state legislation to limit such hours of labor.[21] Four years later President James C. Wilson told a lawyer friend that there were "many reasons why an adult should work, as you and I habitually do, more than eight hours a day, but no reason why any adult should compel a child of fourteen or sixteen years of age to exceed the eight hour limit." Wilson put his views more strongly to the governor and several members of the Pennsylvania legislature in 1915. "From the point of view of the physician interested in sociological matters," he wrote, no measure before the Assembly was more important than the eight-hour day for children under sixteen:

> Upon one point you may feel entirely satisfied—that is, that the medical profession as a body is in full accord upon this subject. Of another thing you may feel confident—that sooner or later it has got to come.[22]

Such concerns were, of course, not without precedent in the College's history. Promotion of public health had been one of the founders' purposes. From time to time in the nineteenth century, the College had offered its views on matters of sanitation and public health, and city and state boards of health had invited its recommendations. As recently as 1910 the state board had sought the College's opinion whether tetanus anti-toxin should be available at no charge to victims of gunshot, fire-cracker, and similar wounds.[23] Anticipating indifference and resistance, the advocates of public health measures, would remind conservative Fellows of this history. In any case, most physicians understood what poverty, malnutrition, inadequate housing, and want of education meant for the health of ordinary people. How or whether any particular physician reacted was uncertain; and institutions responded more slowly than individuals. But individuals moved institutions. In the decades of its most active concern with public health, the principal figure in the College was James M. Anders.[24]

A descendant of Schwenkfelders of Montgomery County, Pennsylvania, and a graduate of the University of Pennsylvania Medical School in 1877, Anders had a long career as professor and dean of the Medico-Chirurgical College and the University's Graduate School of Medicine. For sixteen years he was a member of the Advisory Board of the Philadelphia Department of Health; he was a leader in campaigns to control tuberculosis, abate noise, and purify air, "and, in general," his memorialist wrote, "seemed to foresee the needs of our City regarding public health in advance of most men." Anders was president of the County Medical Society, the American College of Physicians, and the Pennsylvania Society for the Prevention of Tuberculosis. In 1924 he gave the College $5,000 to promote the cause of public health and preventive medicine. In addition to paying the expenses and honoraria of "noted speakers from a distance," the income was to be used to make surveys of hygienic and sanitary conditions, conduct original research in preventive medicine, and, should it ever be sufficient, "to employ a research worker in public, preventive medicine."[25] This was another expression of the hope once cherished by Mitchell and some others that the College might one day support a scholarly research institute like the Rockefeller Institute in New York. In 1925 Anders presented another idea—that the College establish a standing committee on medical education to provide, among other services, information to hospitals on interns, and information to American physicians intending to study abroad and to foreign doctors wishing to study in the United States. "Philadelphia should keep the lead in medical education in this country," he concluded. "The formation of a standing committee by the College would become an agency for good in that direction."[26] Such a committee, he urged, would enable the College to "arrange for a systematic campaign of education among the laity," principally by means of authoritative lectures.

In response to Anders' prompting, the Committee on Public Health and Preventive Medicine was established in 1912. Despite some resentment that Anders' proposal implied that the College had neglected hygiene and public health in the past, the Council agreed that such a committee "would add to the usefulness of the

College and further the original object for which the College was organized." The College approved the proposal and the by-laws were amended accordingly:[27]

> It shall be the duty of the Committee to investigate matters of special importance concerning the Public Health, to report upon the same to the College and to recommend methods of dealing with them.
>
> The Committee shall also inform the College of all steps of an unusual nature taken by the Federal, State or Municipal Governments in connection with the problems of public health and acquaint the College with the character and purpose of proposed legislation relating to health and disease.
>
> The Committee on Public Health and Preventive Medicine shall, when the necessity arises and subject to the approval of the College, make such arrangements as may render the Expert Knowledge of the College upon Hygiene, Sanitary Science and Preventive Medicine available for the uses of the Public Authorities.
>
> It shall also arrange, subject to the approval of the College, for occasional Authoritative Popular Lectures to be delivered within the College Building, the expence of which shall be defrayed by the College.

The new committee lost no time in getting to work. It was constantly before the College or Council with a recommendation or resolution about some public health measure or policy in the city or state. In general, Anders preferred to present his resolutions to the College, where he was more likely to receive a sympathetic hearing, than to pass them through the Council, as the by-laws seemed to direct. And, as the Council recommended, he worked closely with the Committee on Scientific Business to bring speakers on public health to the College under the joint auspices of his committee and the College.

Only a few months after it was created, the Committee, through Anders, proposed that the College endorse a bill in City Councils forbidding the use of night soil as fertilizer, as was still the practice in Philadelphia, unless it was first treated for "infectivity." After some delay the College approved the resolution, and also "registered its emphatic protest" against keeping hogs within

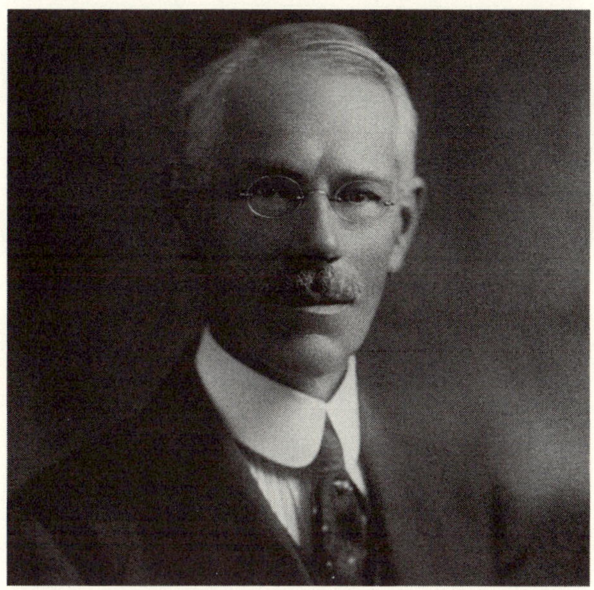

John B. Roberts, (1852–1924). Photograph by Marceau, Philadelphia.

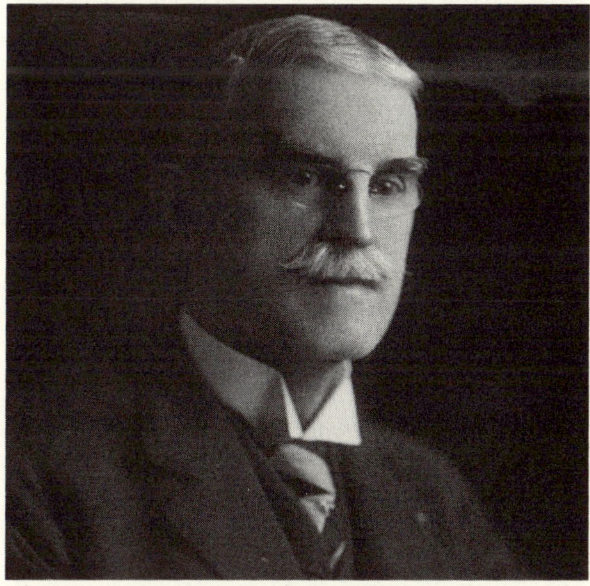

James M. Anders, (1854–1936). Photograph by Eugene O'Connor, Philadelphia.

the city limits.[28] The condition of the streets was another inescapable and constant concern. The College devoted one of its stated meetings to the subject in 1917. Apparently the physicians and the sanitarians could not agree on the definition of a *clean* street; but, as Alexander C. Abbott remarked, any one who had walked around Philadelphia knew what an *unclean* street was.[29]

A simple listing of the measures the College endorsed is a measure of Anders' activity and the breadth of support for his committee's work. At the local level, the committee and College usually supported the successive directors of public health in their programs.[30] In 1921 it commended the director for introducing radium treatment into the Philadelphia General Hospital and for installing "a radium plant" there. In 1924 it offered him help in compiling existing legislation into a health code "in simple language." In 1930 it agreed with him that the number of beds for tuberculosis patients in the city should not be reduced, but that a four-hundred bed hospital was necessary and should be built. In 1923, like almost every other group concerned with civic health and improvement, the College spoke out on the city's water supply. In 1918 the College endorsed regulations for wet nurses drafted by the Babies' Welfare Association. Shocked by the prevalence of puerperal fever among the poor, it voted in 1924 that professors should instruct their students in these realities, that practitioners should develop "an aseptic conscience," and that pregnant women should be made aware of the advantages of maternity hospitals. The College was even willing to join other institutions in inquiries into sanitary conditions and medical care in the city's House of Correction and the Water Bureau. It responded at once to an angry letter from Arthur H. Lea, publisher and civic leader and later a benefactor of the College, which called attention to pollution by oil refineries: a committee sent out to smell the air in 1933 confirmed Lea's charges, and the College recommended that the Department of Health use its powers to abate the nuisance.

Issues with implications for public health beyond Philadelphia were also considered and acted upon. When it appeared in 1914 that Pennsylvania's compulsory vaccination law might be repealed, the College sent a protest to Harrisburg; and when the same threat appeared again in 1924 the College again responded with a strong statement that "universal vaccination is the only certain, known measure of protecting the public against smallpox." A proposal in the state legislature in 1921 to establish a system of compulsory health insurance was condemned as demoralizing, un-American, and inimical to the best interests of the people and the medical profession. The College opposed licensing osteopaths in 1923 and optometrists in 1937. Disturbed by radio advertising of proprietary medicines, but admittedly uncertain whether anything could be done, the College in 1930 endorsed any efforts that might be undertaken to suppress it. In 1928 it agreed to cooperate with the Law Association in the latter's efforts to reduce the abuse of accident litigation by asking the court to establish a panel of qualified medical men from whom only expert testimony might be heard.

By the mid-thirties, however, the Committee's zeal seems to have cooled. So at least one may infer from the Council's request to the chairman in 1937 "to watch for opportunities which he may call to the attention of the Council in which by resolution or otherwise the College may use it influence to further sound public policy."[31] Charles W. Burr promptly pointed to the city's water supply as such an opportunity.

Anders was no less successful in educating the general public, especially through the schools. This took many forms. "Health Day," which he was instrumental in establishing, was one. The College, other medical and civic bodies, and the public schools joined in 1917 to sponsor the observance, and the College continued its support, albeit intermittently, for several years. *The Evening Bulletin* commended the institution for such activities, and the city's Director of Health, a Fellow of the College, was equally pleased—and a little surprised—that "the conservative College of Physicians" should be taking an interest in public health.[32]

To Anders, his committee, and others who took a long view of the nation's health, it was clear that the success of public health reform lay with the young people. R. Tait McKenzie in a paper to the College in 1913 advocated a program of physical education in the schools. So did a representative of the Philadelphia school system, who also addressed the College. Anders agreed: "Compared with the time devoted to the mental training of the child and student, it must be obvious to us as physicians that too little attention is still paid to physical education."[33]

Using statistics gleaned from examinations of recruits in the World War, McKenzie in 1920 again discussed the physical condition of the nation's young people. This time the College urged the Philadelphia Board of Education to institute a program of systematic daily instruction in personal hygiene in the schools and to provide "an adequate number of recreation and community centres."[34] The Board acted, and in 1923 the Superintendent of Schools was able to make an encouraging report: special classes were offered for tubercular students, those with orthopedic problems, those whose sight or hearing was impaired, and the undernourished (17,000 half pints of milk were consumed daily in the elementary schools). By instituting safety patrols, the number of accidents had been reduced. Thirty playgrounds were in operation the year round, with seventy more open in the summer months. Furthermore, the College supported the Board of Health in seeking more public health nurses, school nurses, and oral hygienists "to meet the needs of the normal increase of population." "If our laws demand that children should go to school," Alexander C. Abbott observed in discussing the Superintendent's paper, "then, I believe, it is our duty to see that those children are in physical condition to profit by going to school."[35]

How "modern" the outlook of some of the Fellows was in these matters is suggested by another observation on a paper in 1923 that spoke of preventive medicine as an "opportunity" for the private physician. In essential agreement, Abbott wondered aloud whether "possibly in the future the practitioner may be paid not only for helping the sick to get well, but for such advice as will prevent the well from getting sick."[36]

All this made the College better known. That was gratifying to many Fellows, who recalled the frequent appeals by their presidents to that end. To consider what more might be done, a Committee on Extending Public Usefulness and Influence was formed, with Alfred Stengel of the University of Pennsylvania as chairman. It concluded that public usefulness and influence might best be extended by the Committee on Public Health itself, that special meetings be held for physicians who were not Fellows and for laymen, and that the first two such meetings be on food inspection and distribution in Philadelphia and on midwifery among the poor. Other topics proposed by Stengel's committee for discussion included child welfare, street cleaning, sewerage disposal, smoke nuisance, quarantine regulations, milk supply, housing, the management of social diseases, and a survey of Philadelphia medical and social agencies.[37] Significantly the Committee on Public

Health was renamed the Committee on Public Health, Preventive Medicine and Public Relations in 1935.

With this encouragement from Stengel's committee, Anders invited Seneca Egbert, professor of hygiene in the University of Pennsylvania, to report on the local food supply. Egbert found conditions generally satisfactory, although he cited particular bakeries, bottling plants, food shops, and push-cart markets, where food and beverages were "exposed to the dust of the streets, flies, promiscuous handling by unclean customers, etc." His recommendations ranged from increasing the number of milk and meat inspectors (and their salaries) to inaugurating an educational campaign for both food handlers and the public at large. "When the latter are fully impressed with the importance of the subject in general," Egbert predicted, "they will, in all probability, make the former appreciate the direct economic advantage of it to themselves." On Anders' motion, the Council endorsed the recommendations.[38]

Another of Anders' campaigns resulted in the formation of a city commission on ventilation in public and semi-public buildings and in public conveyances. The College not only named two of its Fellows to the commission but also contributed to its expenses. On the other hand, it declined to endorse efforts to control noise on public streets from automobiles, their sirens and klaxons, from street vendors and newsboys crying their wares, and from other sources.[39]

### *Other Public Relations*

Other issues of general public concern were brought to the College from time to time. The response was often determined by the force or reputation of the sponsor; although some concerns, though admirable, were rejected because they lay outside the institution's scope, and a few were turned down "on advice of counsel" (who, however, was sometimes more "liberal" in his interpretation of the powers of the College than some of the Fellows). Thus, although David Riesman argued in 1917 that the death penalty was "no longer in keeping with the spirit of the times," the College declined to endorse a bill in the legislature to abolish it.[40] However, on a motion of William W. Keen, it strongly protested a bill in Congress in 1921 that would have have allowed Yellowstone Lake in Yellowstone Park to be dammed, and permitted commercial use of national parks and monuments:[41]

> For fifty years, successive Congresses have prevented the invasion of our national parks by commercial companies and have retained them for the use of the nation as reservations of unique scientific value and museums and laboratories of original research, as well as areas of high educative and recreational importance to the whole nation.

At the request of the Civic Club of Philadelphia in 1930 the College formally supported a bill in the legislature to strengthen anti-pollution measures in streams and water. It endorsed the metric system in 1921 and requested that henceforth temperatures, weights, and measurements in the *Transactions* be given in centigrade or metric, although English and Fahrenheit equivalents might be added "in parenthesis." The Fellows repeatedly expressed opposition to those parts of the Volstead Act that limited physicians' discretion in prescribing wine, whisky, and brandy.[42]

## *"Thunder in Philadelphia"*

In 1932 a national commission, headed by Ray Lyman Wilbur, was completing a five-year study of the cost of medical care in the United States. Physicians, hospitals, and medical societies, eagerly awaiting its report, had already begun to discuss subjects they knew the commission had examined. Thus in January and February 1932 several papers—one by a member of the commission—were presented at College meetings describing briefly the work of the commission and also the health systems of Great Britain and Germany and the organization and possible influence of the newly-opened Curtis Clinic in Philadelphia.

The national commission's report, published late in 1932, argued that the American people were not getting the medical care they needed, both because the cost was beyond their reach and because adequate medical care was not available in many parts of the country. To remedy these conditions, the commission recommmended group practice, the extension of basic public health services, payment through insurance or by public funds or both, and the coordination of medical services, especially of rural with urban services. Such services should preferably be organized around hospitals in order to maintain standards, and it was important to preserve or develop "a personal relation between patient and physician."[43] Such thoughts excited instant controversy.

Nine members of the commission—among them Arthur C. Morgan, emeritus professor of clinical medicine at Temple University and a Fellow of the College—in a minority statement rejected the recommendations of group practice and insurance. Morris Fishbein, the editor of the *Journal of the American Medical Association,* in a long editorial on December 3, 1932, denounced the report, which he said was supported by "the great foundations, public health officialdom, social theory—even socialism and communism—inciting to revolution." In this atmosphere of lively controversy, the American Academy of Political and Social Science decided to organize a meeting on the subject, and invited Alfred Stengel, professor of medicine in the University of Pennyslvania and incoming president of the College, to preside. Stengel at first declined, feeling that the report had been received with too much excitement and loose talk; but a few months later he proposed instead that the Academy and the College should hold a joint meeting on the "Medical Profession and the Public." The Council gave a grudging assent, and Stengel put a program together. The meeting proved to be one of the most explosive in the College's long history.

James H. S. Bossard, a sociologist at the University of Pennsylvania, opened the session, which was held on February 7, 1934. Ninety-four Fellows were present. Citing the public's experience with physical examinations and health care in the schools, the army in the World War, veterans' hospitals, and the programs of some industries, Bossard declared that popular attitudes toward free health services were changing. Adequate medical care, he went on, was now seen as a "social necessity," even a social and personal right. Standing against this feeling, he charged, was the attitude of the medical profession, too many of whose leaders were reluctant to change. Such entrenched conservatism, he warned, could lead only to violent reaction, "that a refusal to socialize medical services is to ride directly into the storm of state medicine."

Similar challenges were thrown down by others on the pro-

# Thunder in Philadelphia

## M.D.'S AND SOCIOLOGISTS HOLD STORMY SESSION

ERNEST M. PATTERSON, Ph.D.
President, American Academy of Political and Social Science

HENRY E. SIGERIST, M.D.
Professor of Medical History
Johns Hopkins University

ALFRED STENGEL, M.D.
Professor of Medicine, University of Pa. School of Medicine

THOUGH held in Philadelphia, it was decidedly *not* a Quaker meeting!

Now that it's all over, we might suggest another title for that symposium on February 7 which was staged as a joint conference of the College of Physicians of Philadelphia and the American Academy of Political Science.

Various celebrities representing the medical profession and the laity shared the platform in beautiful Irvine Auditorium at the University of Pennsylvania to discuss the socialization of medical care.

"The Medical Profession and the Public: Currents and Counter-Currents" was the general subject of the conference.

"Sociologists and the Medical Profession: Attack and Counter-Attack" describes somewhat more accurately the actual proceedings.

When all was said and done, though several speakers toyed around the fringe of the subject, so to speak, nobody had adequately presented anything approaching a specific program for carrying out the general idea of taking care of all the thousands of persons needing but unable to pay for good medical care.

Early in the day it became painfully apparent that the conference was made up of two openly hostile groups. Divided sharply into the two schools of thought which have obtained since the epochal publication of reports of the Committee on the Costs of Medical Care, conference speakers in a number of instances handled their opposition without gloves.

Aspersion and recrimination, charge and counter-charge furnished the highlights of the entire meeting. They were, in fact, too numerous and too sharp to fit in, quite, with one's notion of a proper Quaker holiday.

Indeed, as the day wore on toward the close, a number of Philadelphia physicians were declaring that the conference "seemed to have been stacked against the medical profession."

Certainly Dr. Morris Fishbein, editor of the *Journal of the American Medical Association*, had some grounds for feeling that it had been stacked against him personally, his publication, and his organization.

Four of the ten speakers on the all-day program were especially critical of the present organization of medical practice in the United States. They were James H. S. Bossard, Ph.D., professor of sociology at the University of Pennsylvania; Edgar Sydenstricker, director of research for the Milbank Memorial Fund; Michael M. Davis, Ph.D., director of medical services for the Julius Rosenwald Fund; and William Trufant Foster, LL.D., economist.

Dr. Bossard began the skirmish with the opening paper of the conference, "A Sociologist Looks at the Doctors," in which he referred critically to the attitude of many leaders of the medical profession.

"Being well entrenched," he said, "with no difficulties of earning a livelihood, they are reluctant to face any change. They are interested in maintaining the status quo.

"The danger is that they may be too arbitrary. This would be unfortunate. If the sociologist's

[*Continued on page* 85]

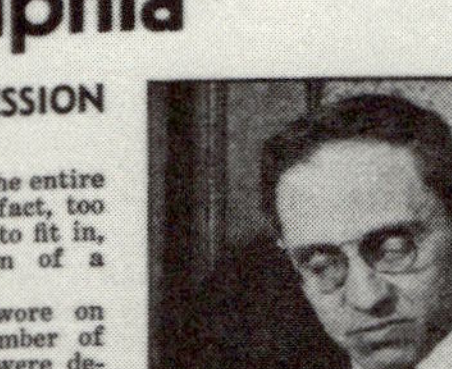

MICHAEL M. DAVIS, Ph.D.
Director for Medical Services
Julius Rosenwald Fund

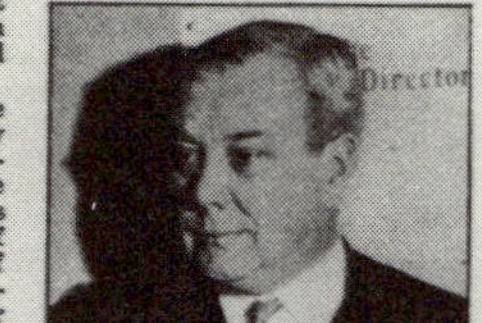



ROGER I. LEE, M.D.
Professor of Hygiene
Harvard Medical School

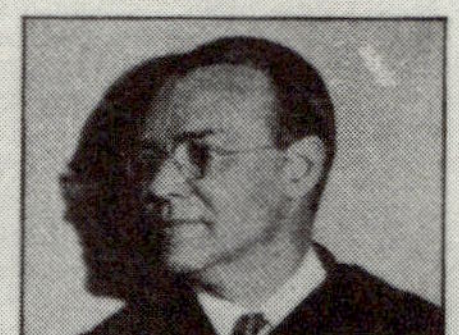

GEORGE P. MULLER, M.D.
Professor of Clinical Surgery
University of Pa. Medical School

24 25

"Thunder in Philadelphia," *Medical Economics,* XI (1934), 24.

gram, and by still others the challenges were thrown back. Thomas Parran, Jr., commissioner of health of New York state, appealed to doctors to accept the reality of social change and to speak and act as good citizens. "When we speak as doctors alone," he explained, "we have been suspected of self-interest." Fishbein, apparently taken aback by the criticisms of Bossard and others, hastily rewrote part of his paper to refute them. He rejected, sometimes in sarcastic tones, charges against his association, and asserted categorically "that no other group except physicians is really entitled to say how medicine should be practiced"—which was not the issue, as yet another speaker promptly pointed out: "What the public demands is the right to say, not how medicine shall be *practiced* but how it shall be *purchased* and *paid for.*"[44]

The uproar was intensified by the local medical press, which reported the meeting in unabashed partisan tones. Samuel H. Browne, a Fellow of the College, in the weekly publication of the County Medical Society, which he edited, called one speaker a "comedian," characterized another as a "nasty kind of bird," said of a third that the subject of his paper was trivial, and declared that the professional credentials of a fourth were dubious. Three days after the meeting, the County Medical Society formally repudiated the views expressed by "certain sociologists" at the meeting.[45]

Needless to say, after so much thunder and anger the Fellows were extremely wary of a repeat performance. Yet such topics as medical costs, health insurance, group practice, and the like, emotion-charged though they were, could not be ignored. Professional journals commented on them, newspapers and magazines discussed them, they were the subjects of political study, debate, and advocacy. In no gathering of physicians, were they long overlooked. In 1937 Esmond Long, director of the Phipps Institute, moved that the College consider its "possible relations . . . to the problem of hospital group insurance." Accordingly President Muller named himself and O. H. Perry Pepper to represent the College on the governing board of the proposed Hospital Group Insurance Plan of Pennsylvania.

About the same time the Section on Public Health requested approval for a meeting on February 6, 1939, to be devoted to "a dignified consideration" of health insurance in Germany, Great Britain, and Pennsylvania. "As a safeguard against undesirable controversy," the Section assured the Council, each speaker would be required to submit his paper to the clerk well before the meeting. The Council gave its approval, but imposed an additional safeguard, "that there shall be no open discussion from the floor." Under these constraints the papers were presented, presumably in frustrated but decorous silence; they were not printed in the *Transactions,* either in full or in abstract.

### *By-laws, 1925*

Yet, despite the activity in the College and its sections, many Fellows were uneasy. It was not simply that the financial situation did not improve, that attendance at meetings was less than it might have been, or that fewer papers were presented than before the War. The feeling was growing that the College was falling behind as a scientific institution. One Fellow, described as "of mature years, but not old, of much prominence as a teacher, and known as the author of standard medical literature," voiced the sentiment at a regular meeting. "This courageous and truthful statement," commented a colleague, "flashed out like a rocket in a dark night." The resulting illumination revealed unsuspected restlessness and dissatisfaction. In particular the College appeared to many Fellows to be controlled by an "old guard," who, having held the offices and committee appointments uninterruptedly for years, were unresponsive to, if not unaware of, the needs and opportunities of the profession and the College.[47]

One of the most outspoken critics was John B. Roberts, a surgeon successful and bold enough to deplore the modern haste to operate and to remind his colleagues of "the value of scientific doubt in surgical analysis."[48] Roberts was a political progressive, who had run for public office on reform tickets. He was especially active in the County Medical Society, of which he was president in 1891 and 1892. In the College he had repeatedly, but vainly, sought to enliven meetings by limiting the length of papers, and to invite new ideas by restricting presidents' terms to two years. When a committee to amend the by-laws was appointed in 1923, Roberts hoped for a *"real revision."* The old rules, he declared in a circular letter to the Fellows, had "prevented scientific development of the organization and have not transferred executive activities sufficiently to younger Fellows."

But the committee on the by-laws was composed entirely of

members of the Council. No radical change, therefore, could be expected. To present the issue squarely to the Fellowship, Roberts, with forty-five Fellows supporting him, moved that the bylaws include a provision that no Fellow might serve more than three years in succession as president or member of the Council, or more than ten years in succession on any committee. Although it claimed to favor rotation in office,[49] the Council recommended rejection of Roberts' motion, explaining that such matters were currently under discussion by the committee.

Undaunted, Roberts brought forward another proposal.[50] Many Fellows, he asserted, took little interest in the scientific papers and discussions, and even less in the business affairs of the College. "Probably not over 1½%" attended the former, not more than half that number the latter. Accordingly, he moved that the annual reports of the secretary and the treasurer be printed and sent to all the Fellows before the annual business meeting in December. The secretary promptly pointed out that Roberts' percentages were wrong, but offered no reply to the basic allegation. As for publishing the annual reports, Roberts was reminded that the Council had considered and rejected that notion in 1917; Fellows could always ask to see them in the College office. Roberts' motion was laid on the table by a vote of thirty to one.

Most of the meetings in 1924 were taken up by the work of revision. Every paragraph and sentence, almost every word, was considered, debated, and rephrased, until finally on Febrary 4, 1925, the new rules were approved. They were not very different from the old ones; they embodied few of Roberts' suggestions; and, like most by-laws everywhere, would take their character and effect from the character and intentions of future officers and Fellows.

Only two classes of members were recognized—Fellows, who must live in Philadelphia or within thirty miles of the city in the state of Pennsylvania (no one from New Jersey was eligible for election), and Associate Fellows, who were chosen from those living beyond the thirty-mile limit.[51] The order of Corresponding Fellow was eliminated, those in that class becoming Associate Fellows. Regularly elected Fellows who moved outside the thirty-mile limit became Non-Resident Fellows without the right to vote or participate in College business unless they continued to pay the regular annual dues. More important was the requirement—aimed at what was perceived to be the practice of electing youthful scions of old Philadelphia—that candidates for the Fellowship should be judged by their "actual achievements rather than by any promise of future accomplishment."

The entrance fee was set at $30 and annual dues at $25. Given the dependence of the College on Fellows' dues, these figures were too low; within a few months an effort was made to raise them to $50 and $30 respectively, but without success. The term of the president was limited to three successive years, as had been the practice for forty years, but no limit was placed on the terms of other officers or of chairmen and members of committees. On the other hand, no member of Council might serve on a standing committee. The considerable power of the president was confirmed and extended, for he had authority to appoint the Committees on Finance, Scientific Business, Public Health, and Entertainments, as well as the executive committees of all the sections and the members of the several prize committees. And although Roberts and others criticized the Council for regarding itself as a board of directors or trustees, when in their view it was "scarcely more than a committee of advice," the new by-laws restated the powers of that body, giving it effective control of all College business. For example, the Council had to approve the annual budget; all propositions for membership had to receive its approval on two separate occasions; all standing committees had to report to it; and any committee recommendations that required College action, had to be laid before the Council first. "Any questions of vital importance concerning the public and professional relations of the College" were also to be submitted to the Council, which might then submit them to the whole College with a recommendation for action. Finally, the power of the Council was increased and extended:

> the Council shall have executive capacity to act upon and dispose of any business of the College not otherwise provided for in the By-laws and shall have power to authorize, at its discretion, the expenditure of any sum of money, from funds not otherwise appropriated by the College . . . . It shall act upon and dispose of any special business authorized or ordered by the College and between the semi-annual business meetings shall have authority to represent the College in any decision involving relations of the College to the public or the medical profession and in

all business transactions not involving the sale or transfer of real estate.

This may have increased the speed and efficiency with which College business could be transacted, but it did so at the expense of interest and participation by the great majority of Fellows. The new by-laws almost completely failed to promote "scientific development" or to give younger Fellows a larger share of the "executive activities" of the College, which is what Roberts had hoped they might do. To be sure, an entirely new Committee on Scientific Business was appointed from which more lively and informative programs were expected. As for the officers and other committees, however, the roster in 1926, the year after the new by-laws were enacted, was hardly different from that in 1924. Three of the four censors continued, including William W. Keen, who had forgotten, or been persuaded to withdraw, the resignation he had submitted as an expression of sympathy with the principle of rotation. The secretary, treasurer, and honorary librarian were unchanged, as was the entire membership of the important standing Committees on Publications, Library, and Hall. The members of the Committee on Public Health in 1926 were the same as in 1925, before the enactment of the new by-laws. Two of the three members of the Committees on Finance, the Mütter Museum, and the Directory of Nurses remained in place, as did three of four members of the Committee on Entertainment and four of five of the prestigious Committee on the Weir Mitchell Oration.

One may sympathize with Roberts' aspirations and frustrations; but one must also recognize that an institution such as the College, with limited means and one full-time clerk, had to depend on the interest and service, freely given, of a few members to discharge its many practical duties, from investing funds to providing daily janitorial services.

### *Financial Constraints*

The new by-laws did nothing for the financial condition of the College. The causes of the continuing distress were apparent to all. The new hall on Twenty-second Street cost more to maintain than the old one, and no provision had been made, when raising funds for it, to defray those increased costs. In addition, the old hall, from which the Fellows still hoped to realize $350,000, remained unsold; and, although it brought in some rental income, the College was deprived of the larger amount it would have received by investing the capital sum the building represented. When the tenant gave up its lease in 1926, the College found itself obligated for taxes, which exceeded what it was ever able to get again in rent. Moreover, in the 1920s all prices rose—salaries, utilities, repairs and other services, books, binding, and printing; but there was no comparable increase in income from endowment, which had been invested conservatively and probably less confidently than economic conditions before 1929 would have justified. A substantial increase of membership, which some Fellows favored, would have brought in several thousand dollars annually, but that recourse was unacceptable to the majority of Fellows. Sentiment was also strongly against raising dues. In these circumstances the College was forced to borrow from the Permanent Fund to balance the annual budgets.

The Council imposed some controls on expenditures, and small economies were realized by such measures as curtailing the binding of books and periodicals, and requiring the sections to pay for printing their meeting notices. Otherwise presidents of the College in the mid-'20s offered only general expressions of hope. "Perhaps," said President Neilson in 1925, "one of you might influence some public-spirited person or persons of means to make such a gift." President Hare two years later agreed, adding that such gifts should preferably be unrestricted.[52]

It remained for John H. Gibbon to sound the alarm in clear and forceful terms. Professor of surgery in Jefferson Medical College since 1907 and recently president of the American Surgical Association, Gibbon had served on many College committees, on the Council, and as vice-president. He knew the College well when he was chosen president in 1928.[53] As long as the old hall was occupied by the Free Library, he explained in his first presidential report in 1929,

> the College received $10,000 per year rent and paid no taxes on the property. Now we are not only receiving no rent, but are paying $10,000 in taxes and losing the interest on the value of the property, which at 5 per cent is $17,500, so that we are actually out more than $25,000 a year. The

> income of the College from all sources, except from endowments and lectureships and from other specific endowments of the Library, is about $15,000, and our expenses about $33,000, not including the $10,000 tax on the old building, which, of course, must be paid and raises our present expense account to $43,000. With these figures before them, let no Fellow imagine that our College is in anything but financial embarrassment.[54]

Repeating his warning the next year, Gibbon demanded, "Shall we go on spending our small principal, hoping, Micawber-like, for something to turn up; or shall we, by increasing our dues or making an assessment on the Fellows, endeavor to make up our deficiency?" The College's expected income in 1930 was $22,000; its projected expenses were $44,000. The difference was made up from the Permanent Fund (accumulated surplus), now nearly exhausted. "If this institution is to function as it has done for nearly one hundred and fifty years," Gibbon declared flatly, "it must have money, and the Fellows must either give it or get it." As he reflected on all the things that ought to be done in the College, Gibbon made a plaintive confession: "If I were asked to state the greatest need of the College today I should say another Weir Mitchell."[55]

The financial crisis of the College worsened as the Depression deepened after 1930. Stocks fell, bonds were defaulted, mortgage interest went unpaid, and principal had to be invested at lower rates of return. Some Fellows, their own income reduced, resigned, unable to pay the annual dues. In 1931 the fellowship was smaller than it had been in 1920. In these circumstances a dinner (paid for out of the Weir Mitchell Entertainment Fund) was held in March 1930 to acquaint the Fellows with the facts and to announce a campaign to raise $500,000 for endowment. The goal was wildly unrealistic; but 143 Fellows and a few lay friends subscribed $48,160, which restored most of what had been borrowed from the Permanent Fund. But when someone suggested making a second appeal, he was told that the 143 could not be expected to make another gift when 342 had given nothing.[56]

Francis R. Packard, elected president in 1931, continued Gibbon's initiatives, and worked even harder to raise money. The son and brother of Fellows and related by blood or marriage to other famous physicians of Philadelphia, including Philip Syng Physick and George Bacon Wood, he was a successful otolaryngologist, teacher, and author of a text on that specialty.[57] Packard was, however, better known as a historian of medicine, gratefully acknowledging throughout life William Osler's influence upon him. He published his first medical historical article in 1897 and four years later, at the age of thirty-one, published a general history of medicine in the United States, which, vastly enlarged, reappeared in a two-volume edition in 1931. He was editor of the *Annals of Medical History* from its founding in 1917 through 1942. Among the Philadelphia institutions that he served, he reserved a special loyalty for the Pennsylvania Hospital (whose history he wrote), the Library Company of Philadelphia, and the College of Physicians, in which he had been a founder and chairman of the Section on Medical History, honorary librarian, secretary, and vice-president.

In several letters Packard gave the Fellows information not only about College finances but also about general College policies. His manifest concern for the institution brought thoughtful and sympathetic responses, each of which he acknowledged personally. From these letters, for example, Packard learned that there was widespread sentiment to enlarge the fellowship, extend the geographical limits of eligibility, and admit researchers without medical degrees, women, and even dentists.[58]

The contributions made in 1930 were welcome, but drastic budget-cutting was required to stabilize the finances. The budget, which had been $32,098 in 1929 and $29,184 in 1930, was cut back to $24,569 in 1932. Every operation of the College was affected. The staff were given summer holidays without pay. Salaries and pensions were cut, the latter by twenty percent. The content and format of the *Transactions* were changed in 1933 in the interest of economy. The Nurses' Directory, which had brought the College nearly $100,000 over half a century but was now losing money, was closed in 1936. The library was especially hard hit. Although income from its restricted funds was not diverted, the appropriation from general College funds was totally eliminated in 1933; and in 1935 the Library Committee's request was cut by thirty percent and the salary it recommended for the librarian was cut by ten percent and, at the mid-year review of finances, that reduced figure was cut by another ten percent.

The financial needs of the College affected the library in another, and unexpected, way. Charles Perry Fisher, as assistant librarian and librarian for nearly half a century, had been tireless,

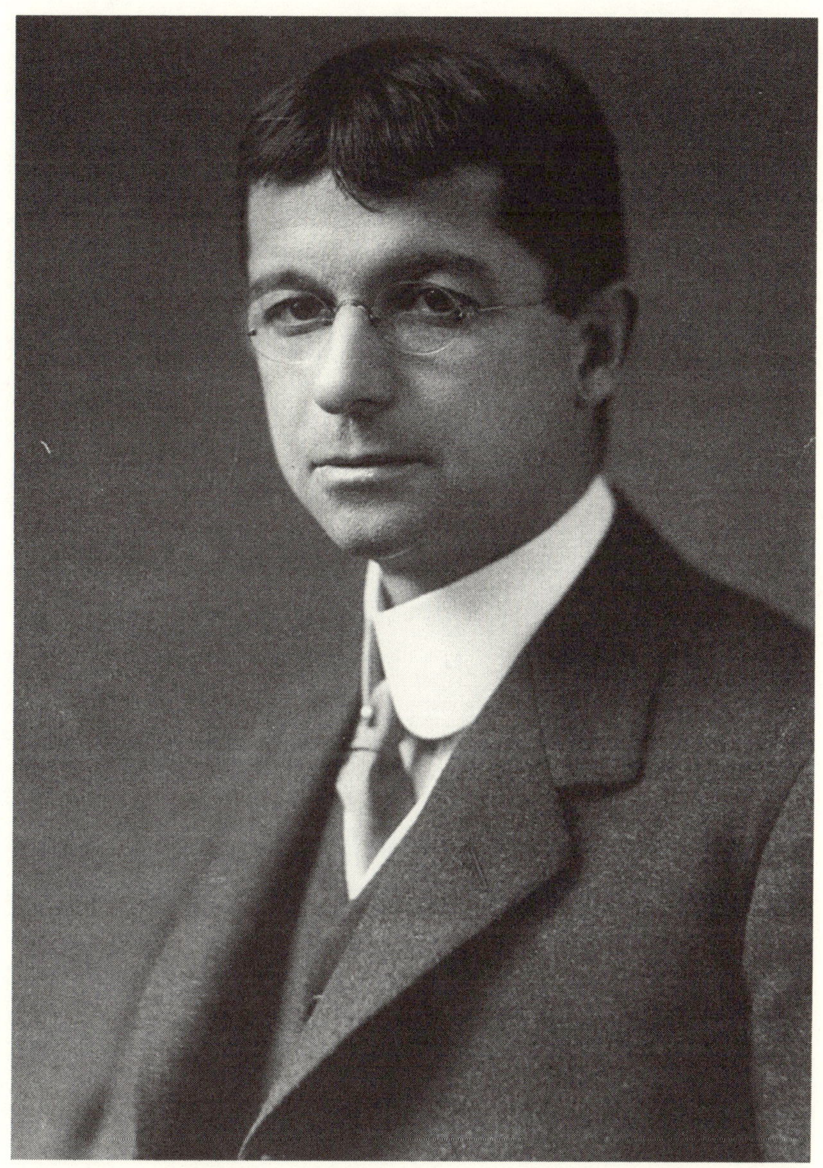

Francis R. Packard, (1870–1950). Photograph by Evans, Philadelphia.

meticulous, and imaginative in the post, and had achieved an enviable reputation for himself and the College among medical libraries and librarians throughout the country. The collection was rich and varied; with Weir Mitchell, William W. Keen, William Osler, and others he had made it so; and he deserved the praise of Archibald Malloch of the New York Academy of Medicine: "To walk about the rooms of the College made me feel as if I should like to go there and read quietly for the rest of my days."[59]

By 1930, however, Fisher had become crotchety. Increasingly possessive of his library, he multiplied rules and regulations on borrowing and the use of the reading room, and enforced them in what many thought a rigid and unfriendly manner. He did not welcome Fellows to his domain, much less strangers; at least once he ordered a reader off a leather couch in the reading room lest the surface be cracked. This attitude was "repellent," especially when the College was trying attract prospective benefactors. Fifty years of service and Fisher's seventieth birthday offered a plausible opportunity, and he was retired, rather abruptly, on June 30, 1932.[60]

He was succeeded by Emlen Wood, a sportsman and graduate of the School of Veterinary Medicine of the University of Pennsylvania, who had recently been appointed assistant librarian and was now made acting librarian. The caution was well-founded, for within a few months the staff was in revolt, Charles W. Burr had resigned as honorary librarian, and the Council was out of patience with the "tangled affairs of the library."[61] Walton B. McDaniel, 2d, a scholar trained in Greek and Latin classics, became librarian on June 1, 1933.

### *Membership*

Financial considerations were also sometimes injected into discussions of membership in the 1920s and 1930s. An increase in the fellowship could easily be justified on strictly professional grounds, but it was also clear that more Fellows would mean more income. Yet there was strong opposition to enlargement. "This College must maintain an isolated position as far as numbers are concerned," declared President Harte. "It was never designed . . . to be a large popular body of medical men."

Objective criteria for election, even when most restrictive, were clear—age, residence, professional conduct, "actual achievement" as a teacher, writer, or practitioner. Personality must also be considered, but this was harder to appraise. Committees and presidents tried to express what the College was and what the ideal Fellow was expected to be; but they produced only generalities which remind a reader of the stated admission requirements of a social club or fraternity—which, of course, in one view, is what the College was. "What is the College?" asked President Hare in 1925, then offered his own answer:

> . . . it is a place in which is found something equivalent to the nucleus of a cell; a place in which the nucleus of our profession is nourished by its surroundings and protected as well from envy, hatred and malice; . . . a place where high ideals are always at home; a place to which we turn, as does the world in general to some great cathedral, to breathe its atmosphere, to worship at its shrine, and on going out to find that doubts as to what is worthy are scattered and proper professional conduct made clear. It is a place to which the novice in our profession turns for inspiration.[62]

As the number of persons able to support such ideals as these was necessarily limited, the College briefly considered establishing a junior fellowship. This would have two happy consequences: the annual dues would lighten the financial burden, and the juniors (as was contemplated in the original by-laws of 1787) would form a pool from which regular Fellows could be selected. The change was not made, although the College did offer library privileges at a small fee to medical students, scholars, and researchers in medicine.

Membership in the College had always been by election; it was never offered routinely to every qualified physician. In earliest times persons applied for membership; after 1834 they had to be formally proposed by four Fellows and, after due deliberation, they might be admitted by vote of the whole College. Most of the Fellows liked it that way, and some even took a certain satisfaction in rejecting nominees they thought unworthy. Candidates not known to four councillors were led around the city by their sponsors to meet them. The election process took at least nine months and could require fifteen or more. Some candidates found the

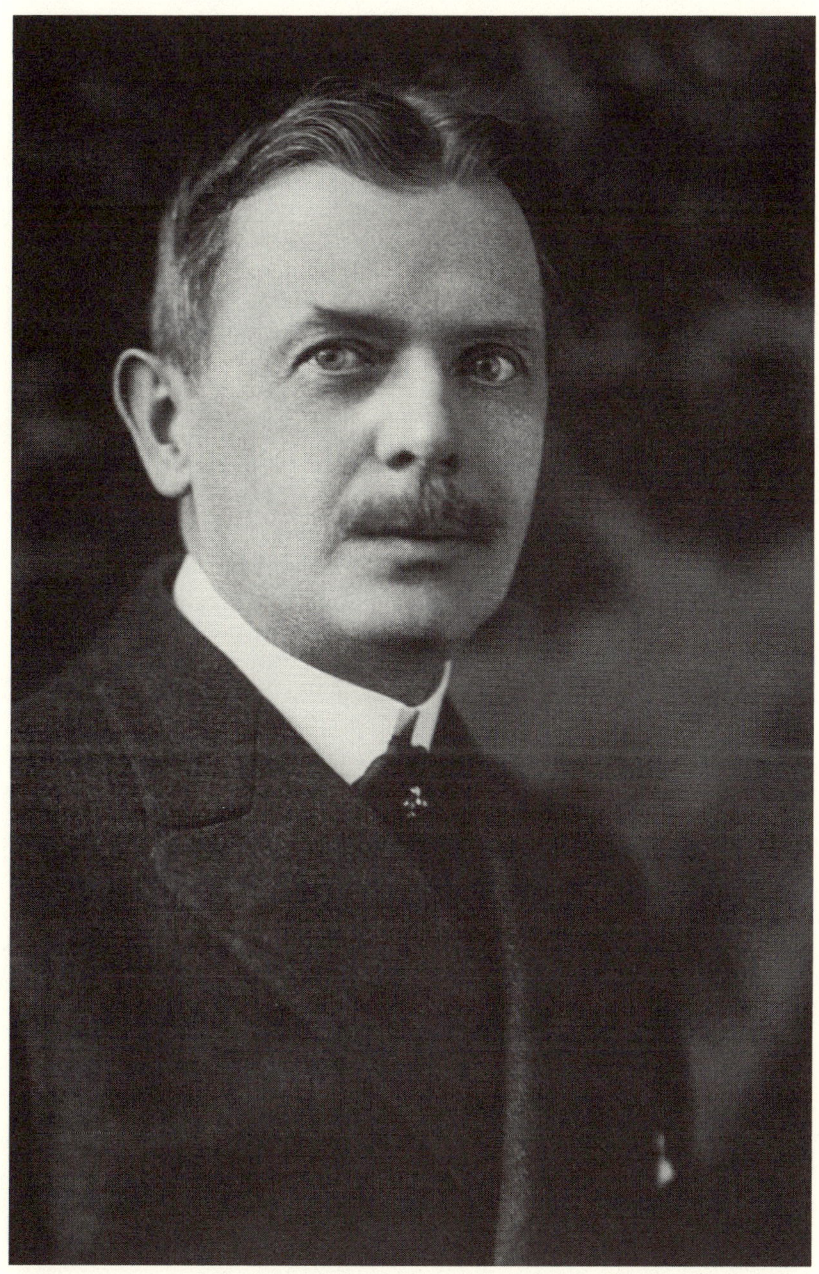

Charles Perry Fisher, (1857–1940). Photograph by Eugene O'Connor, Philadelphia.

ritual quaint and were amused; others resented it. The procedure was modified in 1935, but sponsors judged it prudent to make sure that the candidate was known personally to members of the Council.

The death of an active member was also recognized with traditional formality. The Censors voted whether a memoir of the deceased Fellow should be written, read, and printed in the *Transactions*, or only written and printed, "or merely his name mentioned in the Annual Address of the President."[63]

To many Fellows and most non-Fellows in the decades just after the First World War, the College semed a quintessential "old Philadelphia institution," filled with, or at least controlled by, "old Philadelphians"—terms often spoken with amused contempt or irritation by those who alternately condemned and envied the distinction. The Fellows' roll in 1930 did indeed contain old Philadelphia names—Gibbon, Hewson, Norris, Packard, Pemberton, Pepper, Vaux, many of them sons, grandsons, or nephews of earlier Fellows. A more careful examination of the roll, however, would have shown that many other "old Philadelphians" were in fact not so old. Coming to Philadelphia as medical students, they had stayed on, made their careers in the city, and slowly over the years become "old Philadelphians" by faithfully and unselfishly serving such institutions as the College (as John Bell, Nathaniel Chapman, Charles D. Meigs, the elder John K. Mitchell, Thomas D. Mütter, Joseph Nancrede, Henry Neill, and many others had done a century before). Being born in Philadelphia was not enough, marriage might help, but ability, energy, character, and personality were essential and became increasingly decisive as the standards of medical science and practice rose.

Alfred Stengel, president of the College from 1934 to 1937, was an example. Born in Pittsburgh, the son of German immigrant parents, he never attended college but entered the University of Pennsylvania Medical School in 1886 and graduated in 1889. He obtained an internship at Philadelphia General Hospital, augmented his slender income by quizzing, and in 1892 was invited by William Pepper, professor of medicine and provost of the University of Pennsylvania, to become his office assistant. When Pepper died in 1898, his son William, Jr., who had just completed his internship, invited Stengel to join him as a partner in carrying on the elder Pepper's office practice, an arrangement that continued until 1912, when the younger Pepper became dean of the University Medical School. For about ten years Stengel lived with the Peppers "practically as a member of our family," Pepper recalled; and he spent his summer vacations with them at the house of the elder Mrs. Pepper at Northeast Harbor, Maine. In 1909, at the age of forty-one, he married Martha Otis Pepper, daughter of the elder Pepper's first cousin. Usually identified in any discussion of Medical School or College policy as one of "the Peppers," Stengel was sometimes thought to have owed his success to this connection. It is more likely that he became one of "the Peppers" because they were confident that he would achieve success in his profession. William Pepper, Jr., summarized his friend's career briefly: "the youthful, penurious, untrained boy who came to Philadelphia unknown, without friends or relations. . . by his own effort, brains and native intelligence rose to a commanding position in medicine in this country. . . ."[64]

From the answers to his letters to the Fellows asking for comments on the College, Packard learned that a majority were willing to change the membership requirements, partly for financial reasons, more particularly because the medical profession itself had changed and grown.[65] Accordingly the residency requirement was extended in 1932 from thirty to seventy-five miles and the exception of New Jersey was eliminated. Associate Membership was changed to Honorary Fellowship, and persons working in sciences allied to medicine were declared eligible. Thus in 1936 A. Newton Richards, the distinguished pharmacological researcher at the University of Pennsylvania, but not an M.D., who had first been suggested for election twenty-five years before, was elected an Honorary Fellow.[66] And the bar against women was lifted.

### *Women in the College II*

Half a century had passed since 1868, when the College tried to prevent its Fellows from accepting appointments in women's medical colleges or consulting with the staff and graduates of such institutions. But women were now members of county, state, and national medical societies. They were to be found in research laboratories and departments of public health and in such specialties as gynecology and pediatrics, as well as in general practice. Philadelphia's Woman's Medical College had survived despite poverty and prejudice—and with crucial support from male leaders of the profession. The Johns Hopkins Medical School had admitted women since its inception in 1893. It was only a matter of time before the question of women's admission to the College was pressed.

First, however, the College had to be willing to include qualified women in its programs. The first cautious step was taken in 1913 when David Riesman suggested that Maude Slye of the University of Chicago, who had been studying genetic factors in cancer, be invited to speak at a conference he hoped to organize. The matter was referred to the Council, which, after some deliberation and on motion of William W. Keen, authorized the Committee on Scientific Business to extend the invitation. The situation was without precedent: the Council was uncertain even how to refer to a woman doctor, its minutes speaking of her as "(Doctor) Miss Maude Slye," thus distinguishing (and elevating) her character as a woman above her professional role as a physician.[67] As it turned out, the cancer conference was not held; but the Council's action respecting Doctor Miss Slye provided an unarguable precedent a few months later, when S. Josephine Baker, director of the pioneering Bureau of Child Hygiene in New York City, was invited to speak in a symposium on municipal hygiene on May 6, 1914. The Fellows received her and her paper, President Wilson reported, "in such a way that we may now be prepared to welcome anyone who has a real message of science or applied science to bring, regardless of sex."[68]

In the next ten years, as other women physicians and medical scientists appeared before the College or its sections,[69] more Fellows came to regard the traditional bar against them as an anachronism. By 1930 the majority favored their admission. "After thinking it over carefully," Richard A. Kern told Edward B. Krumbhaar in April 1931, "my only reaction is, why not?"[70] The opposition, however, though small, was determined and resourceful. They raised legal objections; but legal counsel assured the Council there was no impediment: "he" in the charter and by-laws, was generic, applying to men and women equally. Accepting the view that the election of women might be legal, opponents then moved that it was "inadvisable," but the motion was lost.[71] Finally they called for a special vote on the question, perhaps in the hope that this would bring out a hitherto silent majority in opposition. In fact, only fifty-four Fellows attended, and the proposal to admit women was passed on October 7, 1931, by a vote of forty-two to eight.

In the following January Catharine Macfarlane, professor of gynecology in Woman's Medical College, was elected a Fellow.[72] Two years later Martha Tracy, dean of that institution and a member of the Philadelphia Board of Health, was admitted. Before 1940 eleven more women were chosen Fellows, and in 1972 a woman was elected president.

### *Celebration in 1937*

By 1937 the College appeared to have survived or circumvented its worst problems. President Muller in his annual report in January 1938 announced that finances were "now in excellent condition," but he could have meant only that the budget, by dint of deep cuts even into essential functions like the library, was balanced.[73] Attendance at stated meetings remained level, but membership increased—a paradox explained by the reputation of the College and the half-joking, half-cynical advice older Fellows gave their juniors, that they should join "before you make enemies who might keep you out." The public lectures, on various topics directed to no particular audience, were well attended. The officers continued to hope that public agencies would call for the College's advice and assistance, thus helping it to define its purpose.

The on-going scholarly work of the College was invigorated by the new librarian.[74] A man of energy and imagination, with a self-deprecatory humor, McDaniel proved resourceful in coping with restrictions imposed by the precarious financial conditions. By staggering staff vacations, for example, he was able to keep the library open more hours than before, even on Sunday afternoons. Bravely attacking a long-deferred task, he had three thousand books oiled and repaired in his first year. He compiled an updated handlist of the incunabula, revised de Schweinitz' short history of the College to mark the twenty-fifth anniversary of the hall, prepared an analytical index of the *Transactions,* and used his annual reports not simply to list acquisitions, but also especially to instruct the Fellows in the purposes, technologies, and needs of a modern medical library. As a humanist, however, McDaniel was, he wrote in one of his first reports, "acutely conscious of the essential absurdity of gauging the contents of libraries by mathematical measurements"—he believed such measurements "vague and characterless."[75]

McDaniel stimulated the Fellows' appreciation of their institution and its book collection by means of an occasional mimeographed publication called "Fugitive Leaves from the Library," which displayed the range and quality of the collection. It contained, in President Muller's words, "delightful little journeys into the by-ways of the library," that is to say, historical and bibliographical notes that were always informative, usually original, sometimes curious or amusing.[76] Favorably impressed by the College's new librarian and his early improvements, Charles W. Burr in 1934 established a small group of "Friends of the Library," whose first gifts included a copy of Adam Thomson's *Discourse on the Preparation of the Body for the Small-Pox,* printed by Benjamin Franklin in 1750. In 1939 Burr gave the library a microfilm reader. Another warm supporter of the library in these years was Edward B. Krumbhaar, professor of pathology in the University of Pennsylvania, translator of Castiglioni's history of medicine, and editor of a series of useful handbooks under the title *Clio Medica.* Like Burr, Krumbhaar had added many rare volumes to the College collection, which he enjoyed showing visitors; and in 1941 he suggested that the library serve tea every afternoon as a way to bring interested Fellows together for an hour of bookish talk before going home.

Like a balanced budget and fresh activities in the library, a new policy and format adopted for the *Transactions* in the 1930s inspired some confidence in the future. Since the 1920s the *Transactions* had been an increasing worry. Published as a stout volume once a year in a world of quarterly, monthly, even weekly national specialized journals, it made an uncertain contribution. It had no clear editorial policy. Its editor could give it his attention for only brief periods taken from a busy practice. Printing costs rose. A few believed the *Transactions* had no other reason to exist than that it was the oldest medical publication in the country, published (with some interruptions) since 1793.

A new series—the fourth—was begun in 1933. Its limited editorial content and modest format reflected both the financial stringency of the time and the reduced scientific contributions by Fellows. On the other hand, it appeared in two numbers annually, and thus brought scientific papers to the Fellows and others more promptly than an annual volume could. But cost was decisive. By 1937 the *Transactions* had shrunk to ninety-six pages containing only lists of Fellows, officers, and committee members, the annual address of the president, and the report of the Library Committee. Papers read to the College were listed by title only.

In this situation, with the leadership and financial support of Charles W. Burr, and with the librarian, McDaniel, as editor, the *Transactions* underwent another change in policy and format in 1938. It became a quarterly, which meant that papers read to the College would become available even more promptly; and its title was expanded to include "Studies," which signaled that it was open to papers not read at meetings, especially historical and bibliographical essays based on the library's collections. McDaniel's first volume, of respectable size and dignified design, included articles by himself, Krumbhaar, and Richard H. Shryock, author of a pioneering and perceptive study, *The Development of Modern Medicine,* who had just come to the University of Pennsylvania as professor of American history.

Thus, as the College paused in the spring of 1937 to celebrate its sesqui-centennial anniversary, the Fellows could look on themselves as "still a sturdy band of physicians determined to use its immeasurably increased facilities for the purpose for which it was founded." They could also view the future with modest confidence, for, it seemed likely, as McDaniel put it in the anniversary record he prepared, that contemporary conditions of medical science and medical practice would call the College back into "a more public sphere of activity. It becomes increasingly evident," he continued, "that multiplying public health problems may again demand the attention of a medical institution so uniquely favored [as the College] in its constitution and equipment."[77]

CHAPTER XI

# *Problems and Opportunities*

ALMOST without exception in the middle years of the twentieth century, the annual report of the presidents of the College addressed, in varying degrees of urgency, the proper size and character of its Fellowship, the claims of the library, the need for better internal organization, relations with the medical profession and the public—and, again and always, finances. These concerns were not new. They had engaged the Fellows', especially the officers', attention for thirty years; on some of these topics Mitchell, DaCosta, and Agnew had expressed views as long ago as the 1880s. Each subject influenced, and was influenced by, the others, and together all affected every substantial College activity from programs of meetings and the growth of the library to building maintenance and care of the Sinkler Garden.

Annual income from all sources hardly covered necessary expenses; there was no surplus for any additional activity. Furthermore, new proposals, even if financially feasible, were likely to be lost or postponed for want of clear objectives and priorities by which to judge them, and for lack of determination to pursue a chosen course over several years or a decade. Thus the appeals and wistful hopes of one president's report sounded much like those of another's. Devoted to the institution though they were, the officers and other leaders of the College, fully occupied with teaching and practice, lacked the time to carry out changes and reforms that were not always obvious to committee chairmen and members of the large and expanding Council. Without an administrative system or an executive secretary to focus on essential business, secure a decision, and carry it through, the Council and the committees exhausted their members' time, energy, and patience. When, for example, the Women's Committee in 1940 suggested that a garden party be held for the benefit of the Sinkler Garden, the Council felt impelled to get a ruling from its legal counsel before giving permission.[1] Younger Fellows were impatient with this sort of thing; others were frustrated when their ideas were treated with apparent indifference. One dubbed the College "a marble mausoleum."[2]

With annual budgets balanced usually by only one or two hundred dollars, the financial condition, as President Muller told the Fellows in 1939, was "hazardous."[3] With the coming of World War II, it worsened: the College lost $5,000 when it remitted a portion of the dues of Fellows in military service, and income from the still unsold parking lot at Thirteenth and Locust Streets fell. As every president and treasurer had warned and pleaded for twenty years, the College needed a much larger unrestricted endowment.

Nor did it help that the College, an ancient Philadelphia institution housed in a richly-appointed edifice, was widely assumed to be rich. That it contrived to live within its income only offset efforts to present its needs and meager means to both its own Fellows and a wider public.

Muller suggested ways to achieve economies and financial benefits. If the College endowments and other funds were consolidated (to the extent legally permissible) and the income apportioned (in accordance with the donor's wishes), budgeting would be simpler, and the statement of accounts clearer. These changes were eventually made (but not in response to Muller's suggestion), and they increased the income. An investment counsellor, Muller continued, would benefit the College by bringing fuller information and closer attention to the portfolio than its own physician-treasurer and Finance Committee could give. Nor was this suggestion adopted at this time. Another suggestion that was coolly received was that members of elected committees should serve for specific terms. "The tendency has been to renominate year after year for an indefinite period, and we thus lose the infusion of new ideas."[4] Indifference to Muller's recommendations was probably an expression of both the institution's long-standing aversion to change and the officers' and committee chairmen's unwillingness to surrender any of their authority and prestige. Similar motives had prevailed in earlier years to reject motions to appoint a comptroller, to centralize accounts and payments in the treasurer's office, and to require an annual audit of the books.

There were two possible additional ways to raise income and endowment. The first was to increase the number of Fellows, whose entrance fees were added to the permanent endowment and whose annual dues defrayed operating expenses. Membership in the late 1930s, however, was virtually static and, given the reluctance of the Fellows to increase it suddenly, that solution of the budget crisis was unlikely, even unthinkable. As for raising dues, that course was understandably unpopular, especially in a time of financial depression. Eventually, however, both membership and annual dues were increased.

### *College Business*

Despite chronic financial problems, however, the scholarly activities of the College continued, little altered, into the early war years. The library, which Muller called "the pride and glory of the College," received 1,184 journals and periodicals in 1938 and contained 150,033 catalogued volumes and 309,177 "unaccessioned" items. The next year the latter figures were, respectively, 152,454 and approximately 316,000. In 1940 Samuel B. Sturgis gave the library his extensive collection of medical art, which was extended the next year when William N. Bradley gave fifteen bound volumes of photographs of works of art representing Philadelphia doctors. Use of the library also grew steadily: 10,500 visits by non-Fellows, and 2,300 by Fellows were reported in 1940; and these visitors called for some 50,000 titles and borrowed 8,524, not counting reference books consulted at reading-room shelves without a call-slip or librarian's intervention. Researchers for commercial drug firms were a new category of user in these years; and the companies expressed their appreciation of the services they received by monetary gifts.

Presenting papers at stated meetings and special lectures was a principal continuing scientific activity, and an important way in which the College met the public, an objective never long out of the officers' minds. Attendance in 1938 ranged from 550 to 121, with an average of 326. Of this number Fellows accounted for an average of only 47. They found greater stimulation and satisfaction in the sections, which, except for that on medical history, met without interruption even during the war.

Particularly appealing to large lay audiences was a series of lectures delivered in 1938–39. The first was given by Alfred Stengel, former president of the College, on "Currents and Counter-Currents in the Progress of Medicine," and others were by O. H. Perry Pepper, professor of medicine in the University of Pennsylvania, on "Medical Problems of Advancing Age," and Earl D. Bond, director of the Institute of the Pennsylvania Hospital, on "The Modern Interpretation of Mental Disorders." With an average attendance of 227, the series was judged a success, and a second series was offered the next year. Chevalier Jackson of Temple University, inventor of the bronchoscope, which he employed successfully in many well-publicized cases, attracted an audience of 450, "overflowing through the doors of Mitchell Hall." Not only did the lectures give the public useful and authoritative information on medical subjects, President Krumbhaar believed, but they also made the College better known to the citizens generally. However, because of the war the lectures were given up in 1942 at the close of the fourth series.[5]

To be consulted and to advise on public health was yet another way the College attained recognition, something it had yearned for since the days of Weir Mitchell half a century before.[6] In this role the College would be seen most clearly to contribute to the public good.

Accordingly, the work of the Committee on Public Health, Preventive Medicine, and Public Relations usually received special mention in the presidents' reports in the 1940s.[7] The Committee, headed by Joseph Stokes, Jr., joined a similar committee of the County Medical Society to investigate the city hospital at Byberry; as a result of the joint committee's findings and recommendations, the hospital was taken into the state system. On invitation from the city authorities, the joint committee also studied the coroner's office and aspects of the operations of the Board of Health for a proposed revision of the city charter. Water supply and sewage disposal repeatedly were objects of College and County Society attention. So were pasteurization of milk, air pollution, the reporting of premature births, and the health of food handlers. In 1942 the Council gave the College's committee an unusual assignment: to study "an apparent inadequacy" in the teaching of mathematics and science in the public schools. There was in fact so much to do that President Krumbhaar wished the College could add a full-time expert on public health problems and education to its staff.

The Section on Public Health was no less active than the committee and sometimes brought the College more attention. This could be embarrassing, for the Section was less closely controlled by the College than the Committee, and the public did not always recognize the difference between committee and section. On the one hand, the College was pleased when the publicity was favorable; on the other, it feared that Section programs might generate unwelcome controversy. Thus, after suggesting that the Section increase attendance by advertising its meetings on hospital bulletin boards and in newspapers, one president warned that "in this event . . . floor discussion of controversial subjects should be carefully guarded against." Partly with this in mind, the officers of the Section were urged to plan its programs in cooperation with the College's Committee on Scientific Business. Fear of controversy may have been exaggerated, however, at least one meeting on the politics of "medical economics" in 1940 brought out only thirty-four Fellows and, apparently, only mild rumbles of light thunder.[8]

## *World War II*

The war that engulfed the United States in 1940–41 interrupted the life of the College, aggravated some of its problems, and altered a few outward practices. Many Fellows were drawn into the armed services, others engaged in the war work of national and local committees and commissions. In January 1942, only a month after war had been declared, at least twenty-five Fellows were already on active duty; before the end of the year, the number exceeded one hundred. Programs of the stated meetings were prepared with reference to their relevance to war needs. Even a historical lecture to the public on superstition and medical progress was discussed "in Relation to the Present World Emergency." Ballotting by mail was instituted to reduce unnecessary travel. To save energy, avoid duplication, and reach the largest possible audience, the College and the County Medical Society met jointly from 1942 to 1947. The combined meeting seldom drew fewer than two hundred; the average in 1943–44 was 240; and 495 attended at a lecture on hypertension in 1944.[9]

After the summer of 1940 it was clear that the United States would eventually enter the war. Accordingly, in September, at the request of President Krumbhaar, Arthur P. Hitchens, professor of public health and preventive medicine in the University of Pennsylvania, who was already on active duty in the army, offered the College suggestions "looking toward medical preparedness for the possible national emergency," with special reference to the health of the civilian population.[10] As the County Medical Society had already inaugurated weekly meetings on this subject, the College had only to endorse the program and promise cooperation. A few months later, in April 1941, concerned that the supply of doctors for both military and civilian requirements should be adequate, the College formally called on the president of the United States, the Selective Service System, and the surgeons-general of the army, navy, and public health service not to induct into ordinary training medical students and interns "who give reasonable promise of becoming acceptable physicians."[11] These representations were thought to have influenced the government's decision to defer the military service of such persons.

As in the First World War, British physicians and medical scientists brought to the United States the results of their observations and experiences. Thus Francis J. W. Roughton of Cambridge University spoke at the College on blood storage and shock; E. D. (later Lord) Adrian, also of Cambridge, on brain injuries; and the chief psychiatrist of the R. A. F. on psychoneuroses in peace and war. American doctors, as well, discussed such other war-related topics as tetanus, physiological problems of aviation, control of venereal disease, and nutrition in Occupied France.

Sometimes lectures had to be scheduled or re-scheduled at odd times, or even cancelled on short notice, to meet a speaker's obligations elsewhere. John F. Fulton of the Yale Medical School, for example, was to deliver a Weir Mitchell lecture on neurology and war in November 1940, but was unexpectedly sent to London on war business; however, he had a finished manuscript, which he gave the editor of the *Transactions* for publication.[12]

This is not to say that the attention of the College and County Medical Society in their joint meetings was exclusively on military topics. In 1942 the Benjamin Musser lecture was on "The Heart that is Ageing," the Hatfield lecture on "Nutrition, Ageing and

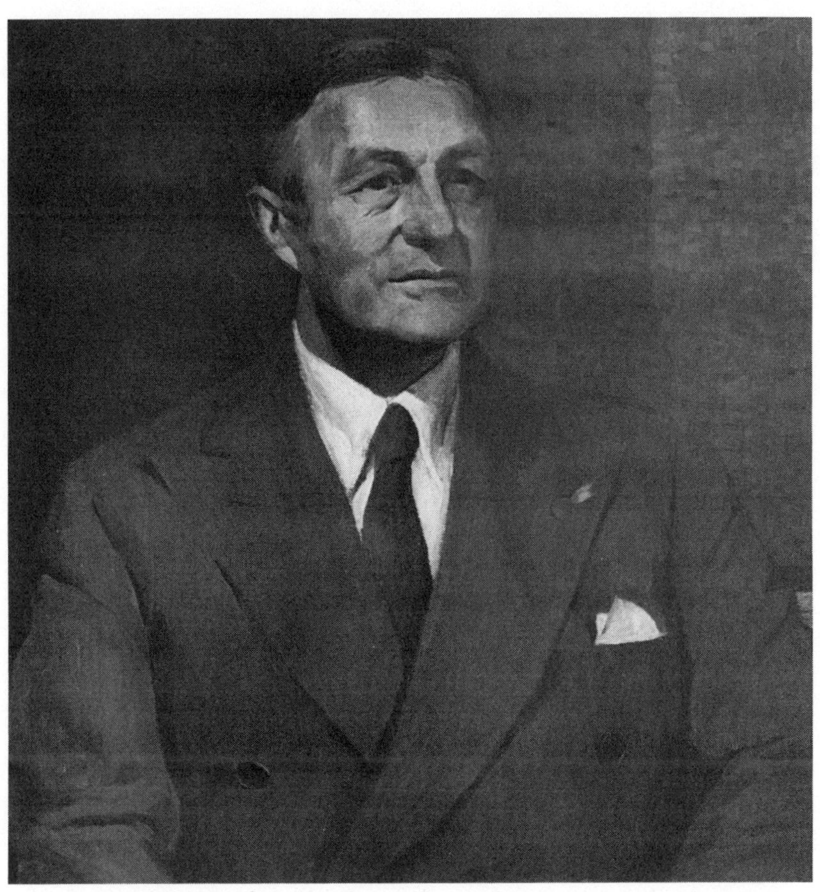

Edward B. Krumbhaar, (1882–1966). Portrait by Daniel Garber.

Longevity," and the Anders lecture on "Fatigue." There were papers on anemia, cancer, infantile paralysis, mumps, tuberculosis, rheumatic fever, and the Rh factor. Yet even subjects of general medical interest often had a wartime origin or military dimension. On February 7, 1945, Chester B. Keefer of the Harvard Medical School, addressing an audience of 385, described penicillin, which was producing such astonishing results in military hospitals. A year later knowledge from another source was revealed —on "Atomic Energy and Cancer" by Lieutenant Colonel Hymer L. Friedell of the Station Hospital at Oak Ridge, Tennessee, and on "The Atomic Bomb Experiments in the Pacific, with a Consideration of the Relationship of Such Tests to the Future of Medicine" by Eugene P. Pendergrass, radiologist of the University of Pennsylvania Medical School.

In October 1946, in accordance with tradition, 139 resident and non-resident Fellows were welcomed home from the armed services at a dinner in the hall of the College. Not every detail of the customary affair, however, had survived the changes of the years intact: a note on the engraved invitations read "Dress optional."[13]

### *Post-war Pressures*

More than social formalities were changing. At the close of his three years in office in 1943, President Krumbhaar attempted to describe the new spirit he sensed moving in the College:

> a further expansion of the trend toward greater liberality and flexibility—a library developed more for use and service than as merely a cherished possession, broader but no lower standards of Fellowship eligibility, more liberal loan of our halls to other organizations, more concern with the public health of our city and state, more cooperation with other medical societies, always with maintenance of the highest possible levels of scientific programs and membership and additions to our possessions.[14]

Not that the old, slow, cautious ways were given up at once. As if in reply to Krumbhaar, his successor as president, O. H. Perry Pepper, likened the College to a geriatric patient whose regimen should not be changed abruptly: "The College of Physicians is a long established dignified organization; no great change should be expected of it in any one year or even in one decade."[15]

But there could be no return to pre-war normality, even if the College's concerns remained unchanged—finances, membership, the roles of its library, meetings, and publications. Outside the College new institutions were arising, new pressures and attitudes developing, that deeply affected medicine and medical institutions. The federal government, for example, was regulating medical practice, and creating agencies with staffs of their own for medical care, research, and administration. These federal agencies called for advice—if they called at all—on the Fellows as individuals, not on the College as a whole. The College, too, had become too large, various, and complicated to be run entirely by volunteer Fellows out of their professional offices in Spruce and Pine Streets. Perry Pepper, leaving office as president in 1946, suggested that the College needed additional salaried staff, "including perhaps a full-time medical secretary."[16]

"There is," President Schaeffer told the Fellows in 1947, reciting the familiar litany,

> an urgent and immediate demand for additional income so as to enable the College to aid more adequately the Library. Every effort must be made to keep our great Library at the forefront of medical libraries . . . .[17]

To this end some internal changes were made. Dues were raised in 1948 from $30 to $50, thus increasing annual income by about $15,000. A conscious effort was made to increase membership for the College's financial benefit. Accounting procedures were reformed; an annual audit was instituted; and, after long delay, the College's many small trusts were consolidated into two common funds. A grant for library cataloguing was received from the American Philosophical Society, but an appeal for voluntary contributions from the Fellows was only "moderately successful." These were at best only temporary expedients, as Schaeffer and the Council knew. What was required was an informed policy, with a decision on practicable means for achieving specific goals. Accordingly, the Council authorized appointment of a committee in 1948 on "the present and probable early future needs of the College," with T. Grier Miller as chairman.[18] The College was so lacking in free funds that it had to call on the Fellows for contributions to pay the committee's architectural and engineering consultants.

Miller was widely respected as a wise counsellor. He was a native of North Carolina and a graduate of the University of Pennsylvania, where he was now professor of medicine with a specialty in gastro-enterology. With A. Newton Richards he had surveyed the medical school and hospital of the university at the request of President Thomas S. Gates, who wanted a guide for the institution's development. Like other Fellows, Miller knew what the College needed. He was also prepared to do something about it.

Miller's committee made two principal recommendations—to open a campaign for funds to extend the library's book stacks, improve its reading room facilities, and increase the unrestricted endowment; and to engage a full-time medical executive secretary, as Perry Pepper had suggested in 1946. Miller repeated these proposals after he became president of the College in 1949.[19]

Of the two recommendations, appointment of an executive secretary was the easier to effect. J. Harold Austin, who had served the College ten years as its secretary and had recently retired as director of the department of research medicine in the University of Pennsylvania, took up the duties of the new office on May 1, 1949. In a short time he organized and rationalized internal administrative practices. Under his lead the College established a pension fund for employees. He also worked out a system of life membership on actuarial bases, which attracted thirty-three subscribers within a year. Unfortunately, Austin died suddenly (on one of his beloved nature walks) after only three years in his post.[20] Not for seventeen years was a successor appointed.

The College income, as everyone knew, was woefully inadequate, even for minimal customary services. As they inspected the Hall, which was now forty years old, Miller's committee had discovered eroding water pipes, a leaking roof over Mitchell Hall, loosening plaster, and a defective boiler. The need for maintenance and repair was urgent, and the cost was rising. As for the library, prices of books and binding had doubled since the war, foreign journals were accumulating faster than the staff could catalogue them, and new journals were being established every month and must be acquired if the library was to retain its preeminence. Some Fellows proposed solutions that were cheap, immediate, and sounded scientific and modern; but Miller and his successor made it clear that little-used volumes would not be sold or warehoused, nor would the collection be reduced to microfilm.

To introduce the College to the public, Miller invited influential laymen to College meetings. Although few accepted, some became interested in the College, and from these and others Miller formed a committee to advise him on fund-raising that was composed of bankers, lawyers, and civic leaders led by Martin W. Clement, president of the Pennsylvania Railroad, and John A. Diemand, president of the Insurance Company of North America. Miller also appointed a new College committee on fund-raising, under Richard A. Kern, which succeeded the committee that Miller had chaired in 1948. Clement lent it the services of an experienced fund-raiser on his own staff. Miller prepared a plain, succinct statement of what the College was and did and what its current needs were. The "memorandum" was directed to individuals, corporations, and foundations "with an understanding of medical problems" and the role of special libraries, appreciated the need for adequate tools of medical research, and had "a genuine interest in maintaining the effectiveness of a great center of medical culture, education and research."[21]

But Miller's hopes remained unrealized. As his term ended in 1952, he could only repeat the needs he had cited three years before and list hopefully some "new opportunities for service" by the College—further educational activities for medical students and young physicians, closer cooperation with, and service to, the medical school libraries, the use of radio and television and of public lectures to educate the public in matters of health and preventive medicine, and more complete service to drug companies and other industrial organizations with medical interests.[22] But, like extended accommodations for the library, these proposals, too, would cost money.

## *Fund-Raising for the Library*

The fund-raising campaign Miller began was pressed vigorously by his successor, Richard A. Kern, professor of medicine at Temple University.[23] The goal was set at $1,500,000—$800,000 for library stacks, $700,000 for endowment; and it was expected that at least $1,250,000 of this sum, including the amount on hand, would be raised within two years. "These figures," Kern conceded, "to many may seem staggering, nay, fantastic." They did, indeed, for at that time the College had collected only $106,000. The offer of $100,000 from the Donner Foundation of Philadelphia on condition that the College raise $1,250,000, must have seemed a mockery.

By mid-1953, five years after Miller made his first appeal, only $131,000 had been collected. Then in November 1953 a representative of the Pew Memorial Foundation, asking anonymity, offered $100,000 on condition that the College raise $400,000 by December 31, 1954, and begin construction of the library addition in 1955. Despite this encouragement and Kern's best efforts, money only trickled in; on September 20 the total stood at $195,000, less than half the Pew goal. Success seemed beyond reach.

Within two weeks, however, the prospect had changed. On September 30 the Donner Foundation, probably in response to a personal appeal by Miller, reduced its challenge to $400,000. On October 2 the Kresge Foundation of Detroit, which had offered $250,000 provided the College first raised $1,000,000, upon representation by Martin Clement reduced its offer and requirement to $100,000 and $400,000 respectively, provided that the building be free of debt upon completion. And on October 5 the Pew Foundation, apprised of these actions, informed the College that it might have $100,000 forthwith, provided work on the building started in 1955, as originally stipulated. Thus, as of October 5, the College was assured of $295,000, but had to raise $105,000 before the end of the year—that is, within three months—in order to get the $200,000 offered by Donner and Kresge. "This threw our machine into high gear," Kern observed afterwards.

On November 30, when the College was still $69,000 short of its goal, Clements and his advisory committee invited thirty business leaders and wealthy citizens to a dinner, where officers of the College presented its case. As a result contributions were made by the Philadelphia Savings Fund Society, the Philadelphia Electric Company, the Smith, Kline & French Foundation, and several insurance companies, including John Diemand's Insurance Company of North America, as well as by several individuals. "A last frantic appeal" went out to the Fellows, who responded "magnificently." On the afternoon of December 29, with less than seventy-two hours to spare, the goal of $400,000 was reached. Telegrams were despatched, phone calls were made to announce the victory. Before the close of the year two days later, $12,000 more came in.

From all sources the grand total was $640,724.35, including pledges of $28,193. Eighty-two per cent of the Fellows had contributed to the result, some more than once.

The fund-raising effort had cost $7,500; but as the gifts, put in short-term investments as they came in, had earned $9,700 in interest, the College was able to put into the building fund not only every cent given for the purpose, but $2,200 more as well. "This," President Kern remarked with satisfaction, "sets something of a record in contemporary fund-raising."

The new stacks were ready to receive books in the spring of 1956. As the Fellows inspected this valuable addition to the College facilities on the day of reception and "open house," they might have reflected with satisfaction on their joint achievement, but probably took little note that none of the hoped-for $700,000 of endowment had been raised. The new stacks answered the College's pressing need for space for its books, library staff, and readers; nothing had been done for its general financial condition.

Day-to-day financial problems continued to nag. Each year's president's report was devoted principally, sometimes exclusively, to money and how to get it. "The financial worries of the College . . . are not new," President Lewis C. Scheffey warned in his first report in 1956, "but have become more acute and our concern is grave." For the first time the budget started to show a deficit—$4,673 in 1956, $16,235 in 1957. To offset the gap, dues were raised from $50 to $60, which brought in an additional $10,000; a special committee was named to generate nominations for membership; and, as usual, ways to augment the permanent endowment were discussed. But appeals to the Fellows for contributions, never strongly pressed, were not successful. Nor did the Fellows respond to urgings that they put the College in their wills: of sixty-nine who died between 1949 and 1953 only one left the College anything.[24] Nonetheless, in 1957 the College managed to buy for $158,905 the garage on an adjoining property so that Fellows might be assured of convenient parking.

### *Above the Bottom Line*

Jonathan E. Rhoads, professor of surgery in the University of Pennsylvania, elected president of the College in 1958, brought to the office and its tasks both wide knowledge of the institution—he had been chairman of a Committee on Policy named by Miller—and sound financial judgment. On the night he was elected, Rhoads told the Fellows he hoped to revive the "sagging" interest in the College, which some regarded as "a dying institution."[25] He gave a clear explanation of the budget and a full account of the College's financial position. An objective of the next decade, he said, should be to increase the endowment by $1,000,000; to make this goal seem less daunting, he pointed out that this meant only $100,000 a year. A small beginning to this end was the response to a proposal by George I. Blumstein, later a president of the College, that Fellows should give $1,000 to endow a journal: within a year thirty-three did so, the number nearly doubled the second year, and eventually exceeded 150.[26]

Taking a larger view of the College and of his role as its president, Rhoads expressed a quiet willingness to re-examine and redirect policies and activities within the limits of the institution's traditions and abilities:

> As the College faces the future, should its purposes either change or undergo a shift in emphasis? If we acccept its basic purposes as a joint effort of this medical community to improve professionally not only its membership, but the entire medical profession for the greater good of the society we serve, I believe that we would want to reaffirm this central purpose. However, when we review the specific and detailed objectives of the various programs instituted to further our basic purpose, there may be more room for revision.[27]

Among Rhoads' specific suggestions were that the library might be opened to members of the County Medical Society if the Society were to make a per capita payment for the service; and that the College might invite distinguished foreign physicians and medical scientists to this country.

Departing from tradition in subsequent reports and speaking in a scientific session, where attendance would be larger than in the January business meeting, Rhoads discussed some of the larger concerns of the medical profession. Thus in his second address he spoke sensibly on the increased cost—and value—of medical care. Citing improvements made within his own lifetime and in the experience of other Fellows, he pointed out that

> it can be demonstrated that medical science has contributed importantly to the quality of life as well as to its length. For these reasons, among others, I do not believe that we, as physicians, should apologize for the increased cost of medical care. We have a product that is different from the one our medical forebears could offer. It is vastly better, and to my mind it is worth its cost many times over both in terms of human values and in terms of economic values.[28]

"Any means," Rhoads concluded, "that permits men to turn money into health—by which I mean real health, qualitatively as well as quantitatively—is a potential boon to mankind."

Rhoads' successor, Thomas M. Durant, professor of internal medicine at Temple University, no less concerned than his predecessors with material things, nonetheless, like Rhoads, tried to make the Fellows think of their opportunities. The College, he said, was "primarily, and almost solely, an educational institution," with a unique role, "adhesive" and counteractive to the fragmentation of medicine by specialization.[29] Although he was not the first to express this idea, Durant made some concrete suggestions to promote it—that the College create an "Interspecialty Forum" to consider such problems as headache, low back pain, and fluid balance; that it make its facilities more generally available to medical schools and other institutions for the discussion of common academic and other problems. He returned to these ideas in his final report in 1964:

> Do we not then possess a golden opportunity to act as a *centripetal* influence in opposition to the *centrifugal* forces driving the various groups farther and farther from each other, and each group, in turn, into further fragmentation? . . . I find great hope in noting that a unifying force has arisen amongst the basic science medical specialists—the new science of molecular biology—which is bringing into a brotherhood with common language the physiological chemist, the microbiologist, the physiologist, the geneticist, and the pharmacologist.[30]

As if in gratifying response to Durant's view for the College, the United States Department of State called on it, in cooperation with four medical schools in Philadelphia, to study the feasibility of establishing a medical school on the American pattern in Ghana. The College was also asked to provide information on the financial status of medical interns and residents in the Philadelphia area for the Pew Foundation, which was considering establishing a revolving loan fund to assist such young doctors. And the College brought together persons from several specialities in the Greater Philadelphia Committee for Medical-Pharmaceutical Sciences, which developed policies and guidelines for drug-testing and drug safety in the wake of the thalidomide tragedy. The Philadelphians' recommendations were later adopted in Chicago and elsewhere.

The mid-60s witnessed other evidences of strengthened activity in the College. Dues were increased from $60 to $90, which added $30,000 to annual income. A substantial bequest came from George W. Norris. The parking garage, bought in 1957, which required costly repairs, was demolished, thus saving the cost of renovation as well as lowering taxes and insurance premiums. An organization of Friends of the College Library was established in 1965 to solicit untapped sources of income—although to little effect: it brought in only $800 and quietly faded away. In 1967 the total assets of the College amounted to an unprecedented $3,745,-141 (of which $1,515,747 was real estate), and its annual budget was $435,051.[31] On the whole, it was with some confidence that President John H. Gibbon, Jr., could bring up once more the suggestion that the College inaugurate a series of lectures or television programs for general audiences and renew its efforts to influence the city government on matters of medicine and public health.[32] A committee on future policies received "floods of suggestions," from streamlining Council meetings to establishing a Fellows' club within the building, complete with lounge, bowling alley, bar, and restaurant.[33]

Another area of growing strength in the College was the Section on Medical History. This continued a long tradition of historical writing in Philadelphia. Before the turn of the century histories of Philadelphia medicine had been written by George W. Norris and Frederick P. Henry, of the University of Pennsylvania Medical School by Joseph Carson, of the Philadelphia School of Anatomy by William W. Keen, of the Pennsylvania Hospital by Thomas G. Morton and Frank Woodbury, among others. But it was principally Francis R. Packard who sustained interest in medical history in the College and in Philadelphia. Packard read his first paper, on medical practice in colonial New England, to the Horatio C Wood Society of the University of Pennsylvania Medical School in 1897. Three years later he read two historical papers at the College. Except for anniversary addresses, they were the first purely historical papers presented there. Packard was followed by Weir Mitchell on the Jenner letters in the library, by George B. McClellan on Philip Syng Physick, and by Ward Brinton on Washington's last illness. The Section on Medical History was created in 1905. It drew members generally from Philadelphia physicians and invited papers from laymen as well as doctors. Packard wrote the first general history of medicine in the United States in 1901 and was editor of the *Annals of Medical History* from its establishment in 1917 until it ceased publication in 1942. Among those who shared his enthusiasm for history was Edward B. Krumbhaar, who took the principal part in organizing the American Association of the History of Medicine in 1924–25.[34]

Its operations suspended by World War II, the Section was revived after the war with seventy-seven members. One of its first programs was a series of nine evening public lectures in 1948 on "Highlights of Medical History," and in the next year it was instrumental in getting the five medical schools in the city to support a course of formal lectures for first-year students, taught by Professors Richard H. Shryock and Owsei Temkin of the Institute of the History of Medicine of Johns Hopkins. These lectures in effect substituted for regular courses in the history of medicine in the curricula of the Philadelphia medical schools. Quite as important, they and the ordinary meetings of the Section called attention to the incomparable historical resources of the College and encouraged those interested in medical history, most of them amateurs or truants from conventional disciplines, in a day before medical history had come of age, with its journals, grants, chairs, and tenured professors. One form of encouragement was publication in the *Transactions & Studies.*

Only one or two papers were now read at stated meetings. Many of these were retrospective and general rather than fresh contributions to knowledge, and speakers often declined or neglected to give them to the secretary for publication. Papers in the clinical sections were generally reserved by their authors for specialized journals, as had long been the practice. Financial considerations also affected the size and content of the *Transactions.* For all these reasons, *T. & S.* was a less significant scientific journal than it had been before the First World War. As a result, there was usually room for historical articles both by physician-historians and by the small but growing number of professional historians of medicine and science. Such articles were welcomed by McDaniel and by his successors as editor, Fred B. Rogers and Robert E. Jones, who were all deeply interested in history. Thus the *Transactions* imperceptibly ceased to be primarily a scientific journal and became in effect, at least in part, a journal of medical history.

### *Library*

The library changed dramatically in the quarter of a century after the Second World War. Physical needs were urgent. Journal publications, for example, exploded, so that the stacks were jammed, and book cases and shelves were placed in hallways and on stair landings. Such conditions had led to the financial campaign of 1949–54 and the construction of a book stack at the rear of the Hall. More than this, the acceleration of research in universities and industrial laboratories resulted in heavier demands on the collection, giving the library its opportunity—thrusting upon it, rather, the necessity—to provide for a broader clientele. For three-quarters of a century the Fellows had pointed proudly to the library as the most important of the College's functions. It was that indeed, and never more so than after 1946.

The library in that year contained 165,004 bound volumes, received 1,248 journals, and had 322,240 "unaccessioned" pamphlets, reprints, reports, catalogues, and the like. By 1953 the numbers had increased to 183,991 volumes, 1739 journals, and 324,312 "unaccessioned" items. The library spent between $3,500 and $5,000 annually for new books (the Armed Forces Medical Library spent $22,848) and accessioned between 725 and 1,000 volumes a year, the work being done by one cataloguer and an assistant. Without adequate money, space, and trained staff, making do with limited resources, as it had always done, the library nonetheless made far-reaching changes.

In the summer of 1953 Elliott H. Morse was named librarian, succeeding W. B. McDaniel, 2d, who now became curator of the Historical Collections, where he soon resumed the task of writing and publishing *Fugitive Leaves.* Morse, a professional librarian who had been on the staff of the University of Pennsylvania Library, came to the College as assistant administrative librarian in 1949. During his thirty-two years of service, twenty-eight as librarian, the library was transformed.

He spent much time in his early years making an objective survey and analysis of the collection, its acquisition policies, the amount of use, the character of users, and the cost of delivering a volume to a reader. He learned which journals were most frequently consulted, which holdings supplemented, and which duplicated, those of neighboring medical libraries, and he formulated a statement of the proper role of the College library at mid-century. Old patterns of use and growth continued, of course—Fellows like Krumbhaar and Sturgis continued to donate rare books, and in 1959 more than one thousand old medical books came in from the Franklin Institute, Academy of Natural Sciences, Preston Retreat, and other institutions; but increasingly the library staff was concerned with the new methods of duplication that were now available and the new systems of information storage and retrieval that were on the horizon.

One of these new responses was the Medical Literature Service, a private operation of Mrs. Virginia Beatty, wife of one of the staff members. Opened on October 1, 1953, after a study of similar systems in the New York Academy of Medicine, the John Crerar Library, and the American College of Surgeons, the Service offered for a fee to make bibliographical searches and reference checks, to make abstracts, and to translate from or into foreign languages. Individual Fellows and commercial firms employed the service, and *Biological Abstracts* and the National Institutes of Health soon contracted with it for specific projects. From the start the Medical Literature Service proved successful; it grew each year; and when the Beattys left Philadelphia in 1956 it was taken into the Library as the Medical Documentation Service. Under June Fulton services expanded and produced substantial income for the College.

Morse's study of the library made it clear that the College was providing ever-increasing service and services to the medical community even as the Fellows, who supported it, were a steadily diminishing proportion of the physicians of Philadelphia and the surrounding area.[35] Some relief was offered in 1957 when the local medical schools, recognizing the indispensable nature of College services, began to make a financial contribution to their cost. It was one of the first steps toward medical library cooperation.

Cooperation was obviously necessary. No single institution could hold all the books and journals that might be required or provide all the services that physicians, medical schools, hospitals, and laboratories had come to expect. Morse began to plan for such cooperation. From 1959 onward the concept can be seen taking shape in his reports. The medical institutions of the area were interdependent; a single regional center of bibliographical literature and information was essential; and such a center required broader financial support than the Fellows of the College could provide, especially since the College made no charge for its reference service.

In 1962 Morse refined his ideas, discussing regional cooperation in reference to the functions of the recently-created National Library of Medicine. Philadelphia, with its complex of medical, scientific, and general libraries linked by a union catalogue, had a special opportunity to create a regional system. "We have steadfastly preferred to assume," Morse wrote,

> that the major function of this regional research library is to pursue a dynamic, internationally comprehensive acquisition policy to the end that when the call comes for this material—however often or seldom, soon or late, for whatever reason, from whatever level of medical or paramedical competence—the book or journal will be here for Philadelphia's physicians . . . and medical leaders, . . . who have kept this library great, whatever the changing demands of the times.[36]

Thereafter things moved rapidly.[37] The director of the National Library of Medicine ordered a report made of the status and needs of medical school libraries in the country. The deans of the Philadelphia schools asked their librarians to evaluate their respective libraries in the light of the national survey. Their memorandum in reply, produced in November 1962, while not disputing the National Library's conclusions, focussed rather on the special needs and strengths of the Philadelphia institutions. The "Philadelphia Plan" was presented at a conference of "regional-minded" librarians at Harvard University in February 1963. The next year, at the request of the Philadelphia deans, President Gibbon of the College appointed a Regional Medical Library Committee, under the chairmanship of John F. Huber, formerly chairman of the College Library Committee. Its task was to keep abreast of national developments.

A strong impetus to the movement was given in 1965, when a bill was introduced into Congress to authorize the establishment of a regional library system. Morse and others of the College lobbied for the bill, which was enacted into law on October 23, 1965, as the Health Sciences Library Assistance Act. No money, however, had been appropriated; and the College, not sure it could count on federal funds, continued to develop its own plan. In October the College's Committee on Library, its thoughts and wishes "unhampered by limitations of budget, space, and personnel," as Morse put it, came up with a nine-point program that included a training program with Drexel School of Library Science, rehabilitation and expansion of physical facilities (air-conditioning, humidity control, an adequate staff lounge), a new department to explore machine techniques, facsimile transmission, regional messenger service, and "publications of an historical and teaching center."[38]

In January 1967 the College "officially and publicly" affirmed its intention to support and expand its regional library functions, "whether or not officially so designated."[39] Thus empowered, President Wood and a committee paid a visit to the National Library. In 1967 the College applied for designation as a regional library. The College library then contained 240,000 volumes, received 3,210 journals, and was lending over 27,000 volumes a year to 300 libraries in thirty-three states.

Wood, Morse, and others appreciated that designation as a regional library would vastly increase the College's administrative responsibilities. Should the federal government become involved, expectations would be raised and controls and guide-lines would be imposed that could not be evaded or left to annual exhortations or other short-term expedients. Appreciating the need, Wood obtained the appointment of John K. Clark, a Fellow, as special assistant to the president; and in 1967 W. Wallace Dyer, another Fellow, was named to the post—unfilled since Austin's death—of executive secretary. Soon afterwards a comptroller (first proposed by John B. Roberts in 1915) was added to the staff. The College was thus reasonably well situated when Congress in 1968 appropriated funds for the regional system, and the College was designated as the library for the mid-Atlantic region. In Morse's words, this was only recognition of "the fortress-like strength of its collections and the reputation for community services which have been guaranteed by many generations of librarians with the strong moral and financial support of concerned Fellows of the College."[40] In the first three months of operation the regional library received five thousand requests, of which it filled ninety percent from its own holdings and seven per cent from other libraries in the region; two per cent were rejected for obscurity or irrelevance, and only one per cent had to be referred to the National Library.

President Wood believed that the College and its library "at this pivotal moment in its history" needed the guidance of experienced medical librarians and administrators. Accordingly, with the assent of the Council, he appointed a distinguished committee of outsiders. Such persons, he reckoned, would not be intimidated by, perhaps not even recognize, College traditions, precedents, and personalities; and though they might recommend nothing that had not already occurred to Fellows, they might be more closely heeded. The committee was led by George P. Berry, retired dean of the Harvard Medical School. It made its report in December 1969.[41]

The Berry committee directed its attention principally to the library, its internal organization, physical accommodations, services, and relations with other institutions. It recognized that for years the Philadelphia area's medical schools, hospitals, and research laboratories had relied heavily on the College, and that the institution's designation as the regional medical library not only gave formal recognition to this role but would require redefining it as the regional responsibilities developed. The committee made a dozen recommendations, ranging from large questions of policy and capital improvements (a new building for current publications, a renovated old Hall for the older books, medical history, and administrative offices and meeting rooms) to such specific matters as charges for photocopying. At the same time, these and other recommendations involved the College as a whole—simplification of by-laws, better accounting procedures, more effective publicity and public relations. The committee recommended that the College enter more fully into the field of public health and welfare, and noted with approval that symposia had been held or were already scheduled on drug abuse and the prospective "population avalanche." One of its most ambitious suggestions was that the College should establish an institute of the history of medicine, which should emphasize current problems in their historical relations.

Some of these recommendations were already in effect, and others could be adopted at once. Still others required time and negotiations. Many needed money. About this, however, the Berry report had nothing to offer except that, as federal support could not be relied on, the Fellows and their friends must provide the monetary support and other assistance that regional library and expanded College activity would require. "Heroic efforts to 'make do' with inadequate space, facilities, and staff," the committee warned, "will no longer suffice."

The Berry report was a landmark in the College's history. New activities were undertaken with greater confidence because it had recommended them, reforms were more easily made with its authority behind them. Even the institute of the history of medicine, with a large endowment of its own, was established. And a realization spread among the Fellows that the College, as it approached its third century, deserved space, facilities, and staff commensurate with its history and its opportunities.

# *Appendix*

***Other Histories of the College***

W. S. W. Ruschenberger, *An Account of the Institutions and Progress of the College of Physicians of Philadelphia during a Hundred Years, from January, 1787* (Philadelphia, 1887). Also in 3 *Transactions,* IX (1887).

S. Weir Mitchell, "Commemorative Address," 3 *Transactions,* IX (1887), cccxxxvii–ccclxcvi.

Alfred Stillé, "Reminiscences of the College of Physicians of Philadelphia," 3 *Transactions,* IX (1887), ccclxvii–ccclxxix.

J. Norman Henry, "The College of Physicians of Philadelphia," in Frederick P. Henry, ed., *Founders' Week Memorial Volume* (Philadelphia, 1909), 124–52.

James Tyson, "Address . . . on the Dedication of the College," 3 *Transactions,* XXXI (1909), 368–408).

George E. de Schweinitz and W. B. McDaniel, 2d, "An Account of the College of Physicians of Philadelphia," 4 *Transactions,* II, Supplement (1934).

Francis R. Packard, "The College of Physicians from its Centennial in 1887 to 1925," 4 *Transactions,* IV, Supplement (1937), 89–116.

Richard H. Shryock, "The College of Physicians of Philadelphia in Historical Perspective," 4 *Transactions & Studies,* XXVII (1960), 150–57.

Thomas A. Horrocks, "The College of Physicians of Philadelphia: 'Not for Oneself, but for All,' " *Pennsylvania Heritage,* XIII, No.1 (Winter 1987), 32–37.

Julie S. Berkowitz, *The College of Physicians of Philadelphia Portrait Catalogue* (Philadelphia, 1984).

Rudolf Hirsch, ed., *A Catalogue of the Manuscripts and Archives of the Library of the College of Physicians of Philadelphia* (Philadelphia, 1981).

### *Short Titles and Abbreviations*

| | |
|---|---|
| APS | American Philosophical Society, Philadelphia |
| CPP | College of Physicians of Philadelphia |
| Council Minutes | Minutes of the Council of the College of Physicians (manuscript) |
| *D.A.B.* | *Dictionary of American Biography* |
| HSP | Historical Society of Pennsylvania, Philadelphia |
| *JAMA* | *Journal of the American Medical Association* |
| K & B | Howard A. Kelly and Walter L. Burrage, eds., *Dictionary of American Medical Biography* (New York, 1928) |
| Ms. Archives | Miscellaneous documents of the College history (one bound volume) |
| Ms. Minutes | Minutes of the College of Physicians (manuscript) |
| Presidents' Letters | Correspondence files of presidents of the College |
| Ruschenberger | W. S. W. Ruschenberger, *An Account of the Institution and Progress of the College of Physicians of Philadelphia* (Philadelphia, 1887). Also printed in the Centennial Volume and in 3 *Trans.*, IX (1887), xxxiii–cccxxxvi. |
| *Rush Letters* | L. H. Butterfield, ed., *Letters of Benjamin Rush* (2 v., Princeton, 1951). |

*Summary*
*Trans.*
*T. & S.*
*Transactions of the College of Physicians of Philadelphia,* Vol. 1, pt. 1 (1793). Resumed as *Summary of the Transactions of the College of Physicians of Philadelphia* 3 v., 1841–50, and New Series, 4 v., 1850–74. Continued as *Transactions of the College of Physicians of Philadelphia,* Third Series, 54 v., 1875–1932; Fourth Series, 45 v., 1933–78. Title changed to *Transactions & Studies of the College of Physicians of Philadelphia,* Fourth Series, VI (1938–39). Fifth Series, 1979—.

A copy of this book, with references to additional authorities, will be placed in the library of the College of Physicians in 1988.

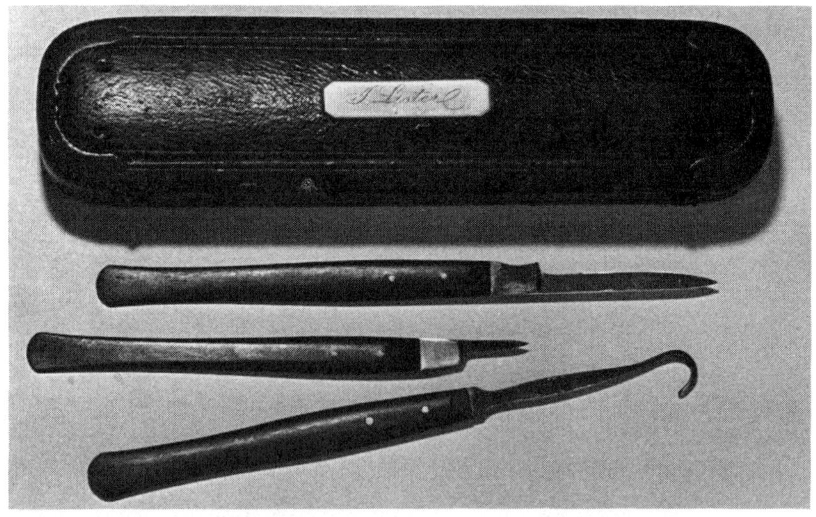

Joseph Lister's Instruments with Case *(Abbe Collection, College of Physicians).*

# *Notes*

## CHAPTER I

1 Rush "A Discourse delivered before the College of Physicians of Philadelphia, Feb. 6th 1787. On the Objects of their Institution," *Trans.*, I, pt. 1 (1793), xix.

2 "Extract of a Letter from a Gentleman in Wilmington, to a Correspondent in Philadelphia," Oct. 21, 1790, *Columbian Magazine,* V (1790), 317–18.

3 Rush, "To the people of the United States," *American Museum,* I (1787), 9–13.

4 Rush, "Discourse," xix.

5 *Boston Gazette,* Oct. 2, 1738, Nov. 10, 1741; Carl Bridenbaugh, ed., *Gentleman's Progress: The Itinerarium of Dr. Alexander Hamilton* (Chapel Hill, N.C., 1948), 115–16, 137.

6 John Bard, "An Essay on the Nature and Cause of Malignant Pleurisy," 1749, *American Medical and Philosophical Register,* I (1811), 409–21; Samuel Bard, *A Discourse upon the Duties of the Physician* (New York, 1769); K & B.

7 8 *Pennsylvania Archives,* IV, 3243.

8 *Connecticut Courant,* Feb. 23, Sept. 7, Nov. 9, 1767, May 8, June 19, 1769, Jan. 15, 1770, Sept. 14, Oct. 26, 1779; James Potter to Benjamin Franklin, New Fairfield, Conn., May 10, 1780; First Medical Society to Royal Medical Society, May 10, 1780; Franklin Papers, LIV, 67, 68 (APS); Potter, *Oration on the Rise and Progress of Physic in America* (Hartford, Conn., 1781).

9 Whitfield J. Bell, Jr., *John Morgan, Continental Doctor* (Philadelphia, 1965), 137–40.

10 Whitfield J. Bell, Jr., "For Mutual Improvement in the Healing Art:

Philadelphia Medical Societies of the 18th Century," *JAMA,* CCXVI (April 5, 1971), 125–29.

11 "Account of the American medical society," *Columbian Magazine,* IV (1790), 206–08; Ruschenberger, 15. The *Columbian Magazine* printed a number of the papers read to the American Medical Society in the 1780s.

12 *The Rise, Minutes, and Proceedings of the New Jersey Medical Society* (Newark, N.J., 1875); Walter L. Burrage, *A History of the Massachusetts Medical Society* (Privately printed, 1923); Creighton Barker, "The Origins of the Connecticut State Medical Society," George Blumer, "Some Remarks on 'Cases and Observations; by the Medical Society of New Haven County,' " *Heritage of Connecticut Medicine* (New Haven, 1942), 1–9, 10–23.

13 Theodore G. Tappert and John W. Doberstein, trans., *The Journals of Henry Melchior Muhlenberg* (3 v., Philadelphia, 1942–58), I, 168, 189–90, II, 68–69, 381–82; Stephen Wickes, *History of Medicine in New Jersey, and of its Medical Men* (Newark, N.J., 1879), 329–30.

14 William Smith, *The History of the Province of New York . . . to the Year M.DCC.XXXII* (London, 1757), 212.

15 See in this connection the 1775 appeal of citizens of Northampton County, Pennsylvania, for legislation requiring physicians to be examined and licensed before being allowed to practice. 8 *Pennsylvania Archives,* VIII, 7197; *Statutes at Large of Pennsylvania,* VIII, 369–77.

16 Griffitts to Rush, London, Aug. 10, 1783, Rush Correspondence, XXI, 94 (HSP).

17 Brodbelt to Rush, Spanish Town, Jamaica, June 25, 1783, *ibid.,* XXV, 69.

18 Lettsom to Rush, London, Aug. 2, 1791, *ibid.,* XXVIII, 18.

19 Lettsom to Rush, London, Sept. 8, 1783, *ibid.,* XXVIII, 3.

20 Rush to Lettsom, Philadelphia, Nov. 15, 1783, *Rush Letters,* I, 312.

21 Lettsom to Rush, London, Feb. 28, 1784, Rush Correspondence, XXVIII, 4 (HSP).

22 Lettsom to Rush, London, Oct. 9, 1784, Feb. 4, 1789, *ibid.,* XXVIII, 6, 11.

23 Lettsom to Rush, London, Sept. 7, 1785, *ibid.,* XXVIII, 7.

24 Rush to Lettsom, Philadelphia, Oct. 26, 1786, Thomas J. Pettigrew, *Memoirs of the Life and Writings of the late John Coakley Lettsom* (2v., London, 1817), II, 428.

25 Ruschenberger, 19–22. Ruschenberger's transcriptions of College minutes and other documents have been checked against the originals.

26 The first draft of the constitution of CPP (Ms. Archives, 3) had a long preamble lamely patterned after the Declaration of Independence: "It having pleased the great Disposer of human events to Separate the

United States from Great Britain, a country from whence a large portion of their knowledge in the arts & sciences was derived, it has become necessary for the members of the republic of letters in America to assume the same powers, in the establishment of literary institutions, which have been exercised by literary associations in the different nations of Europe, from which they are descended." This was cut out, as were references to the reputation for enterprise and industry "which has so long distinguished Pennsylvania in all human pursuits" and to the "harmony which happily subsists among the physicians of Philadelphia."

27 "Constitution," *Trans.*, I, pt. 1 (1793), xiii–xiv.

28 For brief accounts of contemporary British societies, see D'Arcy Power, ed., *British Medical Societies* (London, 1939). See also Lettsom's "Hints for the establishment of a Medical Society in London," June 23, 1773, in his *Hints designed to promote Beneficence, Temperance & Medical Science* (3v., London, 1801), III, 257–61; Medical Society of London, *Memoirs,* I (reprint 1792), iii–xiii; Thomas Hunt, ed., *The Medical Society of London, 1773–1973* (London, 1972); James Gray, *History of the Royal Medical Society, 1737–1937* (Edinburgh, 1952).

29 W. B. McDaniel, 2d, " 'Your Aged Friend and Fellow Servant, John Redman,' " 4 *T. & S.,* IX, (1941), 35–41; Whitfield J. Bell, Jr., "John Redman, Medical Preceptor, 1722–1808," *Pennsylvania Magazine of History and Biography,* LXXXI (1957), 157–69.

30 Redman's address is in CPP Minutes; it is printed in Ruschenberger, 179–83. Redman made a similar address upon his reelection in 1791. *ibid.,* 187–89.

31 Edgar E. Hume, "Surgeon John Jones, U.S Army, Father of American Surgery," *Bulletin of the History of Medicine,* XIII (1943), 10–32; Stephen T. Charles, "John Jones, American Surgeon and Conservative Patriot," *ibid.,* XXXIX (1965), 435–49.

32 Whitfield J. Bell, Jr., "James Hutchinson (1752–1793): A Physician in Politics," Lloyd G. Stevenson and Robert P. Multhauf, eds., *Medicine, Science and Culture: Historical Essays in honor of Owsei Temkin* (Baltimore, 1968), 265–83.

33 Ruschenberger, 43–44.

34 Bell, *John Morgan;* Betsy C. Corner, *William Shippen, Jr., Pioneer in American Medical Education* (Philadelphia, 1951); Marion E. Brown, "Adam Kuhn: Eighteenth Century Physician and Teacher," *Journal of the History of Medicine,* V (1950), 163–77; Nathan G. Goodman, *Benjamin Rush, Physician and Citizen, 1746–1813* (Philadelphia, 1934).

35 John Adams, *Diary* (L. H. Butterfield, ed., Boston, 1961), II, 152; Ruschenberger, 44–48. A future biographer of this engaging person may

find the following references useful: W. Brockbank and F. Kenworthy, eds., *The Diary of Richard Kay, 1716–51* (Manchester, 1968), 48, 52, and Chovet, "Proposals . . .," 1732, Royal Society, Manuscript Letters C.2.88.

36 David Riesman, "Dr. Richard Mead and the Motto of the College of Physicians of Philadelphia," *Medical Life,* XLII (1935), 187–201; [Matthew Maty], *Authentic Memoirs of the Life of Richard Mead, M.D.* (London, 1755), 64.

37 Rush, "Discourse," *Trans.,* I, pt. 1 (1793), xix–xxxi.

38 Francis Hopkinson, "An Oration, which might have been delivered to the Students of Anatomy, on the late Rupture between the Two Schools in this City," *Miscellaneous Essays and Occasional Writings* (3v., Philadelphia, 1792), III, 203–04.

39 Hopkinson, "Account of the grand federal procession in Philadelphia, July 4, 1788," *American Museum,* IV (1788), 57–78.

40 Morgan to CPP, Philadelphia, Dec. 17, 1788, Ms. Archives, 55.

41 Circular Letter, [1789], in CPP (Cage Qb/31).

42 Isaac Senter to CPP, Newport, R.I., Dec. 3, 1789, Ms. Archives, 99; Leverett Hubbard to John Redman, New Haven, July 18, 1790, Committee on the Pharmacopoeia, Papers (CPP).

43 The draft of the memorial to the Pennsylvania legislature, in Rush's hand, Nov. 9, 1787, is in Ms. Archives, 21; the text is printed in Ruschenberger, 183–84. See Rush to Lettsom, Philadelphia, Aug. 16, 1788, *Rush Letters,* I, 480. The memorial to Congress, Dec. 27, 1790, is printed in Ruschenberger, 186; for its reception in the House of Representatives, see *Annals of Congress,* 1st Cong., II, Jan. 5, 1791. Dr. George Logan of Stenton, near Philadelphia, strongly opposed spirituous liquors and testified to the advantages of serving harvest-hands only small beer. Logan to Philadelphia Society for Promoting Agriculture, Stenton, Aug. 1, 1787, Philadelphia Society for Promoting Agriculture, *Memoirs,* VI (1939), 137–38.

44 Philadelphia City Councils, Minutes, I, April 18, 1789.

45 "A Citizen," *Pennsylvania Gazette,* Aug. 27, 1783.

46 Linn to President and Fellows, March 2, 1789, Ms. Archives, 61.

47 William Currie to John Foulke, Nov. 20, 1790, *ibid.,* 139. Statements by Meyer's wife and daughter and others, including Drs. Thomas T. Hewson and William Bache, who had accompanied Foulke when he dressed the leg, are also in Ms. Archives.

48 General Assembly, *Minutes,* 13th Ass., 1st sess. (1787), 141.

49 CPP to John Vaughan, May 11, 1791 (Archives, APS); bills and receipts for the furniture are in Ms. Archives. The prices are most likely given in Pennsylvania currency, in which one pound was the equivalent of 13s. sterling.

50 "Register of Books Borrowed, 1792–1855" (CPP).

51 In a letter to Samuel Powel Griffitts, March 24, 1790 (Ms. Archives, 105), Benjamin Rush wrote that he had received from Benjamin Franklin some time before "a copy of a letter from Dr. Mitchell (a gentleman of a respectable medical Character formerly of Virginia) to a friend containing an Acct. of the Yellow fever, as it appeared in that country abt. 50 Years ago." With Franklin's permission, Rush copied parts of the letter for CPP. "Some of his [Mitchell's] remarks are new, and all of them are calculated to extend our knowledge of the rise & progress of a dangerous disease in the United States." Rush gave Mitchell's letter for publication in *Philadelphia Medical Museum,* I (1804), 1–20. For his account of how he used the letter in 1793, see Rush, *An Account of the Bilious Yellow Fever,* 196–97.

## CHAPTER II

1 The best modern history of the yellow fever epidemic of 1793 is John H. Powell, *Bring Out Your Dead: The Great Plague of Yellow Fever in Philadelphia in 1793* (Philadelphia, 1949). Many of the documents quoted in this chapter, some in manuscript in CPP, were printed in one or more of the principal contemporary accounts: *Proceedings of the College of Physicians of Philadelphia, relative to the Prevention of the Introduction and Spreading of Contagious Diseases* (Philadelphia, 1798); CPP, *Facts and Observations relating to the Nature and Origin of the Pestilential Fever, which prevailed in this City, in 1793, 1797, and 1798* (Philadelphia, 1798); Benjamin Rush, *An Account of the Bilious Remitting Yellow Fever, as it appeared in the City of Philadelphia, in the Year 1793* (Philadelphia, 1794); Mathew Carey, *A Short Account of the Malignant Fever, lately prevalent in Philadelphia* (Philadelphia, 1793).

2 Rush, *Account,* 8–13.

3 Martin S. Pernick, "Politics, Parties, and Pestilence: Epidemic Yellow Fever in Philadelphia and the Rise of the First Party System," 3 *William and Mary Quarterly,* XIX (1972), 559–86.

4 *Rush Letters,* II, 640.

5 CPP, *Proceedings,* 2–3. The manuscript is in Ms. Archives, 233 (CPP). The Recommendations were spread on the Minutes (CPP) and are printed in Ruschenberger, 55–56.

6 *Rush Letters,* II, 642.

7 Redman, "Letter . . . on the Yellow Fever of 1762," Ms. Archives, 235 (CPP). The manuscript was presented to the College by Samuel Lewis in 1865 and was printed in a pamphlet the same year.
8 *Rush Letters,* II, 644–45.
9 Rush, *Account,* 226.
10 *Ibid.,* 227.
11 *Ibid.,* 216–25, 230–32.
12 Carey, *Short Account,* 72.
13 CPP, *Proceedings,* 4.
14 *Ibid.,* 5–6.
15 4 *Pennsylvania Archives,* IV, 267–69.
16 *Rush Letters,* II, 740; Rush, *Autobiography: His 'Travels through Life'* (George W. Corner, ed., Princeton, 1948), 98.
17 Charles Caldwell, *Autobiography* (Philadelphia, 1855), 183–84; Coxe, Commonplace book on yellow fever, 1794–95 (ms., CPP)
18 CPP, *Proceedings,* 7.
19 *Ibid.,* 9–11, 13–14.
20 *Statutes at Large of Pennsylvania,* XV, 119–45, 305–05, 309–12, 456–61.
21 James Stuart to CPP, Aug. 15, 1797, Ms. Archives, 325 (CPP).
22 CPP, *Proceedings,* 17–19; Board of Health, Minutes, I, Aug. 19, 20, 22, 1797. (Philadelphia City Archives).
23 CPP, *Proceedings,* 19.
24 *Ibid.,* 21–22.
25 *Ibid.,* 23.
26 *Ibid.,* 24–25.
27 *Ibid.,* 25–26.
28 *Ibid.,* 27–30.
29 The governor's letter and the Academy's response were reprinted in *The Medical Repository,* I (1797; 3d edit., 1804), 391–98.
30 Academy of Medicine, *Constitution* [and] *Laws* (Philadelphia, 1799); *Rush Letters,* II, 796–97.
31 Board of Health, Minutes, I, Aug. 6, 1798.
32 *Ibid.,* Sept. 1, 15, 1798.
33 *Facts and Observations,* 26–27.
34 Board of Health, Minutes, I, July 2, 1799.
37 *Ibid.,* Aug. 16, 1802.
38 Thomas McKean to Redman, Falls of Schuylkill, Sept. 25, 1799; Redman to McKean, Sept. 26, 1799 (draft). Ms. Archives, 383–385 (CPP).
39 Board of Health, Minutes, I, Nov. 22, 1802.
40 John Haygarth, "An Address to the College of Physicians at Philadelphia, on the prevention of the American Pestilence, " *Medical Transactions,* IV, 143–65. Haygarth derided the evidence put forth by Rush and the Academy of Medicine and made the practical sugges-

tion that the College undertake to determine just how far distant from an infected person the disease polluted the atmosphere. Haygarth sent the College additional testimony supporting his and their view, Oct. 16, 1805. Ms. Archives, 439 (CPP). Albers' letter to CPP, Bremen, March 22, 1805, is *ibid.*, 437.

41 *Rush Letters,* II, 917–18.

42 Robert H. Halsey, *How the President, Thomas Jefferson, and Doctor Benjamin Waterhouse established Vaccination as a Public Health Procedure* (New York, 1936).

43 Coxe, *Practical Observations on Vaccination: or Inoculation for the Cow-Pock* (Philadelphia, 1802), 122.

44 Coxe in *Philadelphia Medical Museum,* I (1805), 22–25.

45 In 1851 the Fellows of the College, other physicians, and the medical students of Philadelphia were solicited for contributions to erect a monument to Jenner in London. *Trans.,* n.s., I (1850–53), 223; Edward R. Squibb, *Journal* (Privately printed, c. 1930), 194, 201.

46 *Rush Letters,* II, 847.

47 Unidentified clipping, April 19, 1803, in Joseph Carson, comp., Scrap book . . . History of the Medical Department of the University of Pennsylvania, III, 141 (CPP).

48 American Philosophical Society, Contract with CPP, April 6, 1798; "Report of Committee on Application of the College of Physicians relative to Rent," Nov. 4, 1814 (APS Archives); APS to CPP, Jan. 3, 1805; John Vaughan to Thomas T. Hewson, Feb. 5, 1811. Ms. Archives, 433, 451 (CPP)

49 CPP to President, APS, July 1815; John Vaughan to Thomas Parke, April 6, 1818 (APS Archives).

50 W.B. McDaniel, 2d, "The First Catalogue of the College Library, 1818," CPP, *Fugitive Leaves from the Library,* n.s., Nos. 48–49 (1961).

51 "Register of Books Borrowed, 1792–1855" (CPP).

52 Caldwell, *Autobiography,* 161–62.

53 *Ibid.,* 121–22, 124; Medical Society of London, *Memoirs,* I (reprinted 1792), 346–49.

54 Samuel X Radbill, "The Philadelphia Medical Society, 1789–1868," 4 *T. & S.,* XX (1952), 103–23; Philadelphia Medical Society, *The Charter of Incorporation and Bye-Laws* (Philadelphia, 1832). Some papers read to the Society are printed in the *American Medical Recorder,* V (1822), 385–86 *et passim.* Minutes of the Society, except one volume in HSP, are in CPP.

55 Currie to CPP, July 1, 1817. Ms. Archives, 483 (CPP).

# CHAPTER III

1 W. B. McDaniel, 2d, "The First Catalogue of the College Library, 1818," CPP, *Fugitive Leaves from the Library,* n.s., Nos. 48–49 (1961).

2 Whitfield J. Bell, Jr., "Thomas Parke, M.B., Physician and Friend," 3 *William and Mary Quarterly,* VI (1949), 569–95.

3 Benjamin Rush, "Discourse . . . On the Objects of their Institution," *Trans.,* I, pt. 1 (1793), xxi.

4 David Hosack and others, Circular, Nov. 21, 1818. Committee on the Pharmacopoeia, Papers (CPP).

5 *The Pharmacopoeia of the United States of America, 1820* (Boston, 1820), 5–16.

6 Thomas Parke and Thomas T. Hewson, Report of the Committee on Pharmacopoeia, Feb. 1, 1820. Committee on the Pharmacopoeia, Papers (CPP).

7 *Boston Medical and Surgical Journal,* IV (1831), 213.

8 *North American Medical and Surgical Journal,* XI (1831), 441–55.

9 *Ibid.,* 178–200; *Boston Medical and Surgical Journal,* IV (1831), 54–55, 230–31.

10 George B. Wood and Franklin Bache, *The Dispensatory of the United States of America* (9th ed., Philadelphia, 1851), "Preface to the First Edition," iii–viii.

11 Ruschenberger, 112–14.

12 *American Medical Recorder,* V (1822), 773. D. Francis Condie to Mayor Joseph Wharton, April 25, 1827. Society Collection (HSP).

13 *Aesculapian Register,* I (1824), 90.

14 CPP, Committee on Small Pox, Minutes, 3 mo. 1828; Benjamin H. Coates, "Medical Essays &c" in Coates-Reynell Papers (HSP). The report of the Philadelphia Medical Society's committee (Edward Jenner Coxe, D. Francis Condie, and Charles D. Meigs) is in *American Medical Recorder,* XIII (1828), 329–47.

15 A.D. Hall, "Memoir of Squier Littell, M.D.," 3 *Trans.,* IX (1887), cdlvii.

16 Governor Andrew Shulze to Thomas Parke, Jan. 17, 1825. Ms. Archives, 569 (CPP).

17 Shulze to Parke, Feb. 18, 1825; George M. Stroud to Joseph Parrish, March 3, 16, 19, 1825; Parrish, Receipt, 6mo. 2, 1825. Ms. Archives, 571, 573, 575, 577, 578.

18 *Medical Examiner,* VII (Jan. 27, 1844), 21.

19 Joseph P. Thompson *et al.* to CPP, Oct. 14, 1833. Committee on the Use of Tobacco, [Papers] (CPP).

20 The fee–bill was printed, with unimportant changes, in *Charter, Ordinances, and By-Laws of the College of Physicians of Philadelphia* (Philadelphia, 1834), 17–18.

21 *Charter, Ordinances, and By-Laws,* (Philadelphia, 1840), 19.
22 W.S.W. Ruschenberger, "A Memory [sic] of Dr. George Fox," 3 *Trans.,* VII (1884), xiv.
23 *American Journal of the Medical Sciences,* X (1832), 197–204, *et passim.* The best account of the cholera epidemics, with special reference to social and cultural relations, is Charles E. Rosenberg, *The Cholera Years: The United States in 1832, 1849, and 1866* (Chicago, 1962).
24 *American Journal of the Medical Sciences,* X (1832), 257–63.
25 *North American Medical and Surgical Journal,* XII (1831), 391–419.
26 Board of Health to ———, March 28, 1832, Letter Book, 1827–36 (City Archives, Philadelphia).
27 Committee on Sickness, Circular Letter, April 9, 1832, *ibid.*
28 *Ibid.*
29 *North American Medical and Surgical Journal,* XII (1831), 391–419.
30 House of Representatives of Pennsylvania, *Report of the Committee appointed to investigate the local causes of Cholera in the Arch Street Prison . . .* (Harrisburg, 1833).
31 CPP, *Report . . . to the Board of Health on Epidemic Cholera* (Philadelphia, 1832); reprinted from standing type in Bell and Condie, *All the Material Facts,* cited below.
32 Philadelphia Medical Society, *Report . . . on Epidemic Cholera* (Philadelphia, 1832).
33 Caspar W. Pennock and William W. Gerhard, "Observations on the Cholera of Paris," *American Journal of the Medical Sciences,* X (1832), 319–90. The paper was dated May 5, 1832.
34 *Report of the Commission appointed by the Sanitary Board . . . to visit Canada, for the Investigation of the Epidemic Cholera, prevailing in Montreal and Quebec* (Philadelphia, 1832). A summary of the Report was submitted to the Board on July 8.
35 Board of Health to the Secretary of the Navy, June 20, 1832; to the Governor of Pennsylvania, July 7, August 5; to the Comptroller of Public Schools, July 11; to the President of the Board of Directors of the Public Schools of Moyamensing, Board of Health, Letter Book, 1827–36 (City Archives, Philadelphia).
36 *Cholera Gazette,* I (Aug. 8, 1832), 80.
37 "Cholera in Philadelphia. Gazette and American Sentinel, 1832." This is a volume of newspaper clippings, with the binder's title "Newspaper Cuttings, 1849" (CPP). Case books of several cholera hospitals are in CPP.
38 *Cholera Gazette,* I (Aug. 15, 1832), 95.
39 William Darrach, Diary, Aug. 20, 1832 (HSP).
40 Samuel Jackson, "Personal Observations and Experiences of Epidemic or Malignant Cholera in the City of Philadelphia," *American*

*Journal of the Medical Sciences,* XI (1832–33), 289–346; Isaac Hays, "On the Pathology of Cholera," *Cholera Gazette,* I (Nov. 21, 1832), 225–43; Jackson, "Report . . . of the Principal facts connected with the prevalence of Malignant Cholera in Philadelphia in 1832," *ibid.,* 244–52. Silver pitchers were presented by the City of Philadelphia to thirteen physicians who had served conspicuously in the epidemic. Nathaniel Chapman's was presented to the College in 1966. Ella N. Wade, "A Silver Pitcher for Dr. Nathaniel Chapman," 4 *T. & S.,* XXXIV (1966–67), 89–90. Of the remaining twelve so honored, eight were, or soon became, Fellows.

41 Hugh L. Hodge, *A Memoir of Thomas C. James, M.D. read before the College of Physicians of Philadelphia* (Philadelphia, 1843), 23.

42 Franklin Bache, "Obituary Notice of the late Dr. Thomas T. Hewson," *Summary,* III (1849–50), 2–10.

43 William Darrach, elected a Fellow in 1828, had attended lectures in Paris, although most of his foreign study was in England and Scotland. James Logan Fisher of Philadelphia, brother of the diarist, died while a medical student in Paris in 1833. On the Americans in Paris in this period, see Russell M. Jones, "American Doctors in Paris, 1820–1861: A Statistical Profile," *Journal of the History of Medicine,* XXV (1970), 143–57.

44 In his *Recherches anatomiques, pathologiques et thérapeutiques sur . . .* [la] *Fièvre typhoide* (2nd ed., I, 1841) Louis mentioned especially, among those who recognized the exactness of his work, Professors Jackson, Shattuck, Holmes, Bowditch, and Enoch Hale of Boston, Gerhard, Stewardson, Pennock, Norris, and Stillé of Philadelphia, and William Power of Baltimore. William Osler's "The Influence of Louis on American Medicine," *An Alabama Student and other Biographical Essays* (New York, 1908), 189–210, is a singularly attractive account of the subject.

45 [Benjamin H. Coates], "Obituary. Dr. J. O'B. Lawrance," *Philadelphia Journal of the Medical and Physical Sciences,* VII (1823), 171–75; Samuel Jackson, "Eulogium commemorative of Jason O'B. Lawrance, M.D.," *ibid.,* 376–98. The *Philadelphia Journal* published notes of the physiological experiments of Lawrance and Coates. See also René La Roche, "Remarks on French Practice," *North American Medical and Surgical Journal,* VIII (1829), 293–318, and "An Account of the Origin, Progress, and Present State of the Medical Schools of Paris," *American Journal of the Medical Sciences,* VIII (1831), 109–24, 401–18; IX (1831), 351–88.

46 *Medical Review and Analectic Journal,* I (1824), 357–83.

47 Eleanor M. Tilton, *Amiable Autocrat: A Biography of Oliver Wendell Holmes* (New York, 1947), 100.

48 Alfred Stillé, "Reminiscences of the College of Physicians of

Philadelphia," *Trans.*, Centennial Volume (1887), 336–37. For a particularly clear exposition and defense of the practice of exact observation and numerical analysis in medicine, see the introductory essay, "Medical Truth: its nature, sources, and means of attainment," in Stillé's *Elements of General Pathology* (Philadelphia, 1848), 25–48.

49 *Charter, Ordinances, and By-Laws of the College of Physicians of Philadelphia* (Philadelphia, 1834).

50 Laurence Turnbull, "Obituary Notice of the late John Bell, M.D., of Philadelphia, 1796–1872," Medical Society of the State of Pennsylvania, *Trans.*, X, pt. 1 (1874), 746–50; Cato, "Sketches of Eminent Living Physicians: No. I. John Bell," *Boston Medical and Surgical Journal*, XL (1849), 99–101, 156–57.

51 *Abt-Garrison History of Pediatrics* (Philadelphia, 1965), 118, 123.

52 K & B.

53 Condie's first "Annual Report on the Diseases of Children," presented March 1, 1842, is in *Summary*, I (1841–46), 36–43. The judgment on milk is in the 1846 report. *Ibid.*, 422.

54 *Boston Medical and Surgical Journal*, XIII (1835–36), 352–353.

55 Togno to President and Fellows, April 1836; Censors, Report, April 27, 1836, Censors, "Reports and Correspondence, 1836–47" (CPP).

56 *Summary*, I (1841–46), 2.

57 *American Journal of the Medical Sciences*, n.s., III (1842), 436.

## CHAPTER IV

1 *Boston Medical and Surgical Journal*, XL (1849), 345.

2 *Summary*, II (1846–49), 281.

3 *Ibid.*, I (1841–46), 272.

4 *Ibid.*, 251–62.

5 *Ibid.*, 50–54.

6 M.W. Wilson, "Notice of a Malignant Epidemic which prevailed in the Lying-in Department of the Philadelphia Hospital (Blockley) in March and April 1842," communicated by Robert M. Huston to *American Journal of the Medical Sciences*, n.s., V (1842), 244–46.

7 *Summary*, I (1841–46), 54–61.

8 *American Journal of the Medical Sciences*, n.s. IV (1842), 410–18.

9 *Summary*, I (1841–46), 71; D.F. C[ondie], review in *American Journal of the Medical Sciences*, n.s., IV (1842), 399–402.

10 *Medical Examiner*, VI (Jan. 21, 1843), 3. Rutter soon afterwards left Philadelphia; he died in Chicago in 1865.

11 Thomas F. Currier and Eleanor M. Tilton, *A Bibliography of Oliver*

*Wendell Holmes* (New York, 1953), 33–35. On this episode, see W. B. McDaniel, 2nd, "Oliver Wendell Holmes and the College of Physicians of Philadelphia," 4 *T. & S.,* XI (1943–44), 15–29; J. Wistar Meigs, "Puerperal Fever and Nineteenth-Century Contagionism: The Obstetrician's Dilemma," *ibid.,* XLII (1974), 273–80; same, "Charles Delucena Meigs, M.D. (1792–1869), as seen by a Great-Great-Grandson," *ibid.,* XLIII (1975–76), 129–35.

12 *Trans.,* n.s., I (1850–53), 330.

13 Charles D. Meigs, *On the Nature, Signs, and Treatment of Childbed Fever* (Philadelphia, 1854), 102–03, 113.

14 *Ibid.,* vii.

15 J. Forsyth Meigs, "Memoir of Charles D. Meigs, M.D.," *Trans.,* n.s., IV (1862–74), 417–48; Samuel D. Gross, *Autobiography* (Philadelphia, 1887), II, 339–47; Cato, "Sketches of Eminent Living Physicians. No. V: Charles D. Meigs," *Boston Medical and Surgical Journal,* XL (1849), 313–15, 333–35.

16 Oliver W. Holmes, "The Contagiousness of Puerperal Fever," *Medical Essays, 1842–1882* (Boston, 1899), 128.

17 *Summary,* II (1846–49), 60–61. In the discussion, recorded in the manuscript minutes but not printed, Alfred Stillé defended Jackson from censure, "assuring the College that he had nothing to do with the patent, which is solely in the name of Dr. Morton." Isaac Hays reported that Jackson had informed Professor Robert Hare of the University of Pennsylvania that the anesthetic agent was pure sulphuric ether.

18 Bigelow's paper (XXXV [Nov. 18, 1846], 309–17) was followed in the ensuing weeks by several others: A.L. Peirson ( *ibid.,* 362–64, 410), John L. Warren ( *ibid.,* 375–79), P.W. Ellsworth ( *ibid.,* 397–98), Samuel Parkman ( *ibid.,* 409–10), A. L. Cox ( *ibid.,* 456–59). Bigelow, J. F. Flagg, and others debated the propriety of Morton's patent. *Ibid.,* 356–59, 379–82, 407–09, 424–25, 440.

19 *Medical News and Library,* IV (Nov. 1846), 108–10.

20 *Summary,* II (1846–49), 61–65; *Medical Examiner,* n.s., VIII (1852), 248; Samuel Jackson (of Northumberland), "Biographical Notice of Dr. Isaac Parrish," *Trans.,* n.s. I (1851–53), 427–51).

21 Isaac Parrish, "Annual Report on Surgery," *Summary,* II (1846–49), 171. The editor of the *Medical Examiner,* Robert M. Huston, then president of the Philadelphia Medical Society, reacted to the news with incredulity and scorn. Six months later he was gratified to notice "a decline of the excitement in relation to it, which prevailed so extensively at first." By March 1848 he had withdrawn from this untenable position. *Medical Examiner,* n.s., II (1846), 719–20; III (1847), 290; IV (1848), 198–99.

22 *Medical Examiner, and Record of Medical Science,* n.s., II (Dec. 1846),

719–20. See also *ibid.*, III (1847), 231–35, 255, 290, 317–28, 331–32, 589–95, 635, *et passim; Medical News and Library,* V (1847), 6, 14–15, 21, 64–67; *American Journal of the Medical Sciences,* n.s., XIII (1847), 260–63; XIV (1847), 512–18.

23 Philip Van Ingen, *The New York Academy of Medicine: Its First Hundred Years* (New York, 1949), 10.

24 Isaac Parrish, "Annual Report on Surgery," *Summary,* II (1846–49), 158.

25 *American Journal of the Medical Sciences,* n.s. XIII (1847), 506.

26 American Medical Association, *Trans.,* (1848), 188–89, 220–21; Isaac Parrish, "Annual Report on Surgery," *Summary,* II (1846–49), 156.

27 *Ibid.,* 165, 171.

28 *Medical Examiner,* n.s., IV (1848), 149, 150, 151. See the editorial comment on Simpson's letter and Meigs' reply, *ibid.,* 198–99.

29 Ms. Minutes, March 7, (1848).

30 *Medical Examiner,* n.s., VIII (1852), 301, 313–14. On anesthesia at the Pennsylvania Hospital, and for the subject of anesthesia generally, see Martin S. Pernick, *A Calculus of Suffering: Pain, Professionalism, and Anesthesia in Nineteenth-Century America* (New York, 1985), 4, 193–94, *et passim.* Pernick states that after the retirement of Edward Peace and George W. Norris from the staff in 1861 and 1863 respectively, use of anesthesia at the Pennsylvania Hospital suddenly increased. However, D. Hayes Agnew ( *The Principles and Practice of Surgery,* Philadelphia, 1881, p.281) says Peace performed the first operation under anesthesia in Philadelphia. Francis R. Packard ("The College of Physicians . . . 1887 to 1925," *Trans.,* IV, suppl., (1937), 106) recorded an anecdote of James Darrach, "a resident physician at the Pennsylvania Hospital in 1846–47," of the first use of ether anesthesia in that institution: "One night a few weeks after Morton had demonstrated ether anaesthesia on October 16, 1846, a man was brought into the Pennsylvania Hospital with a crushed leg requiring amputation. Dr. George W. Norris, the surgeon on duty, told his resident, young Dr. Darrach, to go to the drugstore and get some ether and they would try and use it, neither of them having previously ever witnessed its use. Dr. Darrach soaked a towel with ether, the patient inhaled, and in a few minutes lost consciousness. Dr. Darrach, much alarmed, called to Dr. Norris: 'Sir, the patient has become unconscious.' Dr. Norris replied quickly: 'Take that damned stuff away, Darrach.' " Something like this may have happened, but not to Darrach or not in 1846. James Darrach in that year was sixteen, he received his M.D. degree in 1852, and he was a resident in the Pennsylvania Hospital in 1853–54. That is the year in which anesthetics were first admitted into the Pennsylvania Hospital.

31 John D. Griscom, "Annual Report on Midwifery," *Summary,* II (1846–

49), 323–42; also *ibid.*, 192, 343–47, 403–07 for discussion by D. F. Condie, Henry Bond, Isaac Parrish, Isaac Hays, Samuel Jackson (of Northumberland), and George B. Wood; Isaac Parrish, "Annual Report on Surgery, for 1850," *Trans.*, n.s., I (1850–53), 20–26; also *ibid.*, 225. *Medical News and Library,* X (1852) and XI (1853), *passim,* reported many cases of adverse, even fatal, effects of chloroform.

32 *Medical Examiner,* n.s., VIII (1852), 243–59, 298–320.

33 *Ibid.*, 258.

34 Samuel Jackson (of Northumberland), "Biographical Notice of Dr. Isaac Parrish," *Summary,* n.s., I (1850–53), 427–51.

35 Isaac Parrish, "Report on the Sanitary Condition of Philadelphia," A.M.A., *Trans.*, II (1849), 468, 469–70.

36 *Summary,* I (1841–46), 178–79; Journal of the Select Council, Nov. 23, 1843 (Philadelphia City Archives).

37 *Ibid.*, Sept. 27, 1849; Robley Dunglison, *Autobiographical Ana* (Samuel X Radbill, ed., Philadelphia, 1963), 157–58.

38 Board of Health, Minutes, Feb. 11, 1862 (Philadelphia City Archives); *Report on the Bill to Prevent Salting the Streets* . . . (Philadelphia, 1862).

39 *Summary,* II (1846–49), 272–73.

40 Parrish, "Mortality and Insanity in the Separate Plan Prisons of England and America," *Summary,* n.s., I (1850–53), 173–192.

41 *Ibid.*, n.s., I (1850–53), 362–70.

42 *Ibid.*, 370.

43 *Ibid.*, I (1841–46), 268.

44 Ms. Minutes, March 4, April 1, 1851; *Summary,* n.s., I (1851–53), 80, 95–96.

45 *Ibid.*, III (1857–63), 141.

46 Ms. Minutes, Jan. 6, Feb. 3, 1858.

47 "Cholera in Philadelphia . . . Newspaper Cuttings 1849." (Scrapbook Z10c/18, CPP); *Summary,* II (1846–49), 437–38.

48 *Ibid.*, 429. And see also, *ibid.*, 430–35, 439–42, 442–45, 445–49. It is worth nothing here that on May 7, 1895, one "Dr. Bunting" of Canada, introduced by Francis G. Smith, exhibited to the College Alexis St. Martin, William Beaumont's patient of twenty-five years before. Attendance—thirty-nine fellows—was larger than usual. Smith reported the results of experiments he performed on St. Martin. Smith, "Experiments upon Digestion," *Medical Examiner,* n.s., XII (1856), 385–94, 513–18; *Trans.*, n.s., III (1856–62), 36; Jesse S. Myer, *Life and Letters of Dr. William Beaumont* (St. Louis, 1912), 297; Edward H. Bensley, "Alexis St. Martin and Dr. Bunting," *Bulletin of the History of Medicine,* XLIV (1970), 101–08.

49 Ms. Minutes, Sept. 11, Oct. 4, 1854; John Ward Willson Loose, ed.,

"Cholera in Lancaster and Columbia in 1854," *Journal of the Lancaster County Historical Society,* LXII (1958), 109–46; Philadelphia County Medical Society, *Proc.,* VII (1884–85), 323.

50 Charles D. Meigs to A. Clarkson Smith, Sept. 14, 1854 (CPP Archives).

51 Harford Fraley to "Dr. Wilson [Jewell?]," n.d., (CPP Archives).

52 Ms. Minutes, Oct. 4, 1854.

## CHAPTER V

1 *Summary,* I (1841–46), 373; Nathan Smith Davis, *History of the American Medical Association* (Philadelphia, 1855), 28–31.

2 Morris Fishbein, *A History of the American Medical Association, 1847 to 1947* (Philadelphia, 1947), 19–40.

3 American Medical Association, *Transactions,* I (1848), 16–17.

4 George B. Wood, Journal, III (1836–49). (CPP).

5 Howard K. Petry, ed., *A Century of Medicine, 1848–1948: The History of the Medical Society of the State of Pennsylvania* ([Harrisburg, 1948]), 1–6.

6 *Summary,* II (1846–49), 421.

7 George M. Piersol, "History of the Philadelphia County Medical Society (1849 to 1949)," *100th Anniversary. The Philadelphia County Medical Society, 1849–1949* ([Philadelphia, 1949]), 14–17, 48; John Chalmers DaCosta, "Then and Now," *Selections from the Papers and Speeches* (Philadelphia, 1931), 198–200.

8 Piersol, "History of the Philadelphia County Medical Society," *loc. cit.,* 15–16.

9 Hodge, *An Oration delivered before the Philadelphia Medical Society . . . February 15, 1823* (Philadelphia, 1823), 9–10.

10 A.M.A. *Trans.,* II (1849), 328.

11 *Summary,* I (1841–46), 375.

12 George W. Corner, *Two Centuries of Medicine: A History of the School of Medicine, University of Pennsylvania* (Philadelphia, 1964), 141, 142.

13 A.M.A. *Trans.,* II (1849), 43, 45, 273–74.

14 "Special Committee appointed to prepare 'A Statement of the Facts and Arguments which may be adduced in favour of the prolongation of the Course of Medical Lectures to six months,' " *ibid.,* 359–70.

15 "Register of Books Borrowed, 1792–1855." (CPP).

16 *Medical Examiner,* VI (1843), 79; [Joseph G. Whilden ?], *Address to the Physicians of Philadelphia on the Present Decline of the Medical Character, and the Means of Advancing Professional Respectability*

(n.p., [1825?]); *Philadelphia Medical and Surgical Journal,* IV 1855, 22–24.

17 Committee on the Present Condition of the Medical Profession in Philadelphia, [Report (draft)], March 5, [1839]. (CPP).

18 *Medical Examiner,* II (1839), 140–41, 497, 699–700; IV (1841), 453–54.

19 *Ibid.,* n.s., VI (1843), 115–17.

20 Ms. Minutes, Nov. 3, 1846.

21 *Philadelphia Medical and Surgical Journal,* IV (1855), 114–15.

22 Squier Littell, "Memoir of George B. Wood, M.D., LL.D.," 3 *Trans.,* V (1881) xxv–lxxvi; Henry Hartshorne, "Memoir of George B. Wood, M.D., LL.D.," American Philosophical Society, *Proceedings,* XIX (1880–81), 118–52; Cato, "Sketches of Eminent Living Physicians. No. XIII. George B. Wood, M.D. . . . ," *Boston Medical and Surgical Journal,* XLI (1850) 236–40.

23 Wood, Journal, III, Nov. 13, 1836 (CPP).

24 Samuel D. Gross, *Autobiography* (Philadelphia, 1887), II, 393–98.

25 Nicholas B. Wainwright, ed., *A Philadelphia Perspective: The Diary of Sidney George Fisher* (Philadelphia, 1967), 115.

26 Horatio C Wood, "Reminiscences of an American Pioneer in Experimental Medicine," 3 *Trans.,* XLII (1920), 201–02.

27 For a vivid description of Wood's unnerving mode of examining students, see Astley P.C. Ashhurst, "The Life and Character of John Ashhurst, Jr.," 14–15 (A.P.C. Ashhurst Papers, CPP). See also Samuel C. Busey, *Personal Reminscences and Recollections* (Washington, 1895), 31–37.

28 Mitchell, "Commemorative Address," 3 *Trans.,* IX (1887), ccclxii.

29 Ms. Minutes, April 1, 1879.

30 Ms. Minutes, June 7, 1842.

31 Stillé, "Reminiscences of the College of Physicians of Philadelphia," *Trans.,* Centennial Volume (1887), 345.

32 Isaac Parrish, "Biographical Memoir of John C. Otto, M.D.," *Summary,* I (1841–46), 303–18; also, *ibid.,* 226–27, 228–29.

33 Ms. Minutes, Dec. 4, 1838, Sept. 4, 1840.

34 *Ibid.,* Oct. 6, Nov. 3, 1840, Feb. 2, 1841; Report of the Joint Committee, Sept. 21, 1840 (ms., CPP).

35 Subscription List, Aug. 7, 1845 (Ms. Archives, 625); *Summary,* I (1841–46), 321–22.

36 *Ibid.,* 325, 360–61, 373–74.

37 *Ibid.,* II (1846–49), 60.

38 *Trans.,* n.s., I (1851–53), 330–31.

39 *Philadelphia Medical and Surgical Journal,* III (1854–55), 44.

40 Bache to William Hunt, Oct. 16, 1882, Mütter Museum Archives (CPP). Hunt was Bache's successor as curator of the Mütter Museum.

41 *Trans.,* n.s., II (1853–56), 336, 342.

42 *Ibid.*, III (1856–62), 52–53.
43 Ms. Minutes, Sept. 3, Oct. 1, Nov. 5, 1856, Oct. 7, 1857.
44 *Ibid.*, Dec. 1, 1858.
45 *Ibid.*, Nov. 6, Dec. 4, 1849; Wood, Journal, III, Nov. 10, 1849 (CPP).
46 W. S. W. Ruschenberger, "A Memory [sic] of Dr. George Fox," 3 *Trans.*, VII (1884), xlix–lxix.
47 *Ibid.*, lix.
48 Ruschenberger, 143–48. The Articles of Agreement respecting the Mütter gift are printed in CPP, *Charter, Ordinances and By-Laws* (Philadelphia, 1863), 73–78.
49 Joseph Pancoast, *A Discourse commemorative of the late Professor T. D. Mütter, M.D., LL.D.* (Philadelphia, 1859); Samuel D. Gross, *Autobiography* (Philadelphia, 1887), II, 301–06; *A Philadelphia Perspective: The Diary of Sidney George Fisher* (Philadelphia, 1967), 187.
50 *Report of the Building Committee . . . Appointed December 18, 1864* [sic] ([Philadelphia, 1864]); this is a reprint from the minutes. See also Ms. Minutes, Jan. 5, 1859.
51 Committee of Seven, Minutes (CPP). The editorial was in the *North American;* a clipping, with the Committee's minutes, appears to be dated Oct. 25, 1859. A copy of the printed Circular Letter, April 26 (dated April 13), 1859, is in CPP; it was sent Jan. 19, 1860 to members of the Philadelphia Medical Society, apothecaries, and citizens.
52 Wood to Franklin Bache, March 10, 1861, Wood Papers (CPP); Ms. Minutes, April 4, 1860, June 5, July 3, Sept. 4, 1861.
53 Bache to Wood, Sept. 29, 1861, Wood Papers.
54 Packard to Wood, Oct. 6, 1861; Bache to Wood, Nov. 10, 1861, Wood Papers.
55 Bache to Wood, Dec. 23, 1861, Wood Papers.
56 Packard to Wood, Jan. 5, April 8, 1862; Bache to Wood, Dec. 23, 1861, Wood Papers; Ms. Minutes, May 7, 1862.
57 Bache to Wood, April 20, 1862; Packard to Wood, June 30, 1862, Wood Papers.
58 *Report of the Building Committee,* 124.
59 Medical Society of Pennsylvania, *Transactions,* 3rd ser., pt. 3 (1864), 379–99.

## CHAPTER VI

1 Ms. Minutes, Jan. 6, 1864.
2 The history of each of the portraits, busts, and other paintings in CPP is fully presented in Julie S. Berkowitz, *Portrait Catalogue,* published by the College in 1984.

3 CPP, *Charter, Ordinances and By-Laws* (Philadelphia, 1863), 19.

4 Burton Chance, "Squier Littell, M.D.," *Annals of Medical History*, n.s., I (1929), 53. When Jacob Solis-Cohen began to specialize in laryngology, he was looked upon by some members of the profession "as a sort of *charlatanoid,*" and the medical members of the Academy of Natural Sciences blackballed him for membership. Solis-Cohen, "Remarks," Philadelphia County Medical Society, *75th Anniversary* (Philadelphia, [1924]), 13–14.

5 Edward Shippen, "Memoir of John Neill, M.D.," 3 *Trans.*, V (1881), cxlix–cliii.

6 Frank H. Taylor, *Philadelphia in the Civil War, 1861–1865* (Philadelphia, 1913), 231–35.

7 S. Weir Mitchell, "Some Personal Recollections of the Civil War," 3 *Trans.*, XXVIII (1905), 94; Taylor, *Philadelphia in the Civil War*, 230. Mitchell proudly stated that of 176 Fellows in 1864, 130 served in the war; but the figures are too large. The Fellows numbered 155 in 1864, including twenty–four non–residents.

8 Taylor, *Philadelphia in the Civil War*, 224–30; Burton A. Konkle, *Standard History of the Medical Profession of Philadelphia* (Frederick P. Henry, ed., 2nd ed., New York, 1977), 263–71.

9 Mitchell, *In War Time* (Boston, 1885), 43–45.

10 Addinell Hewson, "Pirogoff's Amputation," *Trans.*, n.s., IV (1863–74), 92–100; John Ashhurst, Jr., "Two Cases of Aneurism," *ibid.*, 137–41; Isaac Norris, "Paraplegia without Discoverable Lesion of the Brain or Spinal Cord," *ibid.*, 204–06.

11 Henry Hartshorne, "On Heart Disease in the Army," *ibid.*, 59–63.

12 W. W. Keen, "Surgical Reminiscences of the Civil War," *ibid.*, 3rd ser., XXVII (1905), 107.

13 Keen, "The History of Surgical Advances in the Past Fifty Years," *ibid.*, XLVIII (1926), 356–59.

14 S. Weir Mitchell, "Some Personal Recollections of the Civil War," *ibid.*, XXVII (1905), 87–94; W. W. Keen, "Surgical Reminscences of the Civil War," *ibid.*, 95–114; John Shaw Billings, "Reminiscences of the Civil War," *ibid.*, 115–21; Horatio C Wood, "Reminiscences of an American Pioneer in Experimental Medicine," *ibid.*, XLIII (1920), 203–04. Mitchell used his wartime hospital experience in his first short story, "The Case of George Dedlow," published in the *Atlantic Monthly* in 1866.

15 William M. Taylor, "Some Experiences of a Confederate Assistant Surgeon," 3 *Trans.*, XXVIII (1906), 91–121; Herbert M. Nash, "Some Reminiscences of a Confederate Surgeon," *ibid.*, 122–44.

16 Mitchell, "The Old College and the New," *ibid.*, XXXI (1909), 415; same, "The Hospitals at Gettysburg," *ibid.*, XXXV (1913), xxvii–xxix; Ms. Minutes, Jan. 1, 1913; editorial in (Philadelphia) *Evening Bulletin*, June 28, 1911.

17 W.W. Keen, "On Medical-Missionary Work with some Notes on the Condition of Medicine in Japan," 3 *Trans.*, IV (1879), 13–25.
18 These reports are in *Trans.*, n.s., IV (1863–74), *passim.*
19 Ms. Minutes, June 2, 1875, March 1, 1876, Nov. 5, 1879.
20 *Ibid.*, March 15, 1871.
21 *Ibid.*, Nov. 5, Dec. 3, 1884.
22 E.B. Shapleigh, "Death from Rattlesnake Bite," *Trans.*, n.s., IV (1863–74), 263–64.
23 John Ashhurst, Jr., "Lacerations produced by a Lion: Death in forty-eight hours from Traumatic Gangrene," *ibid.*, 414–15.
24 Ms. Minutes, March 7, May 2, 1883. On May 7, 1884, Leeds read a paper on "Analyses and Composition of Human Milk." On May 6, 1885, Arthur V. Meigs read a "criticism" of Leeds' paper. The paper of Randolph and A. E. Roussel, "The Nutritive Value of Branny Foods," was read June 4, 1884.
25 Ms. Minutes, Oct. 1, Nov. 5, 1873; Jan.2, Nov. 5, 1884.
26 Irving Wallace and Amy Wallace, *The Two* (New York, 1978), the fullest account of the Twins' career; "Editorial: Chang and Eng," *Philadelphia Medical Times*, IV (Feb. 19, 1874), 327–30.
27 John C. Warren, "An Account of the Siamese Twin Brothers united together from their birth," *American Journal of the Medical Sciences*, V (1829), 253–55.
28 ——— Tucker, "Psychological Observations on the Siamese Twins, Chang and Eng, made in 1836," American Philosophical Society, *Proceedings*, II (1841), 22–28.
29 Ms. Minutes, Feb. 9, 1874.
30 *Ibid.*, Feb. 18, 1874.
31 Harrison Allen, "Report on an Autopsy on the Bodies of Chang and Eng Bunker, commonly known as the Siamese Twins," read on April 1, 1874, and William H. Pancoast, "Report on the Surgical Considerations in regard to the Propriety of an Operation for the Separation of Eng and Chang Bunker," read on May 5, 1875, were printed in 3 *Trans.*, I (1875), 3–46 and 149–69 respectively.
32 "The Siamese Twins at the College of Physicians," *Philadelphia Medical Times*, IX (Feb. 19, 1874), 321–26.
33 Ms. Minutes, April 1, Oct. 7, Nov. 4, 1874.
34 *Ibid.*, Dec. 2, 1874.
35 *Boston Medical and Surgical Journal*, XCIII (Nov. 11, 1875), 565–66.
36 Ms. Minutes, June 3, 1868
37 *Medical News*, XLIX (Oct. 9, 1886), 409.
38 Ms. Minutes, Jan. 7, 1874, June 7, 1882.
39 *Ibid.*, April 3, Dec. 4, 1878, March 5, 1879. On Ludlow, see *D.A.B.*
40 James Bryce, *The American Commonwealth* (2d ed., rev., London, 1891), I, 606–07. See also L.T., "The Water Supply of Philadelphia," *Medical Register*, II (Aug. 6, 1887) 139–41.

41 Ms. Minutes, March 3, 1869, May 1, 1872, Dec. 2, 1874, Oct. 2, 1878, April 4, 1888.

42 *Ibid.*, Dec. 7, 1870. June 7, 1871; Council Minutes, March 29, 1871.

43 Ms. Minutes, Nov. 7, 1877, Feb. 6, 1878, May 7, 1879, July 7, 1880; Rough Draft of Records of Monthly Meetings, Box 2, July-Sept. 1880 (CPP).

44 Ms. Minutes, March 1, 1871.

45 *Ibid.*, Feb. 2, April 5, 1876; Wood to John Shaw Billings, [Jan.? 1876], Billings Papers (New York Public Library).

46 Hamilton, "Thoughts upon Vivisection, with reference to its Restriction by Legislative Action," 3 *Trans.*, V (1881), 103–19; John Ashhurst, Jr., "Biographical Notice of George Hamilton, M.D.," *ibid.*, VIII 1886, xlv–liii. Hamilton's house overflowed with more than 14,000 books and several thousand prints.

47 Ms. Minutes, March 7, 1883, Feb. 4, 1885.

48 Mitchell and Wood, [Report to] *The College of Physicians of Philadelphia*, Nov. 1885. (Printed; photocopy in CPP Pam. 3940); Caroline E. White and others, *A Reply to Certain Charges against the Society for the Restriction of Vivisection* . . . [Jan. 1886]. (Printed, in CPP Pam. 7057).

49 Ms. Minutes, Feb. 3, Mar. 3, April 7, 1886.

50 W. S. Forbes, *History, of the Anatomy Act of Pennsylvania* (Philadelphia, 1898); Ms. Minutes, Feb. 6, April 3, 1867, Jan. 3, Feb. 7, 1883.

51 Forbes, *Anatomy Act,* 13. The first edition of this account (Philadelphia, 1867) was dedicated to the officers of the College of Physicians.

52 Addinell Hewson to James C. Wilson, [April 1914], Presidents' Letters (CPP).

53 [Hiram Corson], *A Brief History of Proceedings in the Medical Society of Pennsylvania . . . to procure the Recognition of Women Physicians* . . . (Philadelphia, 1888), 3–20. Gulielma Fell Alsop, *History of the Woman's Medical College, Philadelphia, Pennsylvania, 1850–1950* (Philadelphia, 1950), 60–74, follows Corson closely.

54 Ms. Minutes, March 4, May 6, 1868.

55 Woman's Medical College, *16th Annual Announcement,* 1865–66; *20th Annual Announcement,* 1869–70. The *31st Annual Announcement,* 1880–81, indicates that W.W. Keen, Horatio C Wood, and Edward T. Bruen, all Fellows of the College, were on the faculty, as were J. Gibbons Hunt and James B. Walker, who were elected Fellows in 1884 and 1885 respectively.

56 Ms. Minutes, July 5, 1871; J. William White, "Memoir of D. Hayes Agnew, M.D., LL.D.," 3 *Trans.,* XV 1893, lvii. White, too, was no friend to women's medical education. Agnes Repplier, *J. William White, M.D.: A Biography* (Boston, 1919), 40–41.

57 *Medical Register,* V (Aug. 18, 1888), 166; *History of the Medical Society of the District of Columbia, 1817–1909* (Washington, 1909), 119–21. The Medical Society of Delaware elected a woman in 1880. *One Hundred and Fiftieth Annual Session of the Medical Society of Delaware, 1789–1939* (Wilmington, 1939), 69. On the effort to admit women into the Massachusetts Medical Society, 1869–84, see Walter L. Burrage, *A History of the Massachusetts Medical Society* ([Boston], 1923), 143–49.

58 Burton A. Konkle, *Standard History of the Medical Profession of Philadelphia* (Frederick P. Henry, ed., 2d ed., New York, 1977), 307–12.

59 Ms. Minutes, March 31, April 7, 1875.

60 The transactions of the Congress, edited by John Ashhurst, Jr., in a stout volume of 1,153 pages, were published the next year. In addition to reports on recent advances in medicine, surgery, and their allied sciences, there were papers, appropriate to the occasion, on the history and accomplishments of medicine in the United States in the preceding century.

61 Keen, "History of Surgical Advances," *loc. cit.,* 356–59.

62 J. Ewing Mears, "Case of Lacerated Wound of the Elbow-Joint, treated successfully by the Antiseptic Method of Professor Lister," 3 *Trans.,* III (1877), 11–15.

63 William J. Taylor, "Address . . . at the Fiftieth Anniversary of . . . the Directory for Nurses," May 14, 1932. Original Documents relating to the establishment of the Nurses' Directory (CPP).

64 Ashhurst's reluctance to adopt antiseptic practices was not the result of ignorance or stubborn pride. A younger colleague, Henry W. Cattell, explained: "the results from his operations—the best of any obtained in the early sixties, owing to careful nursing and the external use of reagents, which were really antiseptics—so far surpassed those of other surgeons that he did not see the need of changing his plan of procedure. Other operators reduced their mortality rates by antisepsis, but even then their results were but slightly better than his." *Public Ledger,* July 9, 1900.

## CHAPTER VII

1 Ella N. Wade, "Letters from Professor Hyrtl Found in a Mütter Museum Scrapbook," 4 *T & S.,* XII (1944–45), 115–18.

2 Bache to William Hunt, Jan. 11, Aug. 18, Sept. 29, 1882. Mütter Museum, Box 1, Letters concerning Purchases (CPP).

3 The terms of the lectureship were changed again in 1901 to provide

for a single lecture annually. "By this means only they [the Mütter Museum Committee] believe that it will be possible to secure a distinguished lecturer and a good audience and thus contribute to the reputation of the College" and the furtherance of Dr. Mütter's intentions. Ms. Minutes, April 3, 1901. The first lecturer in this series was Harvey Cushing of Johns Hopkins. Cushing described his visit to Philadelphia for the lecture in a letter to his father quoted in Fulton, *Cushing,* 211–12.

4 "Remarks Commemorative of Samuel Lewis, M.D.," 3 *Trans.,* XIX (1890), xci–ciii.

5 *Ibid.,* xcix.

6 Ms. Minutes, Jan. 3, 1866.

7 Carson to S. W. Butler, Jan. 27, 1869. Toner Collection, LXXI (Library of Congress).

8 Library Committee, Minutes, Oct. 31, 1884 (CPP).

9 *Ibid.,* Feb. 2, 1885.

10 Frederick Fraley, "History of the Directory for Nurses of the College of Physicians," 4 *Trans.,* IV (1936), xi–xvi.

11 Chadwick to Mitchell, Jan. 22, 1882. "Original Documents relating to the Establishment of the Nurses Directory," (CPP).

12 Keen to Frederick Fraley, April 29, 1932, "Original Documents."

13 A copy of the invoice used by the Directory is in "Original Documents."

14 Committee on the Directory, "To the Fellows of the College of Physicians of Philadelphia," [1890]. Printed handbill, "Original Documents;" D. Hayes Agnew, "Annual Address," 3 *Trans.,* XI (1889), xxx; Arthur V. Meigs, "Annual Address," *ibid.,* XXVII (1905), 2; Council Minutes, Dec. 29, 1896.

15 Philip Van Ingen, *New York Academy of Medicine: Its First Hundred Years* (New York, 1949), 240–41, 296, 302–03; Eugene F. Cordell, *Medical Annals of Maryland, 1799–1899* (Baltimore, 1903), 177, 185, 190–91, 201–02, 259.

16 Council Minutes, Oct. 30, 1900.

17 Ms. Minutes, Jan. 6, 1875; Committee on Hall, Report, 1875.

18 Bache to William Hunt, Oct. 16, 1882. Mütter Museum, Box 1, Letters concerning Purchases (CPP).

19 Ms. Minutes, Feb. 7, March 7, June 6, 1883, Feb. 6, April 2, 1874; Council Minutes, April 3, 1885; Ruschenberger, 149–52. The Mütter Museum income continued to exceed the museum's needs, and as the court had allowed the trustees to contribute $5,000 toward enlargement of the hall, Da Costa raised the question in 1885 whether some of the accumulating surplus might not be applied at some future time to a laboratory of histology and pathological research. "Surely the good which would come would be far greater than from the accumu-

lation of specimens and models . . . ." "Address," 3 *Trans.*, VIII (1886), lvii.

20 Council Minutes, May 24, 1887.

21 Ms. Minutes, March 4, April 1, 8, June 3, 1885.

22 *Ibid.*, June 6, 1888.

23 *Ibid.*, Oct. 7, Dec. 2, 1885, Jan. 6, 1886, April 6, Dec. 7, 1887, Dec. 3, 1890; Committee on Hall, Report, 1896 (CPP).

24 S. Weir Mitchell, "Commemorative Address," 3 *Trans.*, IX (1887), ccclxiii–ccclxiv.

25 Harvey Cushing, *Life of Sir William Osler* (New York, 1940), 239, 277, 1028, 1083, 1279, 1369.

26 See, for example, Ms. Minutes, April 6, 1887, March 7, May 2, 1888. 3 *Trans.*, X (1888), 277.

27 Ms. Minutes, March 1, 1893.

28 *Ibid.*, Feb. 2, 23, 1915.

29 3 *Trans.*, XLII (1920), 118–54.

30 Ms. Minutes, April 2, 1929.

31 John Ashhurst, Jr., "W. S. W. Ruschenberger, M.D.," 3 *Trans.*, XVIII (1896), xxxv–xli.

32 William Osler, "Memoir of Alfred Stillé, M.D.," 3 *Trans.*, XXIV (1902), lviii–lxxi; reprinted in Osler's *An Alabama Student.*

33 Alfred Stillé, "Address delivered at the Close of his Term of Office," *ibid.*, VII (1884), cxxiii–cxxxix.

34 James C. Wilson, "Memoir of J. M. Da Costa, M.D.," *ibid.*, XXIV (1902), lxxxi–xcii.

35 Da Costa, "Address delivered at the Close of his First Term of Office," *ibid.*, VIII (1886), lviii–lix.

## CHAPTER VIII

1 On Mitchell generally see Ernest Earnest, *S. Weir Mitchell: Novelist and Physician* (Philadelphia, 1950); Anna Robson Burr, *Weir Mitchell: His Life and Letters* (New York, 1929); Charles W. Burr, "S. Weir Mitchell: Physician, Man of Science, Man of Letters, Man of Affairs," 3 *Trans.*, XLI (1919), 227–49; and *S. Weir Mitchell, M.D., LL.D., F.R.S. 1829–1914: Memorial Addresses and Resolutions* (Philadelphia, 1914). Osler's recollections and estimate are in *British Medical Journal*, 1914, I, 120–21. I have been unable to find Mitchell's diary, letters, and other papers, which were in possession of the Mitchell family when Professor Earnest used them.

2 Mitchell, *A Catalogue of the Scientific and Literary Work* ([Philadelphia, 1894]).

3 John F. Fulton, *Harvey Cushing: A Biography* (Springfield, Ill., 1946), 226–27.

4 CPP, Centennial Celebration: Ms. Records, 1887; Committee of Arrangements of the Centennial Celebration, Report, Feb. 2, 1887 (CPP, 10c/12); *Trans., Centennial Volume* (1887), *passim.*

5 Ms. Minutes, Oct. 1, 1884.

6 *Ibid.,* June 2, Sept. 1, 1886; CPP, "At a meeting held June 2d . . . Argument" (printed leaflet, 1886).

7 Ruschenberger, *An Account of the Institution and Progress of the College of Physicians of Philadelphia during a Hundred Years, from January, 1787* (Philadelphia, 1887).

8 Gross to Billings, Dec. 12, 1886, Billings Papers (New York Public Library).

9 Ms. Minutes, Jan. 5, 1887.

10 *Medical News,* L (Jan. 8, 1887), 43. The *News* printed Mitchell's "Commemorative Address" in this number.

11 *Ibid.,* (Jan. 22, 1887), 110.

12 Committee to Address Select and Common Councils with regard to the Threatened Invasion of Cholera, Report, 1885 (Ms., CPP Archives). See also Shakespeare's discussion of a paper by Ezra M. Hunt of Trenton, N.J., on "Local and National Preventive Measures against Cholera," May 25, 1885, in Phila. Co. Medical Society, *Proc.,* VII (1884–85), 323.

13 Ms. Minutes, Feb. 4, 1885.

14 *Ibid.,* Nov. 18, 1886; *Medical News,* XLI (Oct. 9, 1886), 407; Shakespeare, *Report on Cholera in Europe and India* (Washington, 1890); Mitchell, "Annual Address," Dec. 3, 1887, 3 *Trans.,* X (1888), lxvii–lxx.

15 Committee . . . to Investigate the Efficiency of our Quarantine Arrangements for the Exclusion of Cholera and other Epidemic Diseases, "Report," Oct. 28, 1887, *ibid.,* 23–45; Ms. Minutes, Oct. 5, 1887.

16 "Address . . . to the Medical Societies of the United States concerning the Dangers to which the Country is Exposed by the Ineffectual Methods of Quarantine at its Ports, and in regard to the Necessity of National Control of Maritime Quarantine," Dec. 14, 1887, *ibid.,* 1–22. Shakespeare continued to urge a national system of quarantine. "The National Government should have Supreme Control of Quarantine on all Frontiers," reprint from *Medical News,* Sept. 10, 1892; Mitchell, "Annual Address," 3 *Trans.,* X (1888), lxvii–lxx.

17 Ms. Minutes, Jan. 4, 1893; Standing Committee on Cholera, Report, Dec. 6, 1893, including printed Circulars, Nos. 1–3 (CPP Archives).

18 James T. Whittaker, "The Bacillus Tuberculosis," 3 *Trans.,* VI (1883), 149–62; Russell M. Maulitz, "Robert Koch and American Medicine," *Annals of Internal Medicine,* XCVII (1982), 761–66.

19 Gross to Billings, [Dec. 12, 1886], Billings Papers (New York Public Library).

20 Ms. Minutes, June 2, 1886.

21 William H. Webb, "Facts serving to prove the Contagiousness of Tuberculosis; with Results of Experiments with Germ Traps used in detecting Tubercle-Bacilli in the Air of Places of Public Resort, and a Description of the Apparatus," 3 *Trans.*, VIII (1886), 71–102.

22 Arthur V. Meigs, "The Contagiousness of Consumption of the Lungs," *ibid.*, XXXIII (1911), 111–19.

23 Edward B. Meigs, "Memoir of Arthur Vincent Meigs, M.D.," *ibid.*, XXXVI (1914), lxxxiii–xciii.

24 Lawrence F. Flick, "Special Hospitals for the Treatment of Tuberculosis," *ibid.*, XII (1890), 39–86.

25 Joseph Walsh, "Memoir of Lawrence F. Flick, M.D.," 4 *T. & S.*, VII (1939–40), 114–19; J. Woodrow Savacool, "Philadelphia and the White Plague," 5 *T. & S.*, VIII (1986), 147–81.

26 Ms. Minutes, Dec. 6, 1893; Council Minutes, Dec. 26, 1893.

27 "Discussion of the Advisability of the Registration of Tuberculosis," 3 *Trans.*, XVI (1894), 1–27. See C.-E. A. Winslow, *The Life of Hermann M. Biggs, M.D., D.Sc., LL.D.* (Philadelphia, 1929), 138–39.

28 Dulles re-asserted the judgment of the majority three years later in a paper entitled "Consumption not Contagious," *ibid.*, XIX (1897), 178–90.

29 Ms. Minutes, Feb. 3, 1915.

30 W. W. Keen, "On Medical Missionary Work. . .," *ibid.*, IV (1879), 13–25; Robert P. Harris, "Foot-Binding in China," *ibid.*, V (1881), 1–17; H. W. Boone, "Medical Matters in China," *ibid.*, X (1888), 69–75; "Leprosy," *ibid.*, XVI (1894), 127–33; Ms. Minutes, Dec. 6, 1899.

31 S.W. Mitchell, "Remarks in regard to Dr. Finlay's Researches with reference to the Bacillus of Yellow Fever," *ibid.*, X (1888), 65–68.

32 Ms. Minutes, Jan. 7, 1903.

33 Reginald H. Fitz, "Perforating Inflammation of the Vermiform Appendix: with Special Reference to its Early Diagnosis and Treatment," *Trans.* Association of American Physicians, I (1886), 107–35; J. Vernon Ellson, "The History of Appendicitis," 3 *Trans.*, XLVII (1925), 557–58; Frank Woodbury, "Cases of Exploratory Laparatomy followed by Appropriate Remedial Operation," *ibid.*, IX (1887), 183–93.

34 John B. Deaver, "Report of 460 Cases of Appendicitis operated upon at the German Hospital in Two Years ending January 1, 1899," 3 *Trans.*, XXI (1899), 138–62. Deaver made the operation "fashionable and a source of revenue." E. E. Montgomery, "Fifty Years in the Practice of Medicine," *ibid.*, XLVII (1925), 109.

35 Francis R. Packard, "The College of Physicians of Philadelphia from its Centennial in 1887 to 1925," 4 *Trans.*, IV, Suppl. (1937), 104.

36 Otto Glasser, *Wilhelm Conrad Röntgen and the Early History of*

*Röntgen Rays* (Springfield, Ill., 1934), 422–79; *Journal of the Franklin Institute,* CXLI (1896), 183–91.

37 W. W. Keen, "The Surgical Treatment of Intracranial Tumors," 3 *Trans.,* XVIII (1896), 56–66. Other papers were by William F. Norris, Charles K. Mills, George E. de Schweinitz, and Charles H. Burnett. On Houston and Kennelly, see *D.A.B.* and *Who Was Who in America* respectively.

38 Arthur W. Goodspeed, "Experiments on the Roentgen Rays," *Science,* III (Feb. 14, 1896), 237; "The Roentgen Phenomenon: A Few Early Results obtained at the University of Pennsylvania," *ibid.* (March 13, 1896), 394; *Medical News,* LXVIII (1896), 7.

39 *Journal of the Franklin Institute,* CXLI (1896), 247–78; American Philosophical Society, *Proceedings,* XXXV (1896), 12, 17–36.

40 3 *Trans.,* XVIII (1896), 97–117.

41 Robert G. Le Conte, "Case of Bullet Imbedded in the Tissues of the Neck, located by Skiagraphy," *ibid.,* 197–98. The term "skiagraphy" was proposed by Henry W. Cattell, demonstrator of morbid anatomy in the University of Pennsylvania and a Fellow of the College.

42 John B. Deaver, "X-Ray Pathology of Fractures about the Elbow, 3 *Trans.,* XIX (1897), 213–17.

43 Charles L. Leonard, "The Röntgen Ray Diagnosis of Renal Calculus," *ibid.,* XXI (1899), 50–63.

44 W. B. McDaniel, 2d, "Recognition of the Specialties in the 'Organic Law' of the College of Physicians," read to the Section on Ophthalmology, 1943, an unpublished paper in CPP, surveys the subject.

45 Philip Van Ingen, *New York Academy of Medicine,* 69.

46 Burton Chance, "Edward Jackson—A Founder of the Section on Ophthalmology of the College of Physicians of Philadelphia," 4 *T. & S.,* XI (1943–44), 32–35. A Chester county Quaker and graduate of the University of Pennsylvania, 1878, Jackson eventually left Philadelphia for Colorado, where he was professor of ophthalmology in the university of that state, 1898–1921.

47 Ms. Minutes, Nov. 5, 1890, Dec. 2, 29, 1891, Jan. 26, 1892.

48 Burton Chance, "Ophthalmology in Philadelphia in the Early Eighteen Nineties," 4 *T. & S.,* XI (1943–44), 77–81; George B. Wood, "The First Fifty Years of the Section on Otolaryngology of the College of Physicians of Philadelphia," *ibid.,* 123–27; A. D. Hall, "Memoir of Squier Littell, M.D.," 3 *Trans.,* IX (1887), cdlv; Mitchell, "Annual Address," *ibid.,* XVI (1894), xxxix–xliii. See the editorial lamenting "the tendency to depreciate the work of the general practitioner as compared with the work of the specialist and professor, the clinical teacher and consultant, the pure physician and the pure surgeon," in *Medical Register,* II (Aug. 13, 1887), 160.

49 Ms. Minutes, Nov. 2, 29, Dec. 7, 1892, Jan. 4, Feb. 21, April 5, 1893.

50 Da Costa, "Annual Address," 3 *Trans.,* XIX (1897), lxxxix–xcv.

51 Da Costa, "Annual Address," *ibid.,* XVII (1895), xlvii–lii; "Annual Address," *ibid.,* XVIII (1896), lix–lx.

52 Ms. Minutes, April 1, Nov. 4, 1896.

53 Francis R. Packard, "The President's Address," 3 *Trans.,* LIV (1932), 5.

54 Kelly records an episode related to him by Dr. Charles H. Mayo, who witnessed it, that throws an unkind light on Price's personality. Because it happened in the College of Physicians (although I have not been able to confirm it), it should be recorded here.

"While Price and his associates in Philadelphia were zealously saving lives by their brilliant operations, a competitor was vaunting his simpler, safer cures of the same conditions by the Apostoli electric treatment. Price soon 'camped on his trail,' as he would express it, and closely followed the work of this man over a series of months. The electro-therapeutist finally announced a paper on his methods before the College of Physicians of Philadelphia. Price significantly asked Dr. Mayo, then visiting him, to be present, as the meeting 'was likely to be interesting.' Before the hour a dray drove up to the hall and a great number of jars containing big and little tumors and specimens were unloaded and deposited on a long table in front of the speaker's desk. Then followed Price, who took a little pad out of his pocket and busied himself writing slips and attaching them to the jars. The electro-therapeutist read his paper and cited the numerous patients cured by his conservative methods. Whenever the initials were given, Price put additional notes on the slips on the jars. The denouement came when the subject was thrown open for discussion. Price arose, one by one named the cases cured and then exhibited the morbid specimens he had afterwards removed from the patients; a big fibroid cut open to show the streaks of the intense cauterization, and the fact that the growth was uninfluenced; in another case he demonstrated that the needles had penetrated the uterine wall at a point remote from the growth; another patient had acquired 'a vicious intestinal adhesion,' jeopardizing the operation. The tubes of a 'cured' pelvic inflammatory mass were picked up and incised and the pus flowed out. The effect was so crushing that the adversary had the pity of the hearers, but his therapeutic procedures were entirely discredited and electrotherapy received its death blow." K & B, 994.

55 "Proceedings against Fellows," Censors' Papers, Box 1 (CPP); A.P.C. Ashhurst, Scrapbook, 33, 79–82 (CPP); Ms. Minutes, June 3, 17, Sept. 2, Oct. 7, Nov. 4, 1891.

56 Edward Martin, "Memoir of Charles B. Penrose, M.D.," 3 *Trans.,* XLVII (1925), lxv–lxxiii.

57 Ms. Minutes, Dec. 2, 1891.

58 Samuel D. Gross, *Autobiography* (2 v., Philadelphia, 1887), I, 40–42, II, 249–50; George Bacon Wood, Journal, III (1836–49) (Ms., CPP); Samuel X Radbill, ed., *Autobiographical Ana of Robley Dunglison, M.D.* (American Philosophical Society, *Trans.*, n.s., LIII, pt. 8 (1963), 84–86.

59 *S. Weir Mitchell, M.D., LL.D., F.R.S., 1829–1914* (Philadelphia, 1914), 26; Mitchell, [Address at the first dinner in the New Building, 1910], Collection of Miscellaneous Brief Manuscripts and Letters, Envelope 10 (CPP).

60 Ruschenberger, 171; Ms. Minutes, Nov. 7, 1877, Jan. 2, 1878, Feb. 7, 1883; John Ashhurst, Jr., "The Surgeon," *Trans., Centennial Volume* (1887), 370. Harvey Cushing attended one of these entertainments in 1903. "Curious performance," he wrote his father. "Does it not strike you so? To have a large banquet once in two–three years. I think Dr. Mitchell gave the original sum whose interest was to be so expended. Object: promotion of good feeling between the members of the College—in the two schools, I presume. Very nice to be invited however . . . . There was much speechifying.—Dr. H. C. Wood—good as usual. Made a strong plea for funds to make up $50,000 for a new building (fire proof) to provide for the growing needs of the library. Some one [Andrew Carnegie] has anon. given $50,000 provided an equal amount is raised . . . . Much tobacco, wine and eats." Fulton, *Cushing,* 228.

61 Mitchell, [Address. . .].

62 (Philadelphia) *Daily Press,* Dec. 18, 1894; "Proceedings against Fellows," Censors' Papers, Box 1 (CPP); Ms. Minutes, Jan. 2, Feb. 6, 1895.

## CHAPTER IX

1 Ms. Minutes, March 9, 1886, Jan. 4, 1893, June 14, 1899, Jan. 7, 1903, Jan. 6, 1909.

2 Arthur V. Meigs, "Annual Address," 3 *Trans.,* XXIX (1907), 2; James Tyson, "Annual Address," *ibid.,* XXX (1908), 5.

3 Council Minutes, Jan. 28, 1902.

4 *Ibid.,* Oct. 24, 1905; March 27, 1906.

5 *Ibid.,* Feb. 25, 1908; Tyson, "Annual Address," 3 *Trans.,* XXX (1908), 5.

6 This aversion to publicity was sometimes carried to absurd lengths. The College refused in 1896 to give the American Medical Association a list of its members, which was wanted in connection with a forth-

coming meeting of the Association in Philadelphia. (The A.M.A. could have found the names and addresses of the Fellows in alphabetical order in the latest volume of *Transactions.*) In 1902 a request from a member of the staff of the Long Island State Hospital in Brooklyn, N.Y., for a copy of the College charter and by-laws involved the thirty-nine Fellows present at the meeting in a series of motions, questions, and discussions (that the request be referred to the Council, that the secretary be instructed to ask why the pamphlet was wanted) before the secretary was directed to mail a copy—which was the burden of the first reaction.

7 Ms. Minutes, Jan. 5, 1898.

8 Council Minutes, April 23, 1907.

9 Ms. Minutes, Feb. 5, 1896.

10 Council Minutes, Feb. 27, 1906.

11 Ms. Minutes, Feb. 6, 1901.

12 *Ibid.,* Oct. 7, 1903; Council Minutes, Dec. 27, 1887, Sept. 25, 1894.

13 J. William White, "Memoir of D. Hayes Agnew, M.D., LL.D.," 3 *Trans.,* XV (1893), xxxiii; Mitchell to George E. de Schweinitz, June 1 [1910], Presidents' Letters; E. B. Krumbhaar, "President's Address," 4 *T. & S.,* X (1942–43), 204.

14 John P. Haines (president, American Society for the Prevention of Cruelty to Animals) to W. W. Keen, July 18, 1893; Keen to Haines, July 20, 1893 (copy); Francis H. Rowley (secretary, American Humane Society, Fall River, Mass.) to Keen, Feb. 20, 1900. Keen Correspondence, Box 2 (CPP).

15 Keen, "Misstatements of Antivivisectionists: Correspondence with American Humane Association," *JAMA,* Feb. 23, 1901.

16 Ms. Minutes, Feb. 7, 1900.

17 Morris Fishbein, *A History of the American Medical Association 1847 to 1947* (Philadelphia, [1947]), 183–84; Jonathan D. Wirtschafter, "The Genesis and Impact of the Medical Lobby: 1898–1906," *Journal of the History of Medicine,* XIII (1958), 17–21.

18 Keen to S. N. Cleghorn, Dec. 18, 1902, Keen Correspondence, Box 1 (CPP).

19 Ms. Minutes, Feb. 3, 1909, April 2, May 7, 1913; James C. Wilson to William L. Rodman, April 7, 1913; Wilson to Wilmer Krusen, April 7, 1913, Presidents' Letters (CPP).

20 William Pepper to James C. Wilson, Oct. 2, 1914, Presidents' Letters (CPP); Ms. Minutes, Nov. 4, 1914, Feb. 3, March 3, 1915. The Council referred the Society's request to the College. The College returned it to the Council "for final action." The Council then appointed a committee with instructions to report back to it. The Committee recommended against the appropriation. Council Minutes, Oct. 27, Nov. 24, 1914, Jan. 26, 1915.

21 Vaughan, "Modern Military Hygiene and Camp Sanitation," 3 *Trans.*, XXXVII (1915), 188–200.

22 Ms. Minutes, June 5, 1918.

23 *Ibid.*, Dec. 6, 1922; Council Minutes, Nov. 28, 1922.

24 *Ibid.*, Oct. 25, 1921; Ms. Minutes, Nov. 2, 1921.

25 Harvey Cushing, *Life of Sir William Osler* (New York, 1940), 239, 343–44.

26 3 *Trans.*, X (1888), lxxii–lxxiii.

27 Mitchell to Billings, Feb. 3, 1886, Billings Papers (New York Public Library).

28 "The President's Address," 3 *Trans.*, XIV (1892), xxix–xxxii.

29 Ms. Minutes, Dec. 2, 1896.

30 J. M. DaCosta, "Annual Address," 3 *Trans.*, XVII (1895), l.

31 Committee on Mütter Museum, Report, 1893 (CPP). The history of the museum may be traced in the Committee's annual reports and in the lists of acquisitions in each volume of the *Transactions.*

32 Ms. Minutes, Dec. 5, 1900.

33 *Ibid.*, Jan. 2, March 6, April 3, May 1, 1901. Jan. 1, 1902.

34 Ms. Minutes, March 4, 1903.

35 [Horatio C Wood], *Report . . . upon Rebuilding,* Feb. 24, 1903; Ms. Minutes, April 1, 1903.

36 Francis R. Packard, "The College of Physicians from . . . 1887 to 1925," 4 *Trans.*, IV, Suppl. (1937), 103.

37 At the announcement to the College of Meigs' death, Mitchell paid tribute to "the perfect courtesy" with which he had presided "during the long period of grave differences of opinion." Ms. Minutes, Jan. 3, 1912; Arthur V. Meigs, "Annual Address," 3 *Trans.*, XXVIII (1906), 5–7; same, "Annual Address," *ibid.*, XXIX (1907), 2–3, Edward B. Meigs, "Memoir of Arthur Vincent Meigs, M.D.," *ibid.*, XXXVI (1914), lxxxvii.

38 Meigs, "Annual Address," *ibid.*, XXVII (1905), 1–7; Charles W. Burr, "S. Weir Mitchell. . .," *ibid.*, XLI (1919), 241.

39 Ms. Minutes, April 1, 1903.

40 *Ibid.*, May 6, 1903.

41 *Ibid.*, May 29, 1903.

42 H. C. Wood, "Annual Address," 3 *Trans.*, XXVI (1904), 5.

43 *Public Ledger,* Aug. 27, 28, 1903.

44 Ernest Earnest, *S. Weir Mitchell, Novelist and Physician* (Philadelphia, 1950), 198.

45 Ms. Minutes, Nov. 2, Dec. 7, 13, 1904.

46 *Ibid.*, Feb. 1, April 5, 1905, May 2, 1906; J. William White and others, [Printed address to] Dear Doctor, Jan. 20, 1905 (CPP).

47 Reviewing these events a few years later, Mitchell observed, "It was well for us that there were some people in the College who were resolute, kept their heads, and saw straight. Surely no more extraordi-

nary example of the difficulty of handling a body of men could be shown . . . ." Mitchell to George E. de Schweinitz, Dec. 9, 1911, Presidents' Letters (CPP).

48 Ms. Minutes, Feb. 6, March 6, 1907.

49 *Ibid.*, May 1, 1907.

50 *Ibid.*, Jan. 1, March 4, 1908, Jan. 6, 1909; Mitchell to William Osler, [Jan. 1909], Cushing Papers, Weir Mitchell Corres. (Yale University School of Medicine).

51 Council Minutes, Dec. 23, 1907.

52 "Exercises on the Occasion of the Dedication of the New Hall . . . ," 3 *Trans.*, XXXI 1909, 327–455; "Papers etc. relating to the laying of the Cornerstone and Dedication of the New Building," 1908–09 (CPP).

53 According to the Philadelphia *Public Ledger,* whose report of the opening of the Hall was on the front page, Nov. 11, 1909, Carnegie's remarks were greeted with "cheers . . . wilder than before. Napkins were thrown in the air, men leaped to their feet and women leaned over the edge of the balcony."

54 The names chosen for the frieze in the Ashhurst reading room were: Hippocrates, Galen, Avicenna, Paré, Vesalius, Harvey, Sydenham, John Hunter, Rush, Jenner, Laennec, Claude-Bernard, Virchow, and Leidy.

55 Mitchell, "Address of Welcome," 3 *Trans.*, XXXI (1909), 443–49.

56 Earnest, *S. Weir Mitchell,* 198; E. T. Stotesbury, [Pledge], Jan. 28, 1910, Presidents' Letters (CPP); James C. Wilson, "Annual Address," 3 *Trans.*, XXXVII (1915), 8.

57 Ms. Minutes, Oct. 7, 1903; Council Minutes, Dec. 23, 1907.

58 *Ibid.*, Jan. 25, 1910, April 24, 1923, Nov. 25, 1925, Nov. 23, 1926, Dec. 27, 1927; Ms. Minutes, Oct. 1, 1924.

59 *Ibid.*, May 6, 1929, May 12, 1930.

60 Finance Committee, "Annual Report for 1938," (CPP).

61 Council Minutes, Feb. 26, Nov. 26, 1946; J. Parsons Schaeffer, "Annual Address," 4 *T. & S.*, XVI (1948–49), 149; George P. Muller, "Annual Address," 4 *Trans.*, V (1937), 5–12.

62 3 *Trans.*, XXXIII (1911), lxxxv–xc.

63 Ms. Minutes, Jan. 5, April 6, Oct. 5, 1910.

64 Mitchell to William Osler, Aug. 14, 1913. Cushing Papers, Weir Mitchell Corres.

65 Charles P. Fisher to George E. de Schweinitz, Oct. 4, 1910; Presidents' Letters (CPP); Ms. Minutes, Nov. 2, Dec. 7, 1910, Feb. 3, April 7, 1915; Council Minutes, Oct. 25, 1910; Committee on the Wearing of Gowns by the Officers at Meetings, Report, Dec. 7, 1910 (CPP); Hobart A. Hare, "Some Suggestions to the Fellows. . .," 3 *Trans.*, XLVII (1925), 13; de Schweinitz to Wilson, Feb. 25, 1916, Presidents' Letters.

66 Council Minutes, Oct. 25, 1910, Dec. 28, 1943; 3 *Trans.*, XLVI (1924), 131–32; *The Custodianship of Rush-Jenner-Pasteur-Lister-Curie Mementos . . . held in Succession by Representative Members of the Medical Profession in the United States* ([Philadelphia, 1923?]).

67 Alfred Stengel to de Schweinitz, April 18, 1910; de Schweinitz to Stengel, April 27, 1910, Presidents' Letters.

68 Richard M. Pearce to de Schweinitz, April 25, [1910], Presidents' Letters.

69 Same to same, April 27, 1910, Presidents' Letters.

70 De Schweinitz to Pearce, April 26, 1910, Presidents' Letters.

71 De Schweinitz to Osler, Jan. 19, 1911, Presidents' Letters.

72 For an appreciation by a distinguished modern architect of the design, construction, materials, and decoration of this splendid, serviceable, and innovative building, see Vincent G. Kling, "Architectural Concepts in 1909 and their Influence on the College Building," 5 *T. & S.*, VIII (1986), 75–87.

73 James Tyson, "Annual Address," 3 *Trans.*, XXXII (1910), 6–7. This echoed a recommendation Mitchell made (but may not have spoken) in an address at the first dinner held in "the New Building": "There ought to be given to us a great endowment by some man in Philadelphia, and it should be independent of the colleges, not asking research work iron men worn out by teaching. It should be called the 'Laboratory of Research' of this College, and should carry on just such work as has been done in New York at the Rockefeller Institute . . . . " Collection of Miscellaneous Brief Manuscripts and Letters, envelope 10 (CPP).

74 Council Minutes, May 26, 1908, March 1, 1910. Mitchell, de Schweinitz, Richard H. Harte, and Wharton Sinkler offered to pay half the purchase price (not exceeding $25,000) if the Swedenborgian Church would purchase the lot.

75 De Schweinitz, "Annual Address," 3 *Trans.*, XXXIV 1912, 11–12; Ms. Minutes, April 6, May 13, June 1, 1910, March 1, Oct. 11, 1911, Jan. 3, 1912.

76 Mitchell to de Schweinitz, Dec. 26, 1911, Presidents' Letters.

77 Same to same, March 7, 1910, Presidents' Letters.

78 Ms. Minutes, Feb. 1, 1882.

79 Da Costa, "Address," Feb. 4, 1885, 3 *Trans.*, VIII (1886), lv–lx.

80 Ms. Minutes, April 8, 1885.

81 *Ibid.*, March 3, 1897; 3 *Trans.*, XIX (1897), 46ff.

82 Council Minutes, Dec. 30, 1885, Jan. 26, 1886.

83 Agnew, "The President's Annual Address," 3 *Trans.*, XIII (1891), xxx–xxxi.

84 Mitchell, "Annual Address," *ibid.*, XV (1893) lxxviii–lxxix.
85 Ms. Minutes, Jan. 2, 1901.
86 Tyson, "Annual Address," 3 *Trans.*, XXXII (1910), 3–4.

## CHAPTER X

1 De Schweinitz, "Annual Address," 3 *Trans.*, XXV (1913), 1–21.
2 Ms. Minutes, Dec. 1, 1911.
3 John T. Carpenter, "Memoir of G. E. de Schweinitz, M.D.," 4 *T. & S.*, VI (1938–39), 344–51; Roberts to de Schweinitz, "Saturday evening" [1911], Presidents' Letters. From Oxford Sir William Osler sent a congratulatory note: "What a change in 25 years!" Osler to de Schweinitz, Jan. 30, 1911, *ibid.* Other Fellows donated silver and glass to the dining room. Hobart A. Hare bequeathed a silver salver given to him by the Nizam of Hyderabad.
4 *Ibid.*, Jan. 6, Oct.26, 1915.
5 Council Minutes, March 27, 1917; Richard H. Harte, "Annual Address," 3 *Trans.*, XXXIX (1917), 14. In 1919 the Finance Committee moved acceptance of a budget although it had not reported what income was expected from the general account. John B. Roberts protested, but the Committee's recommendation prevailed. Ms. Minutes, Jan. 1, 1919.
6 *Public Ledger*, Dec. 16, 1913; Joseph Sailer to James C. Wilson, April 29, 1913; Joseph Leidy to de Schweinitz, [Dec. 1913], Presidents' Letters; Council Minutes, Dec. 30, 1913.
7 De Schweinitz to A. J. O. Kelly, Dec. 14, 1910; Kelly to de Schweinitz, Dec. 15, 19, 1910, Presidents' Letters.
8 Alfred Gordon, "Mendelian Laws of Heredity and Their Application to Eugenics," 3 *Trans.*, XXXVII (1915), 31–36. Gordon was a neurologist on the staff of several Philadelphia hospitals.
9 William H. Arthur, "The Advantages of Military Training for Young Men and the Physical Cultural Value of the Preparedness Movement," Robert T. Morris, "Individualism and Decadence," 3 *Trans.*, XXXVIII (1916), 195–205, 206–210. Dr. Morris thought individualism a "most dangerous trait" and characterized the United States as "a big, helpless, fat, juicy rabbit waiting to be taken. We are too fat to fight." This was before the battles of the Argonne, Château-Thierry, and Belleau Wood.
10 Council Minutes, Feb. 27, 1917.
11 [Francis R. Packard], *History of the Pennsylvania Hospital Unit (Base*

*Hospital No. 10, U.S.A.) in the Great War* (New York, 1921); William J. Taylor, "Annual Address," 3 *Trans.*, XLII (1920), 1.

12 Donald Bateman, *Berkeley Moynihan, Surgeon* (New York, 1940), 217, 220; Council Minutes, Oct. 3, Nov. 17, Dec. 5, 1917.

13 George W. Norris, "Some Medical Impressions of the War," 3 *Trans.*, XLI (1919), 120–28.

14 *Ibid.*, XL (1918), 195–98; Ms. Minutes, Nov. 6, 1918; Council Minutes, Nov. 27, 1918.

15 Richard H. Harte, "Annual Address," 3 *Trans.*, XL (1918), 1–22. The portrait of Harte, presented to the College shortly after the close of his term of office, shows him in military uniform worn under the gown of president of the College.

16 Ms. Minutes, Dec. 3, 1919; 3 *Trans.*, XLIV (1922), 4. Major Alfred Reginald Allen, elected a Fellow in 1903, was described by Francis R. Packard as a brilliant neurologist, who had great mathematical ability and considerable musical talent. He enlisted in the infantry and was killed in action in 1918. Packard, "The College of Physicians from . . . 1887 to 1925," 4 *Trans.*, IV, Suppl. (1937), 116.

17 Hobart A. Hare, "Annual Address," 3 *Trans.*, XLVIII (1926), 1–8; same, "Annual Address," *ibid.*, XLIX (1927), 2–4; also *ibid.*, XLV (1923), 289 and XLVIII (1926), 362–79.

18 Stengel to de Schweinitz, May 12, 1911, Presidents' Letters.

19 Hare, "Annual Address," 3 *Trans.*, XLVIII (1926), 1–8, 14–15. Apathy was not limited to older Fellows. It was reported in 1923 that of sixty-five Fellows elected in the preceding five years, one fifth had not attended a single meeting in that period (forty-five meetings), that twenty-three had attended only once; and that of the entire number only three had attended more than ten meetings. 3 *Trans.*, XLV (1923), 7.

20 Like other medical societies the College had frequently to send representatives to Harrisburg to defend compulsory small pox vaccination against those who would weaken or repeal the law. 3 *Trans.*, XL (1918), 12- 13; Ms. Minutes, Feb. 7, 1923, Nov. 25, 1924. An extreme example of the opposition was the newsletter *Cracks,* edited by one A. B. Clarke, which denounced vaccination in its issue of March 25, 1910, as "the foulest crime of medical history," a "compulsory disease," and "the most far-reaching and despicable Scandal that the world Ever Seen." Although not persuaded by such irrationalities, legislators were not unaware that there were voters who cherished them.

21 Ms. Minutes, Feb. 3, 1909.

22 Wilson to Jasper Y. Brinton, April 8, 1913; Wilson to James V. Lafferty and Samuel W. Salus, March 4, 1915, Presidents' Letters.

23 Committee on the Desirability of Free Distribution of Tetanus Antitoxin, Report, May 4, 1910 (CPP); Ms. Minutes, May 4, 1910.

24 George E. Pfahler, "Memoir of Dr. James M. Anders," 4 *Trans.*, IV (1936), xvii-xx.

25 Ms. Minutes, Feb. 6, 1924.

26 Anders to Hobart A. Hare, Oct. 22, 1925, Council Minutes, Oct. 27, 1925.

27 Ms. Minutes, April 3, Oct. 2, 1912; Anders, "The College of Physicians and the Public Health," 3 *Trans.*, XXXIV (1912), 37–43; George E. de Schweinitz, "Annual Address," *ibid.*, 16–17.

28 Ms. Minutes, April 2, Dec. 3, 1913.

29 *Ibid.*, May 2, June 6, 1917.

30 Anders, "Activities of the Department of Public Health," 3 *Trans.*, XLV (1923), 128–40; Frank H. Caven, "Proposed Plans for a New Water Supply for the City of Philadelphia and Needs for Modern Methods for Disposal of City's Wastes," *ibid.*, 767–92. Caven was Director of Public Works.

31 Council Minutes, May 25, 1937.

32 Ms. Minutes, April 22, 1918; *Evening Bulletin*, July 13, 1916; 3 *Trans.*, XLI (1919), 310.

33 Papers by McKenzie and William A. Stecher of the Philadelphia public schools, with the discussion, are in 3 *Trans.*, XXXV (1913), 183–202. Anders' remarks are on pp. 199–202.

34 Ms. Minutes, June 2, 1920. At this meeting a resolution endorsing the work of school medical inspection and physical education and expressing the sense of the College "that the health of every child be safeguarded in this way" was introduced, but withdrawn.

35 Council Minutes, Sept. 28, 1920; 3 *Trans.*, XLIII (1921), 3, XLV (1923), 124–27; Ms. Minutes, May 2, 1923. It is worth noting here that another Fellow, John H. Girvin, in 1919 proposed that the College urge the Pennsylvania Assembly to enact legislation "to encourage and assist school districts to organize and maintain special education of mentally and physically defective children." Ms. Minutes, April 2, 1919.

36 3 *Trans.*, XLV (1923), 201.

37 Council Minutes, April 29, 1919.

38 Seneca Egbert, "The Food Supply of Philadelphia," 3 *Trans.*, XLI (1919), 287–314.

39 Ms. Minutes, Oct 3, 1900; Committee on Trolley Car Gong and Bell, Report, 1894 (CPP).

40 Ms. Minutes, Feb. 7, March 7, 1917.

41 *Ibid.*, May 4, 1921.

42 Council Minutes, Feb. 25, Mar. 25, May 27, 1930, March 4, 1931.

43 Committee on the Cost of Medical Care, *Final Report: Medical Care for the American People* (Chicago, [1932]); 3 *Trans.*, LIV (1932), 37–68.

44 The addresses were printed, in accordance with the joint sponsors'

agreement, in 4 *Trans.*, II (1934), 1–112, and separately as *The Medical Profession and the Public* (Philadelphia, 1934).

45 *Weekly Roster and Medical Digest,* XXIX (1933–34), 727–33; "Thunder in Philadelphia," *Medical Economics,* XI (March 1934), 24–25 *et seq.*

46 Council Minutes, Dec. 27, 1938.

47 Ms. Minutes, Jan. 2, April 2, 1924; John B. Roberts to "Dear Doctor," May 15, 1924 (copy), Roberts Correspondence (CPP).

48 William E. Robertson, "Memoir of John B. Roberts, M.D.," 3 *Trans.*, XLIX (1927), lxxvii-lxxxii; Roberts, "The Value of Scientific Doubt in Surgical Diagnosis," *ibid.*, XXXVII (1915), 288–307. On the eve of the 1909 local election Roberts appealed to his fellow-citizens to support the reform Penn party: "You know and I know how criminal abortionists flourish in this town; you know and I know how disease and death from vice are spread by low resorts in this community. You can recall how for years typhoid fever killed our fellow citizens because a leader of the Republican Organization delayed the filtration project until he could become a secret partner in the contract." *Public Ledger,* Nov. 1, 1909.

49 Keen initially approved limited terms and announced that he would retire as censor at the next election; his reasons for changing his mind are given in a letter in Ms. Minutes, Feb. 6, 1924.

50 *Ibid.*, April 2, 1924.

51 *Charter, Ordinance and By-Laws of the College of Physicians . . . as amended February 4, 1925* (Philadelphia, 1925).

52 Thomas R. Neilson, "Annual Address," 3 *Trans.,* XLVII (1925), 4; Hobart A. Hare, "Annual Address," *ibid.,* XLIX (1927), 1–2.

53 John B. Flick, "Memoir of John Heysham Gibbon (1871–1956)," 4 *T. & S.,* XXV (1957–58), 116–18.

54 Gibbon, "Annual Address," 3 *Trans.,* L (1928), 2.

55 Gibbon, "Annual Address," *ibid.,* LI (1929), 5; same, "S. Weir Mitchell," *ibid.,* 199; Francis R. Packard, "Annual Address," *ibid.,* LIII (1931), 1–7.

56 Council Minutes, Dec. 23, 1929, Feb. 11, 1930; E. B. Krumbhaar to Packard, March 25, 1931 (copy), Krumbhaar Papers, Box 3 (CPP).

57 W. B. McDaniel, 2d, "Francis R. Packard and his Role in Medical Historiography," *Bulletin of the History of Medicine,* XXV (1951), 66–85; John H. Gibbon, "Memoir of Francis Randolph Packard," 4 *T. & S.,* XVIII (1950–51), 131–32. Three papers on aspects of Packard's career and personality, read to the Section on Medical History, April 19, 1951, are printed *ibid.,* XIX (1951- 52), 75–84.

58 Packard to Krumbhaar, March 21, 1931; Krumbhaar to Packard, March 25, 1931 (copy), Krumbhaar Papers.

59 Malloch to Fisher, April 8, 1926, Fisher & Krumbhaar Correspondence (CPP).

60 Krumbhaar, "Editorial," 4 *T. & S.*, XXIII (1955–56), 38–39; Charles Frankenberger, "Charles Perry Fisher, 1857–1940: A Memoir," *Bulletin of the Medical Library Association,* XXIX (1940), 129–30.

61 Council Minutes, Jan. 24, 1933.

62 Hobart A. Hare, "Some Suggestions to the Fellows of the College by the Newly Elected President," *ibid.*, XLVII (1925), 13; Richard H. Harte, "Annual Address," 3 *Trans.*, XXXIX (1917), 17. See also Council Minutes, Dec. 23, 1935.

63 *Ibid.*, Oct. 27, 1925, Jan. 26, 1926. A study of these distinctions might provide a measure of the reputation the physicians enjoyed among their colleagues.

64 William Pepper, "Memoir of Alfred Stengel, M.D," 4 *T. & S.* VIII (1940- 41), 242–44.

65 Packard, "President's Address," 3 *Trans.*, LIV (1932), 1–10.

66 David Riesman to George E. de Schweinitz, Dec. 2, 1911, Presidents' Letters.

67 James C. Wilson to Riesman, Dec. 13, 1913, Presidents' Letters; Council Minutes, Dec. 30, 1913.

68 Wilson, "Annual Address," 3 *Trans.*, XXXVII (1915), 2–3.

69 Ms. Minutes, March 5, 1915, June 3, 1925; 3 *Trans.*, XLVII (1925), 382.

70 Richard A. Kern to E. B. Krumbhaar, April 20, 1931, Krumbhaar Correspondence, Box 3 (CPP).

71 Council Minutes, March 24, April 28, Sept. 29, 1931.

72 The actions the College took in 1931 occurred with fewer delays and more support from the (male) Fellows than is stated and implied by Dr. Macfarlane in "Women Physicians and the Medical Societies," 4 *T. & S.*, XXVI (1958), 80–83.

73 George P. Muller, "Annual Address," 4 *Trans.*, V (1937), 7.

74 Whitfield J. Bell, Jr., "W. B. McDaniel, 2d (1897–1975)," *Bulletin of the History of Medicine,* XLIX (1975), 428–31.

75 W. B. McDaniel, 2d, "Annual Report. . . 1935;" "Annual Report. . . 1937," 4 *Trans.*, III (1935), xxxviii-li; V (1937), 13–16.

76 Muller, "President's Address," 4 *T. & S.*, VI (1939), 361.

77 *A Record for the Commemoration of the 150th Anniversary . . .* ([Philadelphia], 1937), 2,4.

## CHAPTER XI

1 Council Minutes, April 23, 1940.

2 George E. Farrar, Jr., "Delaware Valley Right or Wrong," *Philadelphia Medicine,* LXII (1966), 743–44.

3 George P. Muller, "President's Address," 4 *T. & S.,* VI (1938–39), 359; Thomas A. Shallow, "Memoir of George P. Muller," *ibid.,* XV (1948), 151–52.

4 Muller, "Annual Address," 4 *Trans.,* V (1937), 5–12.

5 Ms. Minutes, Nov. 18, 1938, Jan. 20, Nov. 15, 1940, Feb. 24, 1942. Pepper noted the long-time, world-wide trend of older age groups to increase in relation to the younger, and described "measures which the layman may take to grow old gracefully, beginning in middle life to work toward health in old age both physically and psychologically. Healthy senescence rather than longevity should be our goal." *Ibid.,* Nov. 17, 1939.

6 In his report to the Fellows at the close of his second term in 1894 Mitchell recommended, among other things, that the College keep in close touch with all public matters affecting the health of the community "and should be ready to assist with advice or influence;" that the Fellows should cultivate the laity; and that papers read to the College "should not be overloaded with long details of cases" and should be limited to thirty minutes. "Annual Address," 3 *Trans.,* XVI (1894), xxxix-xliii. President Tyson in 1908 warned that membership was increasing "too slowly if our College is to continue to exert an influence proportionate to its age and tradition." "Annual Address," *ibid.,* XXX (1908), 1–5.

7 Muller, "President's Address," 4 *T. & S.,* VI (1938–39), 362–63; Council Minutes, Feb. 27, 1940.

8 Muller, "President's Address," 4 *T. & S.,* VII (1939–40), 378–80.

9 E. B. Krumbhaar, "President's Address," *ibid.,* X (1942–43), 202–07; Council Minutes, May 26, 1942. The joint meetings, continued to 1947, were found to be so beneficial and congenial that the two bodies continued to meet jointly twice a year.

10 Council Minutes, Sept. 17, 1940; 4 *T. & S.,* VIII (1940–41), 166–79.

11 Council Minutes, April 29, 1941.

12 Fulton, "Neurology and War," 4 *T. &. S.,* VIII (1940–41), 157–65.

13 Council Minutes, Sept. 24, 1946; Ms. Minutes, Nov. 6, 1946.

14 Krumbhaar, "President's Address," 4 *T. & S.,* X (1942–43), 207.

15 Pepper, "President's Address," *ibid.,* XI (1943–44), 141.

16 Pepper, "Address of the Retiring President," *ibid.,* XIII (1945–46), 144.

17 J. Parsons Schaeffer, "President's Address," *ibid.,* XIV (1946–47), 137.

18 Schaeffer, "President's Address," *ibid.*, XVI (1948–49), 151. On Miller, see Frank P. Brooks, "T. Grier Miller, M.D., 1886–1981," 5 *T. & S.*, IV (1982), 80–83.
19 Miller, "President's Address," 4 *T. & S.*, XVII (1949–50), 147–51.
20 Pepper, "Memoir of James Harold Austin (1883–1952)," *ibid.*, XXI (1953-54), 25–26.
21 See Miller's "President's Addresses" in *ibid.*, XVII (1949–50), 147–50; XVIII (1950–51), 123–25; XIX (1951–52), 152–55.
22 *College of Physicians of Philadelphia: A Memorandum submitted by T. Grier Miller, M.D., President* ([Philadelphia], 1951).
23 Richard A. Kern, "President's Address," 4 *T. & S.*, XXII (1954–55), 113-19.
24 Kern, "President's Address," *ibid.*, XXI (1953–54), 136.
25 Rhoads, "Inaugural Remarks," *ibid.*, XXV (1957–58), 191.
26 Rhoads, "Annual Report," *ibid.*, XXVIII (1960–61), 149–53.
27 Rhoads, "President's Address," *ibid.*, XXVI (1958–59), 168.
28 Rhoads, "The Increasing Value of Medical Care," *ibid.*, XXVII (1959–60), 149–53.
29 Durant, "Annual Report," *ibid.*, XXIX (1961–62), 163.
30 Durant, "The Medical Society in America: Past and Present," *ibid.*, XXXI (1963–64), 282.
31 *Ibid.*, XXXV (1967–68), 208–11. By way of comparison, it may be noted that the endowment of the New York Academy of Medicine in the same year was about $25,000,000 (up from $5,000,000 since 1946), and its annual budget was $1,125,000, of which $475,000 went to the library. Perhaps this is an appropriate place to preserve an anecdote that is related to the College financial condition at this time. A robber entered the building and demanded that Miss Olga Lang, College clerk, give him all the institution's money. She replied that it was not that kind of establishment, that there was no cash drawer. Seeing the safe, the robber threatened Miss Lang, forcing her to open it. The contents were minute books, ledgers, records of all kinds—but no cash. "I told you," Miss Lang told the frustrated thief, "it is a non-profit institution."
32 John H. Gibbon, Jr., "Presidential Address," 4 *T. & S.*, XXXIII (1965-66), 223.
33 Gibbon, "Presidential Address," *ibid.*, XXXIV (1966–67), 125–26.
34 Whitfield J. Bell, Jr., "Practitioners of History: Philadelphia Medical Historians before 1925," *Bulletin of the History of Medicine*, L (1976), 73-92.
35 "Annual Report of the Library," 4 *T. & S.*, XXXI (1963–64), 351–53.
36 "Annual Report on the Library," *ibid.*, XXX (1962–63), 240.
37 "Annual Report of the Committee on Library," *ibid.*, XXXVI (1968–69), 263.

38 "Annual Report on the Library," *ibid.*, XXXV (1967–68), 212.

39 "Annual Report on the Library," *ibid.*, XXXIII (1965–66), 285–90.

40 "Annual Report of the Committee on the Library," *ibid.*, XXXVI (1968–69), 269.

41 George P. Berry, "Report of Visiting Committee to the Library of the College of Physicians of Philadelphia," December 1969 (mimeographed, CPP).

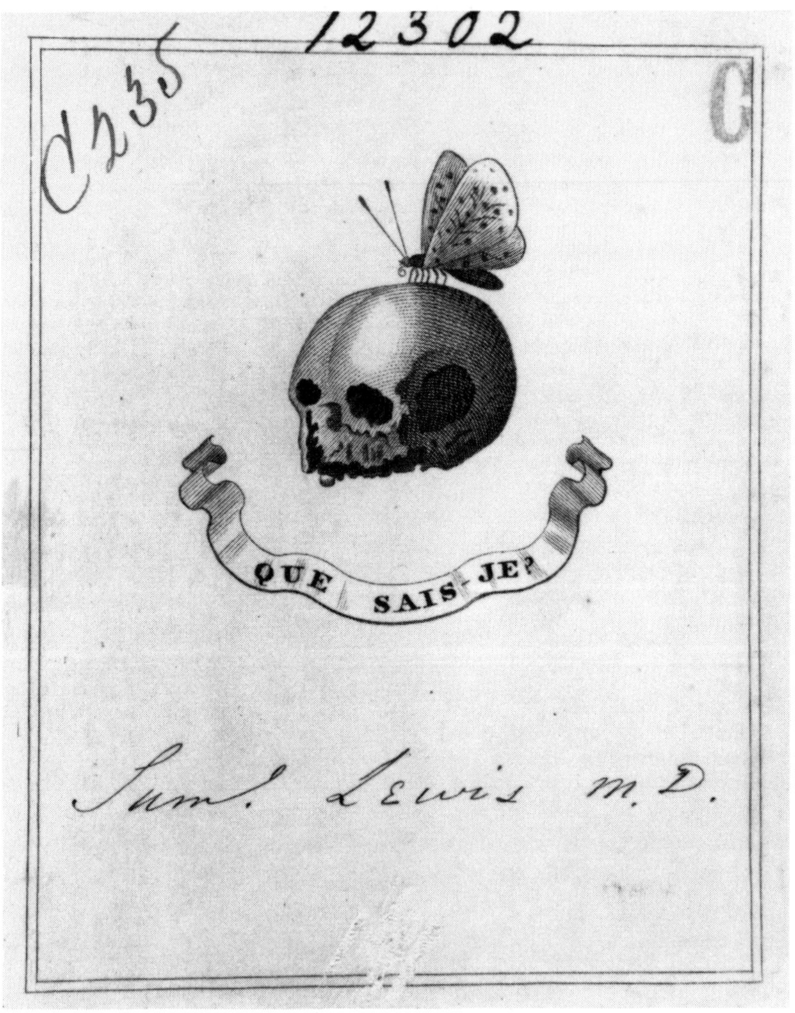


Bookplate of Samuel Lewis, (1813–1890).

# Index

Nos Præses et Vice Præses Col

OMNIBUS AD QUOS

Salu

TESTAMUR Gulielmum

Medicinæ peritum, nostri Collegii Socium

nesque ejus Honores et Privilegia juré ritéqu

hisce Literis, Collegii Sigillo munitis, Nomina

Datum Philadelphiæ die Decimo Qu

Josephus Parrish

Henricus Neill

Johannes C. Otto

Georgius B. Wood

Henricus Bond Secretarius.